Down Syndrome Screening

AF666071

Abhijit Kamat

Down Syndrome Screening

A Practical Guide

Springer

Abhijit Kamat
Dr. Abhijit's Fetal Medicine & Fertility Centre
Ponda, Goa, India

ISBN 978-981-99-7760-4 ISBN 978-981-99-7758-1 (eBook)
https://doi.org/10.1007/978-981-99-7758-1

© The Editor(s) (if applicable) and The Author(s), under exclusive license to Springer Nature Singapore Pte Ltd. 2023
This work is subject to copyright. All rights are solely and exclusively licensed by the Publisher, whether the whole or part of the material is concerned, specifically the rights of translation, reprinting, reuse of illustrations, recitation, broadcasting, reproduction on microfilms or in any other physical way, and transmission or information storage and retrieval, electronic adaptation, computer software, or by similar or dissimilar methodology now known or hereafter developed.
The use of general descriptive names, registered names, trademarks, service marks, etc. in this publication does not imply, even in the absence of a specific statement, that such names are exempt from the relevant protective laws and regulations and therefore free for general use.
The publisher, the authors, and the editors are safe to assume that the advice and information in this book are believed to be true and accurate at the date of publication. Neither the publisher nor the authors or the editors give a warranty, expressed or implied, with respect to the material contained herein or for any errors or omissions that may have been made. The publisher remains neutral with regard to jurisdictional claims in published maps and institutional affiliations.

This Springer imprint is published by the registered company Springer Nature Singapore Pte Ltd.
The registered company address is: 152 Beach Road, #21-01/04 Gateway East, Singapore 189721, Singapore

Paper in this product is recyclable

To Avni and Aarna,
with love.

Foreword

It is indeed a privilege and pleasure to write a foreword for this well-thought-out book, which I am sure will serve as a useful guide for students, practicing clinicians, fetal medicine specialists, and everyone involved in counseling women regarding Down syndrome.

Over the last three decades, tremendous strides have been made in the field of fetal medicine, and there is an unending quest for improving the antenatal detection of fetal anomalies. The recognition of the association of nuchal translucency as a marker for Down syndrome shifted the focus of screening from the second to the first trimester. This first trimester scan has emerged as the "first decision-making milestone" in pregnancy. Further research has identified several other markers like nasal bone, tricuspid regurgitation, and abnormal ductus venosus flow, which, when combined with maternal serum biochemistry, have a high detection rate for identifying fetuses that may potentially have Down syndrome. More recently, the identification of fetal cell-free DNA in the maternal blood has increased the sensitivity of detection of Down syndrome to over 99%.

While several approaches are available for screening, the practicing clinician is often faced with the dilemma of which is the best screening model to use in their practice, and whether the same can be universally applied. A comprehensive book on the various aspects of screening and counseling for Down syndrome was a felt need among obstetricians and fetal medicine specialists alike.

Dr. Abhijit Kamat has put in a significant effort to compile the currently available literature into a comprehensive textbook in an easily understandable form. The chapters are well-thought-out, and the author not only describes the process of screening but has also taken care to include pre-test and post-test counseling. This will help the clinician to explain the available choices to the couple who can then make well-informed decisions.

Including a chapter on examples from real-life practice is a welcome addition which will immensely aid in better understanding of screening. While the book is focused on screening for Down syndrome, Dr. Kamat has also included chapters on screening for preeclampsia and open spina bifida, which should form part of first trimester screening in the current era. This book will be a useful addition in clinical practice and I congratulate the author for putting in the effort to complete this task.

MediScan Systems
Chennai, India

S. Suresh,

Preface

Medical science has made such tremendous progress that there is hardly a healthy human left. —Aldous Huxley, English writer and philosopher

In the summer of 2010, a couple was referred to me at 18 weeks of pregnancy. Two years earlier, their baby was born with tetralogy of Fallot, and despite intervention, the girl succumbed before her first birthday.

This time, I performed a meticulous ultrasound examination, and issued a normal report, except for an isolated echogenic focus in the fetal heart. I explained to the couple that this was likely to be a normal variation, but as she had not undergone aneuploidy screening, I offered her the quadruple marker test. When they failed to report for the screening test even after 4 days, we did a follow-up call. Her partner answered the phone and thanked me profusely for my timely diagnosis of Down syndrome, which had allowed them to abort this baby in time and saved them the trauma of having an abnormal child again. To this day, the guilt of reporting that echogenic focus continues to weigh heavily on my mind.

This book is about prenatal screening for Down syndrome and other aneuploidies. Medical advances have not only improved the efficacy of prenatal screening but have also introduced new complexities. Staying up-to-date with ever-evolving guidelines and recommendations has become an indispensable part of clinical practice. Over the years, I have noticed a worrisome trend: as prenatal screening guidelines get revised, the recommendations tend to become increasingly vague. It is possible that this is influenced by the rising interference by the law in medical practice.

This book is meant for every obstetrician and fetal medicine specialist to be kept in their clinic like the owner's manual kept in the glove box of their car. In case the red engine light starts blinking, you should be able to reach out to a specific section quickly and know how to proceed. Despite referring to numerous guidelines and papers published across the world, I have tried to provide clear pragmatic solutions and management options throughout this book.

The role of the fetal medicine specialist is a strange one. On one hand, he must attempt to pick up all possible findings in the fetus. On the other hand, he must then be able to convince the parents that many of the findings he has picked up are normal variations. Striking this delicate balance becomes increasingly challenging amidst the deluge of digital information available today.

Still, I am hopeful that the day will come when parents are encouraged to look at an echogenic intracardiac focus as their baby's own "beauty spot" and to continue the pregnancy with a positive mindset. If, in writing this book, I can achieve this goal to some extent, I will consider it as my personal journey of repentance.

Ponda, Goa, India Abhijit Kamat

Acknowledgments

To Prof. S. Suresh, everything that I am today is because of you. Also, thank you for writing the foreword to this book.

To my parents, Dr. Jayant Kamat and Mrs. Snehalata Kamat, thank you for your unwavering support.

To my wife, Dr. Bhakti Salelkar, thank you for reading all my chapters (repeatedly!).

To Dr. Padmanabh Rataboli, thank you for guiding me.

To Dr. B. S. Rama Murthy, thank you for believing in me.

To my residents-turned-colleagues-turned-chapter reviewers: Dr. Ankita Sinai Borkar, Dr. Manjunath Hukkeri, Dr. Rohan Fernandes, and Dr. Vikram Dukle, your invaluable feedback made this book so much better.

To Dr. Vishal Kamate, thank you for your academic insights and assistance with the programs.

To Team Springer Nature: Dr. Naren Aggarwal, Ms. Jagjeet Kaur Saini, Ms. Neeraja Padmanabhan, Ms. Machi Sugimoto, Ms. Ellen Seo, and Ms. Safha Shaikh. You were truly professional and a delight to work with!

To my obstetrician colleagues, thank you for your faith in me.

To the expectant mothers who continue to place their trust, and sometimes the lives of their unborn children, in my hands. I am truly grateful for the opportunity to be a part of this incredible chapter in your lives.

Contents

About the Book

Down Syndrome Screening: A Practical Guide is a comprehensive and indispensable resource for all healthcare providers involved in the care of pregnant women. With a focus on practicality and accessibility, this guide aims to equip readers with the knowledge and tools necessary to navigate the complexities of this topic.

Readers will explore the various ultrasound and biochemical markers of aneuploidy, understanding their significance and interpretation. The book then delves into different screening methodologies, including maternal serum screening, noninvasive prenatal testing (NIPT), and second-trimester soft markers. Aneuploidy screening in twins and invasive testing for aneuploidy are thoroughly explained, offering tailored approaches for complex cases. Practical case scenarios aid in the interpretation of normal and abnormal reports, and to manage difficult situations.

Expanding beyond Down syndrome, the book also discusses trisomy 13, trisomy 18, and other aneuploidies. Additionally, it covers screening for preeclampsia and open spina bifida, further broadening the scope of the 11-13+6 weeks scan.

With its practical approach and user-friendly format, *Down Syndrome Screening: A Practical Guide* empowers healthcare professionals to provide pragmatic solutions, support informed decision-making, and, ultimately, enhance patient outcomes. While this book can be read sequentially to get a thorough knowledge on the subject, each chapter completes a specific topic, making this book an essential quick-reference guide for every antenatal clinic.

About the Author

Abhijit Kamat graduated from Goa Medical College with distinction. Following his postgraduation in Obstetrics and Gynecology, he completed his fellowship under Prof. S. Suresh, one of the foremost authorities in the field of fetal medicine in India.

Dr. Abhijit has more than 15 years of experience in ultrasound, infertility, fetal medicine, and fetal therapy, and has performed over 30,000 fetal scans and procedures. Currently, he is the director of Dr. Abhijit's Fetal Medicine and Fertility Centre, Goa, India. He has given numerous lectures on the subject of fetal medicine at national and international conferences.

Abbreviations

AC	Abdominal circumference
ACOG	American College of Obstetricians and Gynecologists
ADAM12	A disintegrin and metalloprotease-12
AFP	Alpha-fetoprotein
AGTR1	Angiotensin II receptor type 1
ALARA	As low as reasonably achievable
ALL	Acute lymphoblastic leukemia
AML	Acute myeloid leukemia
AOS	Aqueduct of Sylvius
APOE	Apolipoprotein E
APP	Amyloid precursor protein
ARSA	Aberrant right subclavian artery
ART	Assisted reproductive technology
BAC	Bacterial artificial chromosome
BACE2	Beta-secretase 2
BOBs	BACs-on-beads
BP	Blood pressure
BPD	Biparietal diameter
BSOB	Brainstem to occipital bone distance
CfDNA	Cell-free deoxyribonucleic acid
CFTR	Cystic fibrosis transmembrane conductance regulator
CHD	Congenital heart defect
CMA	Chromosomal microarray
CNV	Copy number variation

COX	Cyclooxygenase
CPC	Choroid plexus cyst
CPM	Confined placental mosaicism
CRELD1	Cysteine-rich with EGF-like domains 1
CRL	Crown rump length
CSF	Cerebrospinal fluid
CVS	Chorionic villus sampling
DC	Dichorionic
DCDA	Dichorionic-diamniotic
DMR	Differentially methylated region
DNA	Deoxyribonucleic acid
DR	Detection rate
DSCAM	Down syndrome cell adhesion molecule
DV	Ductus venosus
DYRK1A	Dual-specificity tyrosine phosphorylation-regulated kinase 1A
EDTA	Ethylenediaminetetraacetic acid
EDV	End diastolic velocity
EIF	Echogenic intracardiac focus
ET	Embryo transfer
FGR	Fetal growth restriction
FIGO	International Federation of Gynecology and Obstetrics
FISH	Fluorescence in situ hybridization
FL	Femoral length
FMF	Fetal Medicine Foundation
FOGSI	Federation of Obstetric and Gynecological Societies of India
FPR	False positive rate
FTS	First trimester screening
GC	Guanine-cytosine
HC	Head circumference
hCG	Human chorionic gonadotropin
H-hCG	Hyperglycosylated human chorionic gonadotropin
HL	Humeral length
HSA21	Homo sapiens autosome 21
ICSI	Intracytoplasmic sperm injection
IRIA	Indian Radiological and Imaging Association

ISSHP	International Society for the Study of Hypertension in Pregnancy
ISUOG	International Society of Ultrasound in Obstetrics and Gynecology
IT	Intracranial translucency
IUGR	Intrauterine growth restriction
IVC	Inferior vena cava
IVF	In vitro fertilization
LDA	Low-dose aspirin
LR	Likelihood ratio
LV	Lateral ventricle
MAP	Mean arterial pressure
MC	Monochorionic
MCC	Maternal cell contamination
MMIHS	Megacystis-microcolon-intestinal hypoperistalsis syndrome
MoM	Multiples of median
MPSS	Massively parallel shotgun sequencing
MSAFP	Maternal serum alpha-fetoprotein
MTHFR	Methylenetetrahydrofolate reductase
NB	Nasal bone
NGS	Next-generation sequencing
NICE	National Institute for Health and Care Excellence
NIPGT	Noninvasive pre-implantation genetic testing
NIPS	Noninvasive prenatal screening
NIPT	Noninvasive prenatal testing
NPV	Negative predictive value
NT	Nuchal translucency
NTD	Neural tube defect
ONTD	Open neural tube defect
OPU	Ovum pick-up
OSB	Open spina bifida
PAPP-A	Pregnancy-associated plasma protein-A
PCR	Polymerase chain reaction
PE	Preeclampsia
PGD	Pre-implantation genetic diagnosis
PGT	Pre-implantation genetic testing
PI	Pulsatility index

PICALM	Phosphatidylinositol binding clathrin assembly protein
PIV	Pulsatility index for veins
PlGF	Placental growth factor
POC	Products of conception
PPV	Positive predictive value
PRF	Pulse repetition frequency
PSV	Peak systolic velocity
QFPCR	Quantitative fluorescent polymerase chain reaction
RAT	Rare autosomal trisomy
RNA	Ribonucleic acid
RPL	Recurrent pregnancy loss
SCA	Sex chromosome aneuploidy
SFlt-1	Soluble fms-like tyrosine kinase-1
SGD	Single gene disorder
SNP	Single nucleotide polymorphism
SOGC	Society of Obstetricians and Gynaecologists of Canada
STS	Second trimester screening
SUA	Single umbilical artery
TAS	Transabdominal sonography
TAT	Turnaround time
TIFFA	Targeted imaging for fetal anomalies
TNF	Thickened nuchal fold
TORCH	Toxoplasmosis, rubella, cytomegalovirus, and herpes simplex virus
TR	Tricuspid regurgitation
TTTS	Twin-to-twin transfusion syndrome
TVS	Transvaginal sonography
uE3	Unconjugated estriol
USG	Ultrasonography
UtPI	Uterine artery pulsatility index
VACTERL	Vertebral, anal, and cardiac abnormalities, tracheo-esophageal fistula, esophageal atresia, renal, and limb abnormalities
VEGF	Vascular endothelial growth factor
VM	Ventriculomegaly
VOUS	Variant(s) of unknown significance
WHO	World Health Organization
β-hCG	Beta-human chorionic gonadotropin

1 Down Syndrome: Historical, Genetic, Clinical, and Ethical Perspectives

1.1 Introduction

Down syndrome is the commonest genetic condition affecting over five million individuals globally. In this chapter, we look at the fascinating history of how this syndrome came to be discovered and named, and the evolution of prenatal screening tests. We also look at the genetic mechanisms causing Down syndrome, its clinical features, and long-term sequelae. We then examine the social aspects of living with this condition, something that every clinician dealing with anxious parents should know. Finally, we debate whether we are correct in attempting to eradicate Down syndrome from society, or whether we should allow these children to be born. This, in a sense, questions the very existence of this book!

1.2 Historical Background

1.2.1 John Langdon Down (1828–1896)

John Langdon Down (Fig. 1.1) was born on 18 November 1828 in Cornwall, England, the youngest of 7 children of the merchant Thomas Joseph Down. He left school when he was 14 years and

© The Author(s), under exclusive license to Springer Nature Singapore Pte Ltd. 2023
A. Kamat, *Down Syndrome Screening*,
https://doi.org/10.1007/978-981-99-7758-1_1

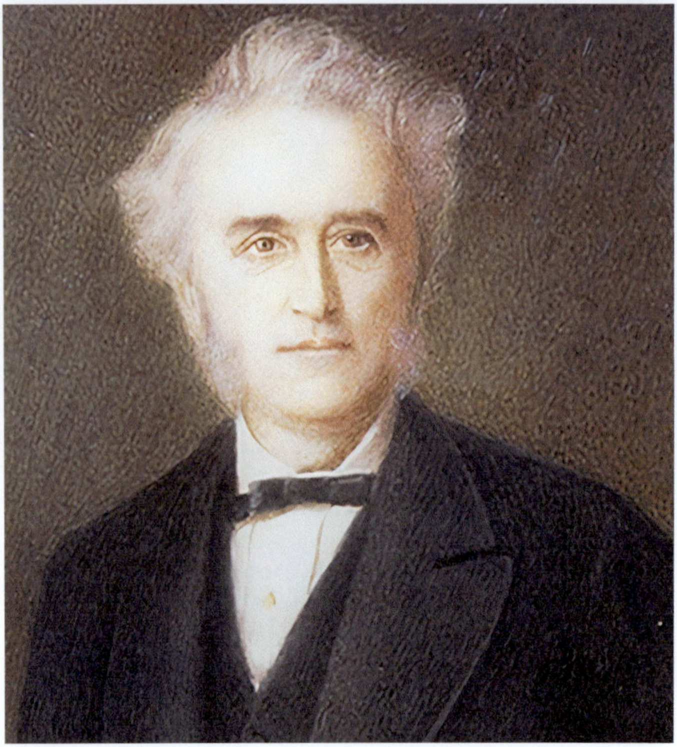

Fig. 1.1 John Langdon Down. Portrait by Sydney Hodges (c. 1870)

joined his father's grocery store. For the next 4 years, he had no formal education [1].

In 1846, he had what he described as a mystical experience. On a hot summer day, John and his family went for a stroll through the fields around Devon when it started raining. The family took off running and sought refuge at a nearby farm, where a strange-looking girl offered them tea. The girl had a flattened face, almond-shaped eyes, and small hands and feet. She could not understand his words, nor could she speak coherently. As he later recalled,

> *I was brought into contact with a feeble-minded girl, who waited on our party and for whom the question haunted me - could nothing for her be done? I had then not entered on a medical student's career but ever and anon... the remembrance of that hapless girl presented itself to me and I longed to do something for her kind.* [1]

Unknown to himself, he had just been introduced to what would later be known as Down syndrome. His encounter with this ill-fated girl awakened in him a deep desire to study medicine. After his father's death in 1853, John applied to the Medical School of the London Hospital, and secured admission there. He was an outstanding learner, winning gold medals in medicine, surgery, and obstetrics, as well as the award for best student in his final year. By this time, he could barely make ends meet, but his sister supported him and provided him lodging in London, where she lived with her husband, Philip Crellin. One day, Philip's sister Mary Crellin came for a visit, and for John, it was love at first sight. After a brief period of courtship, they got married [1].

One of the largest mental institutions in England at the time was the Royal Asylum for Idiots in Earlswood. This asylum was known for its poor health facilities, lack of human dignity, and widespread deaths among patients because of tuberculosis. The 'Lunacy Commission,' a board established to monitor the well-being of the mentally ill, was growing increasingly concerned with the appalling conditions at the asylum. In order to address the problem, they appointed John as the new chief physician and medical superintendent. Supported by his wife, John started a regimen of positive mental stimulation, nutritious food, and occupational training for the inmates. Within a few years, they had completely transformed the asylum into a facility for rehabilitation and recovery. In 1868, after being denied permission to hold an exhibition of his patients' artwork, John resigned from the Royal Asylum and established his own institution at Normansfield [1].

Besides his work on Down syndrome (subsequently named after him), he made several contributions to scientific literature, including the first description of Prader-Willi syndrome [2]. John Langdon Down breathed his last in the autumn of 1896 at the age of 67. Following his death, his sons, Reginald and Percival, assumed responsibility for running his institution. In a cruel twist of irony, Reginald's own son was born in 1905 with Down syndrome.

1.2.2 Observations on an Ethnic Classification of Idiots

While several of the clinical features seen in Down syndrome had been earlier documented by French doctors Jean-Étienne Dominique Esquirol and Édouard Séguin, they did not recognize their occurrence together as a syndrome [3].

In 1866, John Langdon Down published his historic paper titled 'Observations on an Ethnic Classification of Idiots' (Fig. 1.2). He accurately documented several physical traits of Down syndrome and emphasized their similarity to the Mongolian race:

> *A very large number of congenital idiots are typical Mongols… The hair is not black, as in the real Mongol, but of a brownish colour, straight and scanty. The face is flat and broad, and destitute of prominence. The cheeks are roundish, and extended laterally. The eyes are obliquely placed, and the internal canthi more than normally distant from one another… The lips are large and thick with transverse fissures. The tongue is long, thick, and is much roughened. The nose is small.* [4]

He also described typical patterns of behavior in affected children:

> *They are humorous, and a lively sense of the ridiculous often colors their mimicry. This faculty of imitation may be cultivated to a very great extent, and a practical direction given to the results obtained. They are usually able to speak; the speech is thick and indistinct, but may be improved very greatly by a well-directed scheme of tongue gymnastics. The coordinating faculty is abnormal, but not so defective that it cannot be greatly strengthened.* [4]

Many of today's readers may be offended by the use of the word 'idiot' and John's apparently racist reference to Mongolians. This was quite far from the truth. Scientific literature in that era fre-

OBSERVATIONS ON AN ETHNIC CLASSIFICATION OF IDIOTS.

By J. LANGDON H. DOWN, M.D., Lond.

Those who have given any attention to congenital mental lesions, must have been frequently puzzled how to arrange, in any satisfactory way, the different classes of this defect which may have come under their observation. Nor will the difficulty be lessened by an appeal to what has been written on the subject. The systems of classification are generally so vague and artificial, that, not only do they assist but feebly, in any mental arrangement of the phenomena which are presented, but they completely fail in exerting any practical influence on the subject.

The medical practitioner who may be consulted in any given case, has, perhaps in a very early condition of the child's life, to give an opinion on points of vital importance as to the present condition and probable future of the little one. Moreover, he may be pressed as to the question, whether the supposed defect dates from any cause subsequent to the birth or not. Has the nurse dosed the child with opium? Has the little one met with any accident? Has the instrumental interference which maternal safety demanded, been the cause of what seems to the anxious parents, a vacant future? Can it be that when away from the family attendant the calomel powders were judiciously prescribed? Can, in fact, the strange anomalies which the child presents, be attributed to the numerous causes which maternal solicitude conjures to the imagination, in order to account for a condition, for which any cause is sought, rather than hereditary

s 2

Fig. 1.2 Facsimile of the first page of Down's classic paper describing the syndrome

quently used the word 'idiot' to refer to an intellectually subnormal person. John himself believed that all men were created equal, a belief strengthened by his observation of 'Mongolian Idiocy' in people of all races, not only Mongolians [4].

1.2.3 Origin of the Name 'Down Syndrome'

By the turn of the century, 'Mongolism' had become the most widely used term to describe Down syndrome, its exact cause still unknown. The German scientists Schleiden, Virchow, and Bütschli were the first to describe the structure of chromosomes. With the evolution of genetics in the early twentieth century, it became apparent that chromosomes were the carriers of genes. In 1955, Joe Hin Tjio, an Indonesian-born American cytogeneticist, discovered the correct number of chromosomes in human beings. In 1959, Lejeune et al. proved that Down syndrome was caused by the presence of an extra chromosome, which was subsequently labeled as HSA21 (Homo sapiens autosome number 21) [5].

In 1961, a distinguished group of genetic experts wrote to the editor of the Lancet, suggesting that the word 'Mongolism' be replaced with a better scientific term. They suggested four alternatives: (1) Langdon Down Anomaly, (2) Down's Syndrome, (3) Congenital Acromicria, and (4) Trisomy 21 Anomaly. After much deliberation with the scientific community, the editor of the Lancet selected the term Down syndrome. The People's Republic of Mongolia had already petitioned the Director General of the World Health Organization (WHO), expressing displeasure with the usage of the derogatory term 'Mongolian Idiot'. In 1965, the WHO formally ratified the term Down syndrome [6].

1.2.4 Evolution of Screening Tests

As early as 1933, it was recognized that children with Down syndrome were usually born to older mothers [7]. In 1968, Trisomy 21 was diagnosed for the very first time by amniocentesis [8]. By 1972, raised maternal serum alpha fetoprotein (MSAFP) was linked to the risk of open neural tube defects.

In 1983, a pregnant woman underwent MSAFP testing to screen for neural tube defects. The levels were unusually low, and her obstetrician, Dr. Merkatz, assured her that her baby would be normal. Unfortunately, her baby was born with Edwards syndrome. The distressed mother asked Dr. Merkatz whether her low

Table 1.1 Evolution of prenatal aneuploidy screening

Year	Discovery of prenatal screening tests for aneuploidy
1983	Low AFP levels associated with trisomy 18 and trisomy 21
1987	High levels of human chorionic gonadotropin (hCG) associated with trisomy 21
1988	Low unconjugated estriol (uE3) levels associated with trisomy 18 and trisomy 21
1988	Triple marker test developed
1991	Low pregnancy-associated plasma protein-A (PAPP-A) linked to trisomy 21
1992	Increased nuchal translucency (NT) linked to trisomy 21
1996	Addition of inhibin A to the triple test (quadruple test)
1997	Combined first-trimester screening (NT, PAPP-A, and hCG)
1999	Integrated screening in the first and second trimesters
2008	Trisomy detected from cell-free DNA in maternal blood using next-generation sequencing (NGS)
2011	Noninvasive prenatal testing (NIPT) available commercially

AFP levels were related to this syndrome. Dr. Merkatz did not shrug her off. Instead, he collected follow-up data on women who had their AFP levels checked during pregnancy and subsequently gave birth to chromosomally abnormal babies. He was astonished to note that MSAFP levels had indeed been low in 43 out of the 53 women with aneuploidy. Thus, the concept of maternal serum screening for aneuploidy was born [8].

Screening techniques have continued to evolve over the years, with increasing sensitivity and declining false-positive rates. Table 1.1 lists the evolution of prenatal aneuploidy screening over the last 50 years [8, 9].

1.3 Meiosis in Human Germ Cells

Meiosis is a process by which a parent cell duplicates its chromosomal material once before dividing twice, resulting in the formation of four daughter cells (Fig. 1.3). Each daughter cell contains half the number of chromosomes present in the original cell. This process typically occurs in the germ cells of sexually reproducing organisms, including humans.

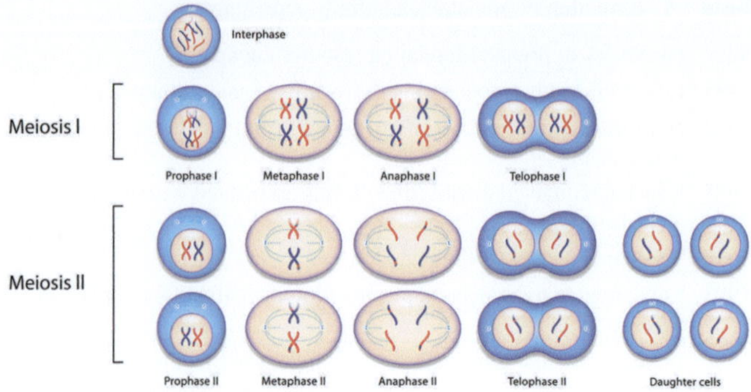

Fig. 1.3 Process of meiosis

The human germ cell contains 2 copies of each of the 23 chromosomes, i.e., 46 chromosomes in all (diploid cell). Meiosis results in the formation of the sperm or the oocyte, which contains a single copy of the 23 chromosomes (haploid cell). The process is divided into meiosis I and meiosis II, each representing one round of cell division. Each of these is further subdivided into four stages called prophase, metaphase, anaphase, and telophase.

A single spermatogonium undergoes meiotic division to form four sperms. In females, the process is slightly different. During meiosis I and meiosis II, one of the resultant cells is much smaller than the other, and gets extruded as a polar body. Thus, one cycle of meiotic cell division produces only one oocyte. Once the oocyte fuses with a sperm, the resulting zygote once again gets two copies of each chromosome (one copy from each parent), and is a diploid cell.

1.3.1 Prophase I

Prophase I is the longest and the most complex stage, and is further subdivided into leptotene, zygotene, pachytene, diplotene, and diakinesis. Chromosomal condensation continues throughout the prophase.

Leptotene The diffuse chromatin within the cell nucleus condenses to form chromosomes. Each chromosome has two sister chromatids and resembles the shape of the letter 'X.'

Zygotene The homologous chromosomes (maternal and paternal) find each other and form stable pairs.

Pachytene The homologous chromosomes come close together, forming synapses. The synapsed chromosomes now resemble tetrads, comprising two sister chromatids from each of the two chromosomes. The chromosomes form cross-overs between non-sister chromatids and exchange genetic information.

Diplotene The synapsed chromosomes move slightly away from each other.

Diakinesis The chromosomes condense further and the four parts of the tetrads are distinctly visible. The nucleoli disappear and the nuclear membrane disintegrates into vesicles.

Spindle formation occurs with microtubules originating from two opposite ends of the cell. The microtubules attach themselves to chromosomes at the centromeres.

1.3.2 Metaphase I

The paired homologous chromosomes move along the metaphase plate and align along an equatorial plane that bisects the spindle.

1.3.3 Anaphase I

The spindle microtubules shorten, pulling homologous chromosomes to the opposite sides of the cell.

1.3.4 Telophase I

The chromosomes reach the poles (half the original number at each pole). The spindle disappears and nuclear membranes form, surrounding the haploid set of chromosomes at each pole. Pinching of the cell membrane divides the cell into two (haploid) daughter cells as the chromosomes uncoil to form chromatin.

1.3.5 Meiosis II

Meiosis II is the second meiotic division and involves the separation of sister chromatids. Mechanically, the process is like mitosis, with each haploid cell further dividing into two (haploid) daughter cells.

Prophase II The nucleoli and the nuclear membrane disappear, and the chromatin condenses. Spindle fibers form again, arising from opposite poles of the cell.

Metaphase II The centromeres attach to spindle fibers again.

Anaphase II The shortening of the spindle fibers pulls apart the sister chromatids which move toward opposite poles.

Telophase II This is like telophase I, and is marked by decondensation of chromosomes to chromatin. Nuclear membranes re-form and the spindle disappears. Cell wall pinching and cytoplasmic division produce four daughter cells, each with a haploid set of chromosomes.

1.3.6 Difference Between Meiosis in Sperms and Oocytes

Spermatogenesis takes approximately 90 days in humans. Primary spermatocytes (containing 46 chromosomes) undergo meiosis I and form 2 secondary spermatocytes (containing 23 chromosomes). Each secondary spermatocyte undergoes meiosis II to form two spermatids each, which subsequently develop into spermatozoa. Thus, one primary spermatocyte gives rise to four sperms.

Human oocytes reach the diplotene stage of prophase I before birth. They remain arrested at this stage until puberty, when hormonal changes trigger the continuation of meiosis until the metaphase II stage. Meiosis II proceeds to completion only after the oocyte has been fertilized by a sperm. Unlike spermatocytes, human oocytes do not have centrosomes to produce the meiotic spindle. Instead, the microtubules forming the spindle arise from microtubule organizing centers at opposite ends of the cell [10]. Each primary oocyte divides twice during the process of meiosis. The first division produces a haploid daughter cell, and a tiny cell called the polar body, which is extruded. In meiosis II, division of the daughter cell again produces a single haploid cell (the ovum) and a second polar body. Therefore, each primary oocyte produces just one mature ovum and two polar bodies.

1.4 Genetic Mechanisms Causing Down Syndrome

Down syndrome is the phenotypic result of an excess of genes originating from chromosome 21. This may be inherited either as a whole extra chromosome or a part of chromosome 21. The exact genetic mechanism responsible for Down syndrome in each case determines not only the recurrence risk, but also the testing protocol to be offered to the woman in subsequent pregnancies.

1.4.1 Human Chromosome 21

Human chromosome 21, also known as HSA21 (Homo sapiens autosome number 21), was the second chromosome to be sequenced after chromosome 22. It is the smallest autosome, with a size of 47 million base pairs and comprising only 1.5% of the human genome. As per the latest Ensembl/GENCODE release [11], HSA21 is known to have 221 protein-coding genes, 447 non-protein-coding genes, and 185 non-functional pseudogenes. Approximately 40% of HSA21 comprises repeat content, which may have a gene compensatory function.

While more genes are likely to be identified in the future, there is no doubt that HSA21 is relatively gene-poor compared to other chromosomes. Then how do we explain the system-wide phenotypic disruption caused by trisomy 21?

1.4.2 Theories of Causation of Phenotype

The following mechanisms have been postulated in order to explain the profound and varied systemic abnormalities in individuals with trisomy 21 [12].

Gene Dosage Imbalance The simplest theory is an excessive expression of HSA21 genes because of an extra chromosome. A classic example is the increased susceptibility to Alzheimer's disease caused by the increased expression of the APP gene which codes for amyloid precursor protein.

Genome-wide Dysregulation It has been suggested that HSA21 genes regulate the expression of genes on other chromosomes as well. For example, endocardial cushion defects seen in Down syndrome have been linked to abnormalities in CRELD1 expression, a gene located on chromosome 3.

Critical Region Hypothesis Individuals with a partial trisomy can also display the typical clinical features of complete trisomy 21. The study of these individuals has led to the identification of a few Down syndrome critical regions on HSA21, comprising only 30 genes, whose disruption is sufficient to cause the expression of the complete phenotype [13].

1.4.3 Possible Genotypes Causing Down Syndrome

Free Trisomy 21 Ninety-five percent of individuals with Down syndrome have an extra copy of chromosome 21 (Fig. 1.4). This occurs because of the failure of homologous chromosomes to separate during meiosis I or failure of sister chromatids to separate during meiosis II, known as nondisjunction. This results in one cell having an extra copy of the chromosome, while the other cell has none.

In 90% of cases, the nondisjunction occurs during oocyte formation. In the rest, it is of paternal origin, or occurs after fertilization (post-zygotic nondisjunction). Nondisjunction is the only mechanism related to maternal age, possibly resulting from prolonged meiotic arrest lasting for 40 years or more.

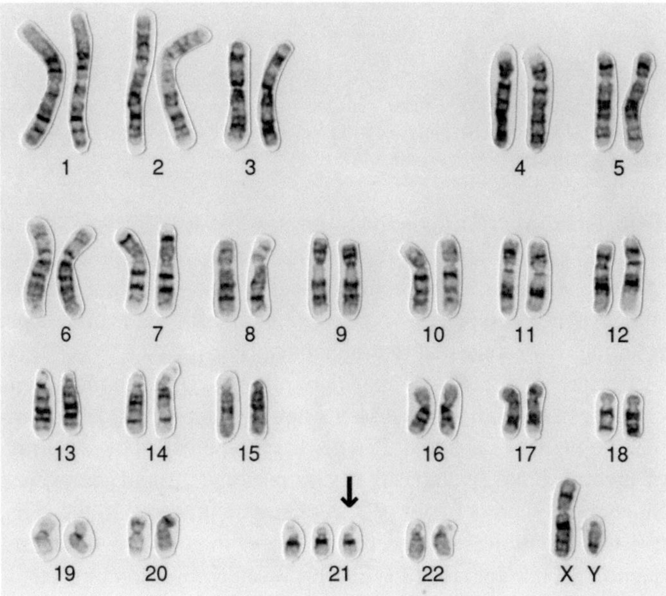

Fig. 1.4 Karyogram of a male with Down syndrome caused by trisomy 21. An extra copy of the complete chromosome 21 is present (*arrow*)

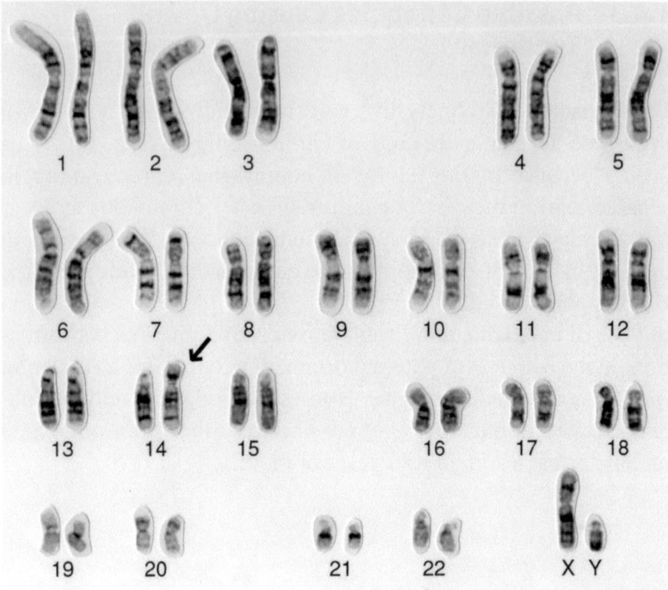

Fig. 1.5 Karyogram of a male with Down syndrome caused by an unbalanced translocation t(14;21). An extra piece (the long arm) of chromosome 21 is seen attached to chromosome 14 (*arrow*)

Translocation Translocation is responsible for less than 5% of cases of Down syndrome [12]. In translocation, a part of one chromosome breaks away and joins another non-homologous chromosome (non-homologous = not belonging to the same pair), resulting in an abnormal rearrangement (Fig. 1.5).

Reciprocal translocation occurs when two non-homologous chromosomes exchange segments among themselves. For example, if a woman has a t(21;22), her karyotype will show a portion of chromosome 21 attached to chromosome 22 and vice versa. Since there is no net gain or loss of genetic material in the cells, this translocation is balanced, and the woman suffers no consequences. If her oocyte (carrying this fused chromosome) is fertilized by a normal sperm, the fetus receives this extra bit of chromosome 21 piggyback riding on the mother's chromosome 22. The translocation now becomes unbalanced, and the fetus exhibits all features of Down syndrome.

A second type of translocation is called Robertsonian translocation. This occurs in acrocentric chromosomes (chromosomes 13, 14, 15, 21, and 22). Acrocentric chromosomes have their centromere near the end of the chromosome, with a great difference in the size of the long (q) and the short (p) arms. In Robertsonian translocation, the long arms of two chromosomes join each other, forming a large chromosome with the loss of short arms of both. Since the short arms of these chromosomes are tiny, they do not contain essential genetic sequences and the individual does not suffer any ill effects. Like reciprocal translocation, Robertsonian translocation causes Down syndrome when it becomes unbalanced in the fetus.

Most translocations causing Down syndrome occur de novo in the fetus, with both parents having a normal karyotype. Nevertheless, an increased number of affected individuals in the family tree hints at the presence of a translocation running in the family. Rarely, translocation may be limited to the gonads of one parent, in which case, the peripheral blood karyotype of both parents will be normal.

Mosaicism An individual with mosaic Down syndrome has a mixture of euploid cells (with 46 chromosomes) and aneuploid cells (with an extra copy of chromosome 21). Both parents typically have normal karyotypes. Two genetic mechanisms can lead to mosaicism. First, nondisjunction of chromosomes in some cells after fertilization can produce aneuploid cell lines. The second mechanism is trisomy rescue, in which some of the embryonic cells expel the extra chromosome in order to become euploid.

Others Other genetic mechanisms include partial trisomy 21, ring chromosome formation, and double centromere. These are seldom encountered in clinical practice.

1.5 Clinical Features and Sequelae

Individuals with free trisomy 21 or translocation Down syndrome have a range of characteristic clinical features and sequelae. In cases with mosaicism or partial trisomy 21, the abnormalities may be milder.

1.5.1 Physical Attributes

The physical features of Down syndrome are so distinctive, that the diagnosis is virtually unmistakable (Table 1.2).

Table 1.2 Range of physical features in a child with Down syndrome

System	Clinical findings
Body contour	Hypotonia, short stature, obesity, hypermobility of the joints
Neurological and behavioral	Mental subnormality, cheerful nature
Craniofacial	Brachycephaly, flat occiput, up-slanting palpebral fissures, inner epicanthal folds, midfacial and sinus hypoplasia, flat nasal bridge
Eyes	Brushfield spots on iris, refractive errors, strabismus, nystagmus, cataract
Ears	Small low-set ears, hearing loss
Mouth	Macroglossia, high arched palate, teething problems
Neck	Short broad webbed neck, atlanto-axial instability
Skin	Dry, rough, inelastic skin
Limbs	Short and broad hands, clinodactyly or hypoplasia of the middle phalanx of the fifth finger, single transverse palmar crease (simian crease), sandal-gap deformity between the first two toes
Genitalia	Cryptorchidism, micropenis, hypospadias

1.5.2 Neurological Problems

Genes implicated: APP (amyloid precursor protein), BACE2 (beta-secretase 2), PICALM (Phosphatidylinositol binding clathrin assembly protein), APOE (Apolipoprotein E), DYRK1A (Dual-specificity tyrosine phosphorylation-regulated kinase 1A) [14].

All children with Down syndrome have a mild-to-moderate learning disability. Epilepsy (commonly infantile spasms) is noted in 10% of affected children and may persist into adulthood. Affected individuals have a high risk of early-onset Alzheimer's disease, with over two-thirds developing dementia by the age of 50 [13, 14].

1.5.3 Musculoskeletal Problems

Hypotonia along with increased joint laxity is common. Joint laxity can cause frequent falls, leading to fractures. Atlantoaxial instability may be present. Abnormal function of the insulin-like growth factor results in short stature and delayed skeletal maturation.

1.5.4 Congenital Heart Disease

Genes implicated: CRELD1 (Cysteine-rich with EGF-like domains 1) on chromosome 3 [12].

Endocardial cushion defects (atrioventricular septal defect, ventricular septal defect) are the commonest lesions, with up to 50% prevalence at birth. The other defects seen are atrial septal defects, tetralogy of Fallot, and patent ductus arteriosus. Secondary pulmonary hypertension occurs in later life [14].

1.5.5 Gastrointestinal Tract Abnormalities

Genes implicated: DSCAM (Down syndrome cell adhesion molecule) implicated in Hirschsprung disease [14].

Trisomy 21 is present in 1 in 3 fetuses with an antenatally diagnosed duodenal atresia, mandating the need for invasive testing in these fetuses. Imperforate anus can be present as an isolated finding or as part of the VACTERL association (vertebral anomalies, anal atresia, cardiac anomalies, tracheoesophageal fistula, esophageal atresia, renal and limb anomalies). Other abnormalities observed are small bowel atresia and annular pancreas.

Hirschsprung disease is characterized by the absence of nerve ganglion cells in a portion of the colon, causing a lack of peristalsis and resulting in functional obstruction. Other functional disorders include gastroesophageal reflux, chronic constipation, recurrent diarrhea, and celiac disease.

1.5.6 Hematological Disorders

Genes implicated: GATA-binding factor 1 [15].

Hematologic abnormalities in newborns with Down syndrome (HANDS) include a triad of neutrophilia, thrombocytopenia, and polycythemia. These abnormalities usually self-correct within 3 weeks of birth. Pediatric onset acute lymphoblastic leukemia (ALL) and acute myeloid leukemia (AML) occur more frequently when compared to normal children [15].

1.5.7 Disorders of Sight and Hearing

Ophthalmic disorders include refractive errors, iris and retinal abnormalities, cataract, strabismus, amblyopia, and nystagmus.

Hearing loss can be sensorineural or conductive (because of anatomical abnormalities in the ear).

1.5.8 Endocrine Disorders

Hypothyroidism and primary hypogonadism are frequently noted.

1.5.9 Reduced Risk of Hypertension and Cardiovascular Disease

Genes implicated: Angiotensin II receptor type 1 (AGTR1) gene [14].

Reduced expression of *AGTR1* gene results in a reduced risk of hypertension and cardiovascular disease. Reduced insulin resistance is seen, particularly in women with Down syndrome, which reduces the risk of atherosclerosis [16].

1.6 Ethics of Prenatal Screening

The best time in history to have been born with Down syndrome is today. Individuals with trisomy 21 are living lifespans of 50–60 years, are independent, and gainfully employed. Termination of an affected pregnancy is no longer a straightforward decision, and many parents choose to continue their pregnancies.

Over the past two decades, researchers have realized that the birth of a Down syndrome child is a stress on the family life rather than a misfortune. At least three factors contribute to this stress: (1) increased demands of parenting role—feeling trapped or overwhelmed, (2) dealing with the child's behavior and temperament, and (3) worries about social and cultural acceptability and the child's future. And just like any other stressor, some families cope well, while others do not [17].

The acceptance rate of screening depends on the counseling offered to women. Although counseling should ideally be nondirective, in reality, it seldom is. Rather, the personal beliefs of the healthcare provider often influence the choices made by patients. In Sweden and Iceland, for example, heavy-handed genetic counseling has resulted in a near elimination of Down syndrome babies. Nevertheless, it is the clinician's duty only to provide prospective parents with clear information on what to expect if they give birth to a baby with Down syndrome. He or she should refrain from participating in the decision to continue or terminate the pregnancy. Before debating whether prenatal screening is ethical, it is imperative that we explore the family dynamics and self-perception in children with Down syndrome.

1.6.1 Parents of Children with Down Syndrome

Parents of Down syndrome children experience a lower sense of satisfaction in life and exhibit higher depressive symptoms than do parents of normally developing children. When compared to children with other disabilities, however, they report fewer negative effects (called 'the Down syndrome advantage').

The mother is usually the primary caregiver for the affected child. Mothers take care of most of the child's needs like hygiene, feeding, dressing, teaching, and taking the child for therapy. Maternal stress levels in early childhood are like that in families with normal children, but as the Down syndrome child grows older, maternal stress rises, probably because of the widening gap between similarly aged peers. Among all, the child's behavioral abnormalities seem to affect mothers more strongly, as seen in cases with coexisting autism. Nevertheless, most mothers seem to cope well, with the main complaint being the inability to have a fulfilling career or gainful employment [17].

Fathers participate mostly in playing, discipline, and decision-making about services. Stress among fathers is lower than in mothers, but fathers tend to worry more about the long-term outlook and social acceptability of their child [17].

Family cohesiveness and marital relationships are close to normal in affected families. One study compared divorce rates among parents of children with Down syndrome, other birth defects, and no identified disability. Divorce rates among couples with a Down syndrome child were the lowest among all three groups [18].

1.6.2 The 'Down Syndrome Advantage'

Mothers of children with Down syndrome report a less pessimistic view of life, greater closeness to the child, and a feeling of reciprocation of love from the child, compared to children with other developmental disabilities. This continues into adolescence and early adulthood.

Several factors have been proposed to account for this 'Down syndrome advantage':

1. Down syndrome children are happier and display fewer behavioral problems.
2. Mothers of Down syndrome children are older and more mature.
3. Availability of specific support groups and social networks for this condition.

The 'Down syndrome advantage' is found to be greatest when the child has no coexisting physical or mental disability, and when early intervention and support are provided to the family [19].

1.6.3 The Sibling Experience

Siblings of children with Down syndrome report a largely positive influence of the child in their life, especially when the affected child is younger than them. They develop greater feelings of empathy, appreciation for individual differences, social adjustment, and sacrifice. Older female siblings are especially seen to provide great comfort and care to the child and often take on a 'maternal' role in the child's life. This close personal contact with the affected sibling continues into adulthood.

Having a brother or sister with Down syndrome also leads to more positive relationships and greater satisfaction in their own lives. Many believe that they have developed additional strengths because of their sibling with Down syndrome [17].

1.6.4 Effect of Early Interventions and Support Groups

Early interventions and introduction to social support groups is the foremost thing that improves the lives of the affected children and their families. Support groups for parents, both professional and non-professional, are present in most parts of the world today, thanks to the impact of social media. Obstetricians need to encourage the parents who choose to continue pregnancies to get in touch with support groups even before their child is born. This ensures a positive birth experience and better bonding with the child right from birth.

1.6.5 Financial Impact

Having a child with Down syndrome has a major impact on family finances. First, the mother usually finds it difficult to do a regular job, at least till the child finishes schooling. Second, many of the affected children have associated health problems, and may need frequent hospitalization. Third, if the family is financially constrained, they may not afford special intervention and support system for their child. This leads to increased difficulties in bringing up the child and the inability of the mother to pursue gainful employment, thus completing the vicious cycle.

1.6.6 Care of the Individual After Parents' Death

As life expectancy among individuals with Down syndrome has increased and many live well until the fifth or sixth decade, the question of care after death of both the parents is an important issue to which we have paid little attention so far. In most cases, it is expected that the elder sibling (often the sister) will continue to take care of the person's needs.

At present, there are few formal support systems for care after the parents' death. If the child has no siblings, life after parents' death can be very difficult and uncertain. Individuals with Down syndrome also have a very high incidence of Alzheimer's disease, which means they can no longer care for themselves (even if they could when they were younger).

1.6.7 Self-Perception of Down Syndrome Individuals

Children with Down syndrome have a very positive outlook about themselves, a trend that continues into early adulthood. They are happy in life and display great love for their family. Surprisingly, their happiness quotient does not depend on their physical or intellectual abilities.

Skotko et al. conducted a cross-cultural epidemiological survey in 2011 among 319 individuals with Down syndrome. They reported that most individuals were happy with their lives, their appearance, and accepted the difference between themselves and normal children. Negative responses were more common in individuals who were staying in group homes rather than with parents. Negative outlook was also more common among children who had just finished high school. This was likely linked to their transition through adolescence, which is an awkward time even for normal teenagers [20].

1.6.8 Is Down Syndrome Screening Ethical?

In a survey involving members of 28 ethics committees in the United Kingdom, questionnaires based on clinical scenarios were generated for 4 unnamed clinical conditions. One of the clinical conditions matched the description of a child with Down syndrome, without labeling it as such. The ethics committee members were asked to opine whether they considered it ethical to perform prenatal screening for the condition described. For a clinical scenario representing Down syndrome, only half the surveyed members considered prenatal screening to be ethical. These numbers reduced even further when procedure-related loss was mentioned as a complication of screening [21].

The following ethical issues have been raised from time to time as arguments against universal screening for Down syndrome:

1. As affected children often have an acceptable quality of life, screening involves conflicting rights and interests between two parties: the unborn child, and the mother/couple seeking the diagnosis. Furthermore, it is not possible to predict the severity of the disorder before birth.
2. The idea of providing equal access to medical care and treatment for all patients is challenging to put into practice due to a shortage of resources. Because of high costs associated with prenatal testing, Down syndrome children are selectively eliminated from high-income families compared to low-income ones. Consequently, couples with lower income and education level are more likely to give birth to these babies, for whom they cannot provide the necessary care.
3. Religious and cultural bias effects screening, especially in communities where there is a religious objection to abortion. Is screening then simply a eugenic exercise?
4. Invasive testing is not 100% safe, and for every Down syndrome baby detected, there is a price to be paid in terms of loss of normal fetuses. Noninvasive prenatal testing has mitigated this concern to some extent.

However, we should not be hasty in labeling prenatal screening as an unethical exercise. Giving birth to a Down syndrome child has its own problems that need to be considered, especially in low or middle-income countries:

1. Children with Down syndrome require an extraordinary amount of dedication and care, including consistent physical, emotional, and mental therapy in order to be able to eventually lead an independent life. Developing countries lack the social infrastructure and formal education systems to care for specially abled children.
2. At an individual level, couples often lack the financial resources required for early intervention, increased medical care, and special education.
3. Many children with Down syndrome have co-existing neurological problems like severe autism.

4. Affected children may also have structural abnormalities which are not picked up before birth.

In conclusion, it is prudent to counsel prospective parents in detail before offering them aneuploidy screening. Clinicians need to provide comprehensive information about the conditions being screened for, the need for further testing, and the risks of invasive testing. The couple's views on termination of pregnancy also need to be considered. Subsequently, the decision of the couple whether to undergo screening should be respected, even if it goes against the belief of the obstetrician.

Image Attributions

Fig. 1.1: Sydney Hodges. Portrait of John Langdon Down (c. 1870). https://en.wikipedia.org/wiki/File:JLHdown.jpg. Public Domain. Accessed May 19, 2023.

Fig. 1.2: John Down. Observations on an ethnic classification of idiots. Source: Wellcome Collection. https://wellcomecollection.org/works/e2wvvdt4. Public domain. Accessed May 19, 2023.

Fig. 1.4: Down syndrome human karyotype 47,XY,+21. Wessex Reg. Genetics Centre. Source: Wellcome Collection. https://wellcomecollection.org/works/wmcdanw6. Attribution 4.0 International (CC BY 4.0). Accessed June 23, 2023.

Fig. 1.5: Unbalanced translocation 46,XY,t(14;21). Wessex Reg. Genetics Centre. Source: Wellcome Collection. https://wellcomecollection.org/works/xpcvauhp. Attribution 4.0 International (CC BY 4.0). Accessed June 23, 2023.

References

1. Ward OC. John Langdon Down: the man and the message. Downs Syndr Res Pract. 1999;6(1):19–24.
2. Down JL. Polysarcia and its treatment. London Hosp Rep. 1864;1:97–103.

3. Mégarbané A, Ravel A, Mircher C, Sturtz F, Grattau Y, Rethoré MO, et al. The 50th anniversary of the discovery of trisomy 21: the past, present, and future of research and treatment of Down syndrome. Genet Med. 2009;11(9):611–6.
4. Down JLH. Observations on an ethnic classification of idiots. London Hosp Rep. 1866;3:259–62.
5. Lejeune J, Turpin R, Gautier M. Le mongolisme, maladie chromosomique. Bull Acad Natl Med. 1959;143(11–12):256–65.
6. Van Robays J. John Langdon Down (1828-1896). Facts Views Vis Obgyn. 2016;8(2):131–6.
7. Penrose LS. The relative effects of paternal and maternal age in mongolism. J Genet. 1933;27(2):219–24.
8. Wald NJ, Kennard A, Hackshaw A, McGuire A. Antenatal screening for Down's syndrome. J Med Screen. 1997;4(4):181–246.
9. Cuckle H, Maymon R. Development of prenatal screening—a historical overview. Semin Perinatol. 2016;40(1):12–22.
10. Severson AF, von Dassow G, Bowerman B. Oocyte meiotic spindle assembly and function. Curr Top Dev Biol. 2016;116:65–98.
11. Cunningham F, Allen JE, Allen J, Alvarez-Jarreta J, Amode MR, Armean IM, et al. Ensembl 2022. Nucleic Acids Res. 2022;50(D1):D988–95.
12. Antonarakis SE, Skotko BG, Rafii MS, Strydom A, Pape SE, Bianchi DW, et al. Down syndrome. Nat Rev Dis Primers. 2020;6(1):9.
13. Aït Yahya-Graison E, Aubert J, Dauphinot L, Rivals I, Prieur M, Golfier G, et al. Classification of human chromosome 21 gene-expression variations in Down syndrome: impact on disease phenotypes. Am J Hum Genet. 2007;81(3):475–91.
14. Asim A, Kumar A, Muthuswamy S, Jain S, Agarwal S. Down syndrome: an insight of the disease. J Biomed Sci. 2015;22(1):41.
15. Choi JK. Hematopoietic disorders in Down syndrome. Int J Clin Exp Pathol. 2008;1(5):387–95.
16. Draheim CC, McCubbin JA, Williams DP. Differences in cardiovascular disease risk between nondiabetic adults with mental retardation with and without Down syndrome. Am J Ment Retard. 2002;107(3):201–11.
17. Hodapp RM. Families of persons with Down syndrome: new perspectives, findings, and research and service needs. Ment Retard Dev Disabil Res Rev. 2007;13(3):279–87.
18. Urbano RC, Hodapp RM. Divorce in families of children with Down syndrome: a population-based study. Am J Ment Retard. 2007;112(4):261–74.
19. Esbensen AJ, Seltzer MM. Accounting for the "Down Syndrome Advantage". Am J Intellect Dev Disabil. 2011;116(1):3–15.
20. Skotko BG, Levine SP, Goldstein R. Self-perceptions from people with Down syndrome. Am J Med Genet A. 2011;155A(10):2360–9.
21. Reynolds TM. Down's syndrome screening is unethical: views of today's research ethics committees. J Clin Pathol. 2003;56(4):268–70.

Ultrasound Markers for Aneuploidy at 11–13 Weeks

2

2.1 Introduction

First-trimester ultrasound was traditionally used for localizing the pregnancy and establishing viability and gestational age. In 1992, Dr. Kypros Nicolaides and coworkers coined the term nuchal translucency (NT), and showed that NT ≥ 3 mm was associated with an increased risk of aneuploidy [1]. Over the years, several other first-trimester ultrasound markers were studied to improve the detection rate of chromosomal defects. Among these, absent nasal bone, tricuspid regurgitation, and abnormal ductus venosus flow are the three markers that have been successfully incorporated into screening algorithms [2]. With improvement in ultrasound resolution, widespread availability of transvaginal probes, and a better understanding of embryology, it is now possible to detect several structural malformations in the first trimester itself. This chapter discusses the first-trimester ultrasound markers that are used to screen for common trisomies. It also enumerates the first-trimester structural abnormalities which are strongly associated with chromosomal defects. Finally, it considers the thermal effects and safety of ultrasound in the first trimester.

© The Author(s), under exclusive license to Springer Nature Singapore Pte Ltd. 2023

A. Kamat, *Down Syndrome Screening*,
https://doi.org/10.1007/978-981-99-7758-1_2

2.2 Increased Nuchal Translucency

Nuchal translucency (NT) refers to the thickness of the fluid layer in the posterior aspect of the fetal neck between 11 and 13 + 6 weeks of gestation. As NT varies in fractions of a millimeter, a slight error in the measurement can have a large effect on the aneuploidy risk which is subsequently calculated. The correct technique of measurement and the regular audit of images obtained by ultrasound operators are important to ensure the success of any screening program. The Fetal Medicine Foundation (FMF) has standardized this technique, and runs a free Internet course to train sonographers across the world.

2.2.1 Technique of Measurement of NT [3]

- The gestational age should be between 11 and 13+ 6 weeks.
- The fetus should be facing upwards. The neck should be in the neutral position (neither flexed nor hyper-extended), which is ensured by a small pocket of fluid between the fetal chin and neck. The image should be zoomed so that only the fetal head and upper part of the fetal thorax are visible. At this magnification, a small movement of the calipers should change the measurement by 0.1 mm only.
- A midsagittal view of the face should be obtained. This is recognized by the nuchal skin posteriorly, the transparent diencephalon in the center, the echogenic tip of the nose anteriorly, and the rectangular form of the palate (Fig. 2.1a).
- The image should be optimized, and the gain reduced as necessary, so that the skin of the neck appears as a thin distinct line separate from the underlying amniotic membrane.
- The calipers should be positioned on-to-on such that the inner border of the horizontal caliper lines should exactly match the inner borders of the lines defining the nuchal space. The calipers should not be within the black nuchal fluid (Fig. 2.1b).

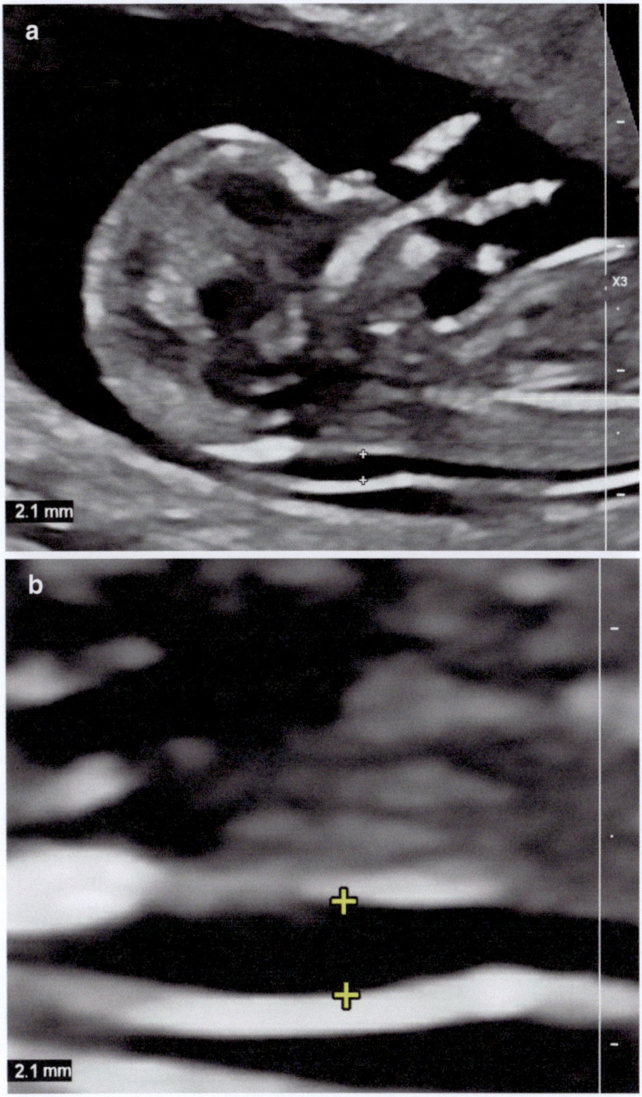

Fig. 2.1 (**a**) Midsagittal view of a fetus at 12 weeks of gestation showing the correct magnification and technique for measurement of nuchal translucency (NT). In this example, the NT measurement is 2.1 mm. (**b**) Magnified image showing the correct 'on to on' placement of calipers. Note that this degree of magnification should not be used when actually measuring the NT

- More than one measurement is recommended, and the highest NT value among them should be selected.
- When there is a cord loop around the neck, NT should be measured above and below the cord, and the average of the two should be considered as the NT value.

2.2.2 Using NT for Down Syndrome Screening

Nuchal translucency is a continuous variable which increases with advancing gestational age. Therefore, it should not be described using terms like 'mildly increased' or 'borderline.' For Down syndrome screening, the NT value should only be interpreted in the context of a combined first-trimester screening test (see Chap. 4). If the woman refuses aneuploidy screening, no further testing should be offered, unless the NT value is ≥3 mm or the fetus has a structural malformation.

2.2.3 Genetic Testing in Fetuses with Raised NT

Nuchal translucency value of 3.0 mm lies above the 95th percentile at any gestation between 11 and 13 + 6 weeks (Fig. 2.2). While a cutoff of 3.5 mm was used for definitive testing in the past, the risk of chromosomal aberrations in the fetus with an NT value between 3.0 and 3.5 is as high as 13.5%. Therefore, invasive testing should be considered in all fetuses with NT above 3.0 mm [4].

There is a debate whether to perform karyotyping or chromosomal microarray (CMA) in fetuses with markedly raised NT. The advantage of CMA is that it can detect submicroscopic abnormalities, thus increasing the yield slightly over and above that achieved with karyotyping. Conversely, CMA cannot detect triploidy and balanced translocations, and it may miss low-level mosaicism. If CMA is used, another rapid aneuploidy test like fluorescence in situ hybridization (FISH) should be performed, primarily to detect triploidy (which commonly presents with a significantly raised NT). Balanced translocations do not result in phenotypic abnormalities; therefore, it is acceptable if they are

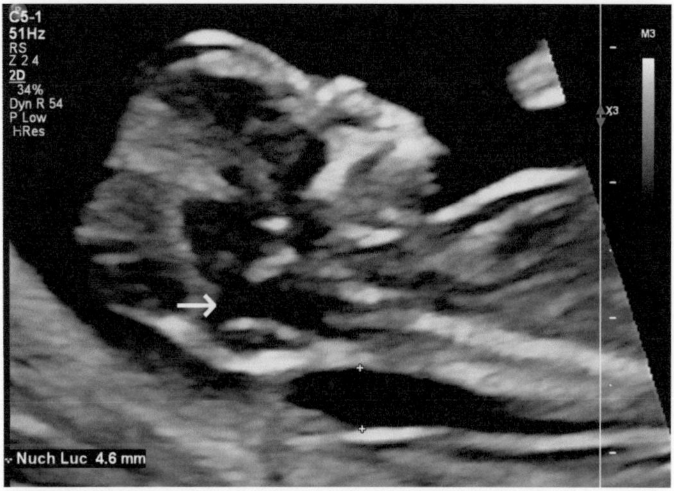

Fig. 2.2 Raised NT in a fetus with trisomy 21. The posterior cranial fossa also appears abnormal (*arrow*)

missed. Two-step testing is a good strategy if logistically possible. In the first step, rapid FISH testing is performed for the common aneuploidies (13, 18, 21, X, and Y). If FISH testing detects an aneuploidy, it is confirmed by karyotyping. If FISH returns a normal result, a high-resolution CMA is done to look for submicroscopic chromosomal aberrations.

Whenever invasive testing is done for raised NT, DNA storage should also be offered. DNA storage is inexpensive, and if the karyotyping or CMA returns a normal result, the stored DNA can be used to subsequently test for rare genetic conditions like Noonan syndrome.

Noninvasive prenatal testing (NIPT) has several limitations when the NT is ≥3.0 mm:

- Since the incidence of chromosomal abnormalities in this group of women is high (approximately 1 in 7), and NIPT screen-positive results require confirmation by invasive testing, many of these women still require CVS or amniocentesis [4].

- Using NIPT as an intermediate screening test increases the time to diagnosis.
- NIPT can miss cases of mosaicism and translocations.
- Most laboratories perform NIPT by the next-generation sequencing or the counting method, which does not detect triploidy (since the relative ratios of the chromosomes remain unaltered).
- NIPT has a low sensitivity and PPV for submicroscopic chromosomal aberrations.

2.2.4 Follow-Up of Euploid Fetuses with Raised NT

Different mechanisms have been proposed as a cause of nuchal edema. Down syndrome fetuses have a higher concentration of hyaluronic acid in the extracellular space, which traps fluid. Alternative mechanisms have been suggested in fetuses who are chromosomally normal. They include abnormal lymphatic drainage, venous congestion in the head or neck, cardiac failure, fetal anemia, and fetal hypoproteinemia [5].

Fetuses with a raised NT and a normal karyotype or CMA are still at risk of adverse pregnancy outcomes, and this risk is directly proportional to the NT value. Problems seen in these fetuses include:

1. Cardiac defects: The most common abnormalities seen are narrowing of aortic isthmus, septal defects, and valvular abnormalities.
2. Other structural malformations.
3. Evolution to hydrops.
4. Genetic conditions like Noonan syndrome.
5. Placental dysfunction, growth restriction, and intrauterine death.

In a study by Souka and coworkers, the chances of the baby being normal at birth were 70% for an NT of 3.5–4.4 mm, 50% for an

NT of 4.5–5.4 mm, 30% for an NT of 5.5–6.4 mm, and 15% for an NT of 6.5 or more. The other indicators of a favorable prognosis were absence of structural malformations, resolving nuchal edema, and a normal growth profile [6].

Women whose fetuses show (an apparently isolated) nuchal edema should undergo an expert evaluation at the time of the anomaly scan with concurrent fetal echocardiography. If no major abnormalities are detected, growth monitoring should begin from 26 to 28 weeks with a review of fetal anatomy in the third trimester. Euploid fetuses with a raised first trimester NT but having normal prenatal and postnatal evaluation do extremely well in the long term. Physical and neurodevelopmental development in these children is comparable to the general population [7, 8].

2.2.5 Raised NT and Noonan Syndrome

Noonan syndrome is an autosomal dominant single-gene disorder seen in approximately 10% of chromosomally normal fetuses with NT > 3.5 mm. Fifty percent of individuals have a mutation in the PTPN11 gene; mutations in other genes have also been implicated [9]. Affected individuals have typical features, such as a prominent forehead, widely spaced eyes, depressed nasal bridge, low-set ears, and a deep philtrum. There is an increased incidence of cardiac defects, musculoskeletal and dermatological problems, problems with eyesight, hearing and speech, subnormal intelligence, and an increased susceptibility to malignancies.

An important point to note is that Noonan syndrome is neither detected by karyotyping, nor by microarray, but requires molecular testing for specific single-gene mutations (available as a 'Noonan syndrome panel' with most genetic labs). In fetuses with raised NT, testing for Noonan syndrome should particularly be considered when a similar finding was reported in an earlier pregnancy and the karyotype was normal.

2.3 Absent Nasal Bone

Nasal bones are two slender bones on either side of the midline in between the orbits. Nasal bones develop through an intramembranous ossification starting at 9–10 weeks of gestation, but are usually not visible on ultrasound until the 11th week [10]. When imaged in the coronal view at 11 weeks, the two bones can be seen separately, with a gap in between. In the mid-sagittal view of the fetal face, the echoes arising from the two bones overlap, giving the appearance of a single echogenic line beneath the skin of the nose. This single line is labeled as the *nasal bone* (NB), essentially an ultrasound finding rather than an anatomical one. When this line is not visualized or appears fainter than the overlying skin, it is reported as an absent nasal bone.

The reported incidence of absent NB in Down syndrome fetuses varies widely; a meta-analysis in 2014 reported absent NB in 36% of trisomy 21 fetuses compared to 0.5% of normal fetuses. Addition of NB to the combined first-trimester screening test achieves a detection rate of 93% with a false-positive rate (FPR) of 2.5% [3, 11, 12]. The following section describes the guidelines set by the Fetal Medicine Foundation (UK) for the certificate of competence in the assessment of the NB.

2.3.1 Technique of First-Trimester Assessment of NB [3]

1. The gestational age should be between 11 and 13 + 6 weeks.
2. The fetus should be facing upward with the neck in the neutral position (i.e., neither flexed nor hyper-extended). This is ensured by a small pocket of fluid between the fetal chin and neck. The image should be zoomed so that only the fetal head and upper part of the fetal thorax are visible.
3. An exact mid-sagittal view of the face should be obtained. This may be recognized by the nuchal skin posteriorly, the transparent diencephalon in the center, the echogenic tip of the nose anteriorly, and the rectangular form of the palate.

4. The ultrasound probe should be held parallel to the direction of the nose and should be gently moved from side to side to ensure that the nasal bone is seen separate from the skin.
5. In the correct section, three distinct lines are seen: the first two lines are horizontal and parallel to each other, resembling an equal sign (=). The top line represents the skin and the bottom one, which is thicker and more echogenic than the overlying skin, represents the nasal bone. A third line, almost in continuity with the skin, but slightly antero-superior, represents the tip of the nose (Fig. 2.3).
6. When the line representing the nasal bone is not visualized, or appears thinner and less echogenic than the overlying skin, it is classified as absent NB (Fig. 2.4).

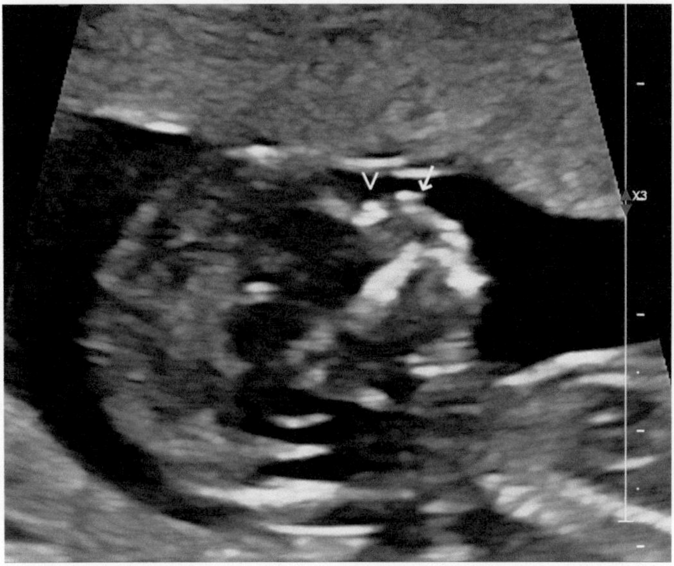

Fig. 2.3 Midsagittal view of a fetus at 13 weeks of gestation showing a normal NB. Note the presence of two proximal lines representing the NB and the nasal skin (*arrowhead*), and the third distal line representing the tip of the nose (*arrow*)

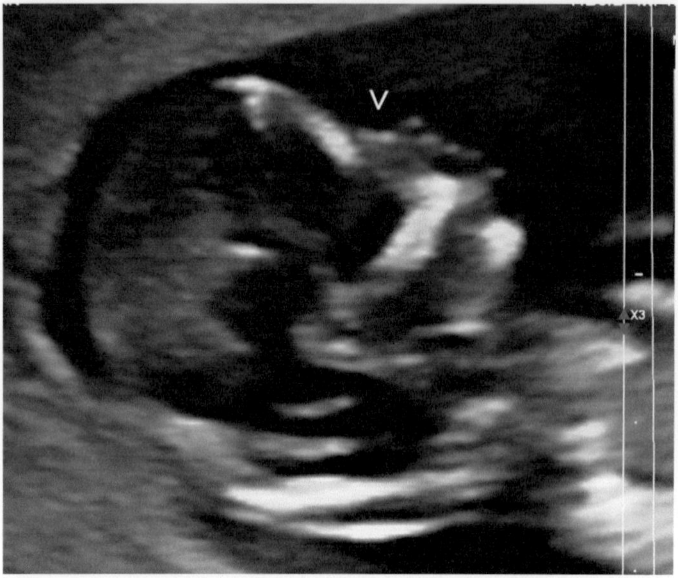

Fig. 2.4 Midsagittal view of a fetus at 13 weeks of gestation showing an absent NB. Note the absence of the equal sign (=) in the nasal region (*arrowhead*). Compare this with Fig. 2.3

2.3.2 Important Pointers Regarding NB Assessment

1. An absent NB in the first trimester should only be considered in the context of combined screening along with NT and serum biochemistry. If the combined screening test shows a low risk, no further testing is necessary, and the NB should be reevaluated in the second trimester.
2. There should be a clear institutional policy about including NB in the screening protocol. If NB is included, it should be used in all pregnant women. Otherwise, it can be used as a part of contingent screening, where it is assessed only in women with an intermediate risk result in the combined screening test (see Chap. 9).

3. The ultrasound operator needs to be specifically certified for NB. An annual audit is mandatory to maintain the quality of assessment.
4. Nasal bone *length* has no significance in the first trimester, and should not be reported.
5. Ossification of NB is a continuous process. The optimal gestation for the first trimester NB evaluation appears to be at a CRL between 65 and 74 mm. In case the NB appears unossified (absent) at 11–12 weeks, the fetus should be reevaluated at 13 completed weeks before making the diagnosis.
6. Individual NBs seen in the coronal view should not be reported, as unilateral hypo-ossification is not validated as a marker for aneuploidy.

Importantly, NB assessment is technically difficult compared to NT. Incorrect assessment can reduce the efficacy of screening, rather than enhance it. It is not a mandatory part of the first trimester scan, and should only be performed in centers having sonographers who are trained and formally certified for NB assessment. Otherwise, first-trimester screening should be performed using only NT combined with maternal age, free β-hCG, and PAPP-A [13].

2.4 Abnormal Ductus Venosus Flow

At 11–13 weeks, the fetal ductus venosus (DV) is a tiny vessel (0.5 mm diameter) connecting the left portal vein to the inferior vena cava. The DV diverts approximately 30% of the blood coming from the placenta to the fetal heart, bypassing the fetal liver. As there is a continuous forward flow from the placenta to the heart, the entire DV waveform remains positive (above the baseline) throughout the cardiac cycle. However, as the DV is intimately connected to the heart, any major alterations in cardiac preload or afterload are reflected in the DV flow.

A normal DV waveform comprises three waves (Fig. 2.5). The first and highest peak (S-wave) corresponds to the ventricular systole, when the right atrium is nearly empty and there is a large

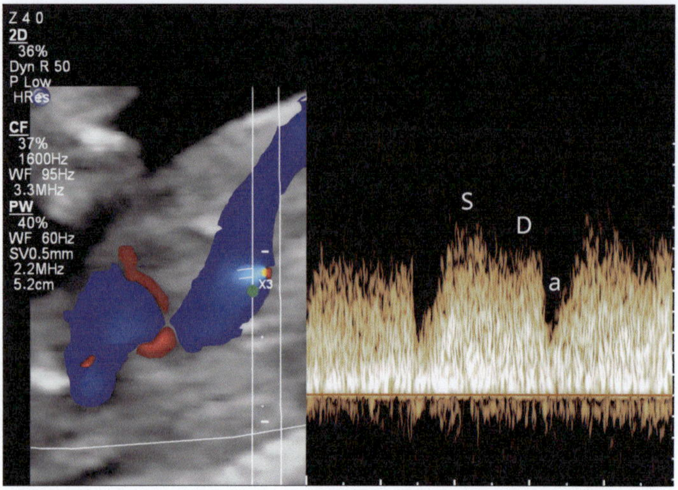

Fig. 2.5 Parasagittal view of fetal thorax and abdomen of a 13-week fetus showing insonation of the DV. Note the small size of the sample volume (*SV, 0.5 mm*) placed in the aliasing area, with the insonation angle parallel to the direction of flow. Also note that there is antegrade flow throughout the cardiac cycle. *S*—ventricular systole, *D*—ventricular early diastole, *a*—atrial contraction

gradient of flow from the umbilical vein to the heart. As the right atrium starts emptying during ventricular early diastole, it produces the second peak (D-wave). The third and the last wave, which occurs during atrial contraction, is called the a-wave. As right atrial pressure is high, it has the smallest magnitude.

2.4.1 Technique of First-Trimester Assessment of DV [3]

1. The gestational age must be 11–13 weeks and 6 days.
2. The image should be zoomed so that the fetal thorax and abdomen occupy the whole image. After obtaining a midsagittal view, the probe should be adjusted to the right of the midline and the color switched on to demonstrate the umbilical vein, DV, and fetal heart.

3. The pulsed wave Doppler sample gate should be less than 1 mm, and it should be placed in the yellowish aliasing area with an insonation angle of less than 30°.
4. A low wall filter frequency (50–70 Hz) and a high sweep speed ensure that the a-wave is clearly visible.
5. The DV can be assessed either for the presence or absence of the a-wave, or the pulsatility index for veins (PIV) can be calculated by tracing the Doppler waveform on the ultrasound machine.

2.4.2 Ductus Venosus Flow and Down Syndrome Screening

Reversed a-wave is seen in only 1.6% of euploid fetuses compared to 24–66% of fetuses with Down syndrome (Fig. 2.6). The mechanisms linking an abnormal DV flow to aneuploidy include

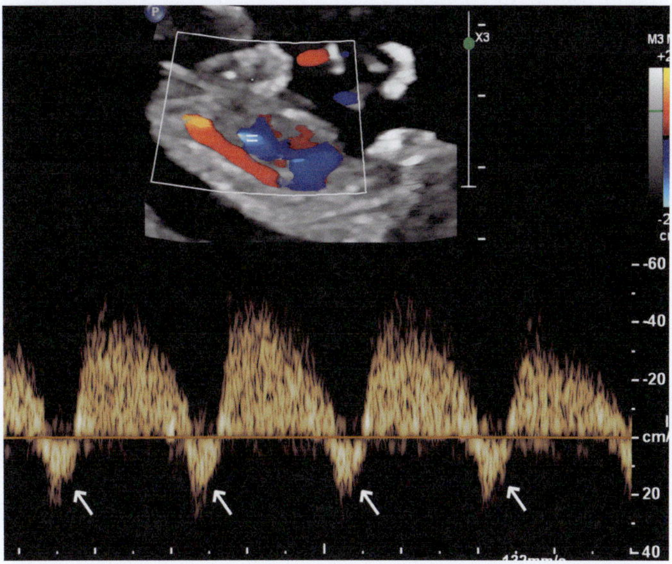

Fig. 2.6 Parasagittal view of the thorax and abdomen of a 13-week fetus with trisomy 21 showing reversal of a-wave in the DV (*arrows*)

cardiac muscle dysfunction with an alteration in preload or afterload, or associated cardiac anomalies. Using DV flow in the contingent or integrated screening model increases the detection rate of Down syndrome to 96% for an FPR of 3% [14, 15].

Instead of subjective assessment of DV for a-wave reversal, the DV pulsatility index for veins (PIV) can be used, and improves the detection rate of aneuploidy. Most ultrasound machines automatically calculate the DV-PIV by tracing the DV waveform. Every 1.0 MoM increase in DV-PIV increases the aneuploidy risk by 4.2 times [16].

2.4.3 Other Abnormalities Detected by DV Insonation

Absence of the DV is a rare condition which may be detected at the 11–13 weeks scan. It is associated with a significant risk of adverse outcomes, including structural malformations, aneuploidy, growth restriction, hydrops, and fetal demise. Fetuses with absent DV should undergo invasive testing, detailed anatomy scan with echocardiography, and careful surveillance throughout pregnancy.

As the DV reflects the pressure changes in the right atrium, the assessment of DV flow serves as a screening tool for early detection of cardiac anomalies. It is yet uncertain whether it provides any additional value for cardiac anomaly detection, over and above that provided by an increased NT.

Finally, in monochorionic twins, abnormal DV flow or discordant DV-PIV is another predictor of twin-to-twin transfusion syndrome, along with discordance in NT and CRL.

2.4.4 Disadvantages of Routine Evaluation of DV at the 11–13 + 6 Weeks Scan

Because of its small size, the correct assessment of DV requires extensive training, certification, and audit. It is prone to false-positive results because of contamination from the nearby veins

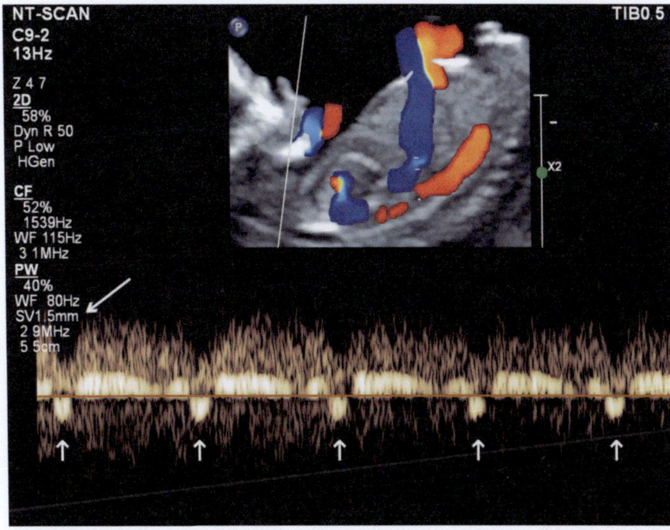

Fig. 2.7 False positive a-wave reversal (*short arrows*) due to contamination by signals from fetal IVC, caused by a large sample volume size of 1.5 mm (*long arrow*). Note the positive IVC waveforms superimposed on the DV waveforms. Also note that the blood flow in the DV remains positive throughout

such as the inferior vena cava (IVC) (Fig. 2.7). Prolonged use of pulsed wave Doppler to insonate the DV also exposes the fetus to unnecessary ultrasonic energy with an increase in thermal index.

Ductus venosus assessment is *not* a part of the routine 11–13 + 6 weeks scan. Sonographers performing DV assessment should undergo specific training and an annual audit. Because changes in the DV flow can occur in euploid fetuses with cardiac defects, and in aneuploid fetuses without cardiac defects, it should not be used as a first-line screening tool for aneuploidy. The problems caused by an incorrectly interpreted DV probably outweigh any benefits of using it in routine clinical practice.

2.5 Tricuspid Regurgitation

Tricuspid regurgitation (TR) in aneuploid fetuses may result from altered tissue hyaluronic acid (as in Down syndrome), or secondary to cardiac malformations. Addition of TR in risk calculation algorithms improves the sensitivity and reduces the FPR.

2.5.1 Technique of First-Trimester Assessment of TR [3]

1. The gestational age must be 11–13 weeks and 6 days. The magnification of the image should be such that the fetal thorax occupies the whole image.
2. A 4-chamber view of the heart should be obtained with the apex either at a 12 o'clock or a 6 o'clock position.
3. The pulsed wave Doppler sample gate of 2–3 mm should be placed across the tricuspid valve with an insonation angle of less than 30° with respect to the inter-ventricular septum (Fig. 2.8).
4. Assessment should be performed thrice. Tricuspid regurgitation is diagnosed if the regurgitant jet has a velocity of over 60 cm/s and is present for at least half the duration of ventricular systole (Fig. 2.9).
5. Sweep speed should be high in order to space out the waveforms.

2.5.2 Tricuspid Regurgitation and Down Syndrome Screening

Tricuspid regurgitation is seen in only 4.4% of euploid fetuses compared to 67% of trisomy 21 fetuses, 33% of trisomy 18 fetuses, and 15% of fetuses with other chromosomal abnormalities [17].

For reasons similar to DV flow assessment (see above), evaluation of tricuspid flow is not routinely recommended at every

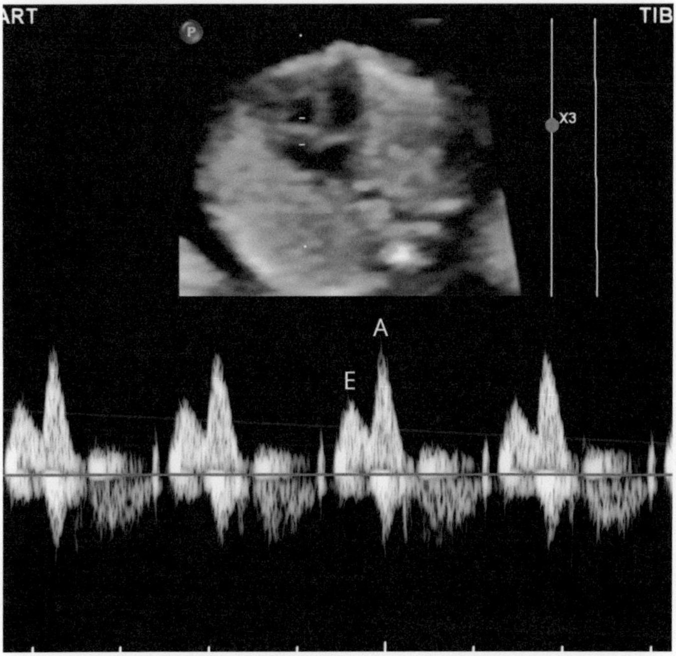

Fig. 2.8 Four-chamber view of the heart in a 13-week fetus showing placement of pulsed Doppler sample volume for tricuspid Doppler flow assessment. The E wave corresponds to early filling, and the A wave corresponds to atrial contraction. There is no TR

first-trimester scan. Rather, it is an option for contingent screening of women who receive an intermediate risk result in the combined first-trimester screening test.

2.5.3 Tricuspid Regurgitation and Congenital Heart Defects (CHD)

The presence of TR increases the odds of the fetus having a CHD. However, this association holds true only in fetuses with additional findings, such as a raised NT or abnormal DV flow. Isolated TR, seen in the first trimester in a low-risk population, is

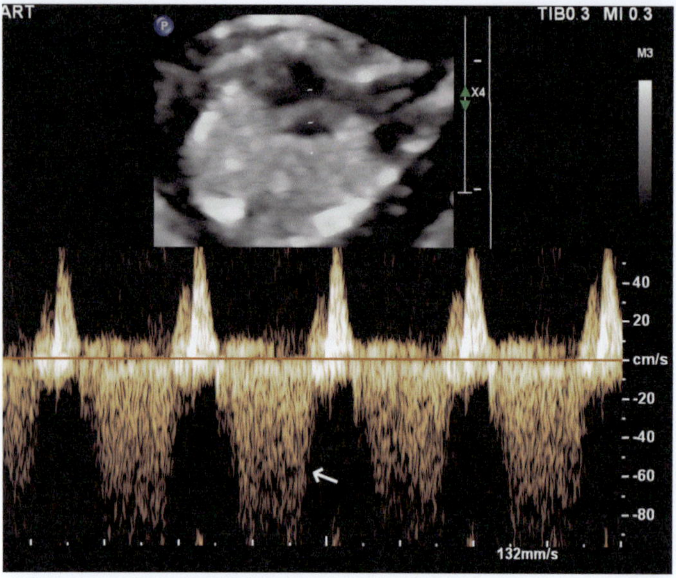

Fig. 2.9 Tricuspid regurgitation (*arrow*) in a fetus with trisomy 21 (same case as Fig. 2.6)

not associated with CHD [18]. Still, fetuses with TR detected in the first trimester should have a formal echocardiography performed at the time of the targeted anomaly scan.

2.6 Fetal Heart Rate (FHR)

In chromosomally normal fetuses, the mean FHR reduces from 170 beats per minute at 10 weeks to 155 beats per minute at 14 weeks. Fetal tachycardia is noted in approximately 10%, 70%, and 50% of fetuses with trisomy 21, trisomy 13, and Turner syndrome, respectively. Its pathophysiology is related to the outflow tract abnormalities seen in these conditions, with the tachycardia being triggered by baroreceptors, secondary to narrowing of the aortic arch. Fetal bradycardia is seen more frequently in association with triploidy and trisomy 18, and may be related to severe growth restriction and impending death in these fetuses [19]. However, because of its inconsistent association with specific aneuploidies, the addition of FHR to combined screening does not improve its performance significantly.

2.7 Structural Abnormalities Associated with Aneuploidy

Several structural abnormalities identifiable in the first trimester are strongly linked to aneuploidy. The most common ones are briefly described below. Detailed discussion on the counseling and management of pregnancy in each case is beyond the scope of this book. However, as a rule, invasive testing should be offered to all women who choose to continue pregnancy.

2.7.1 Cystic Hygroma

Cystic hygromas are macrocystic lymphatic malformations (lymphangiomas) comprised of endothelium-lined cystic spaces with scanty stroma. Most cystic hygromas occur in the nuchal region, and may be difficult to differentiate from other causes of raised NT (Fig. 2.10a). However, cystic hygromas usually have the 'nuchal ligament' separating the two lymphatic sacs on either side (Fig. 2.10b, c). In addition, they may have several septa within the sacs. Other locations include the axilla (Fig. 2.10d) and rarely, the chest.

The commonest genetic abnormalities associated with a cystic hygroma are trisomy 18, Turner syndrome, and trisomy 21, followed by trisomy 13 and Noonan syndrome. Chromosomal microarray may detect additional genetic abnormalities, particularly in cases of septated cystic hygromas.

Earlier studies reported a uniformly poor prognosis, with <20% of fetuses having a normal outcome [20]. A recent cohort study of 410 cases of septated cystic hygromas diagnosed before 14 weeks reported significantly better outcomes. The survival rate

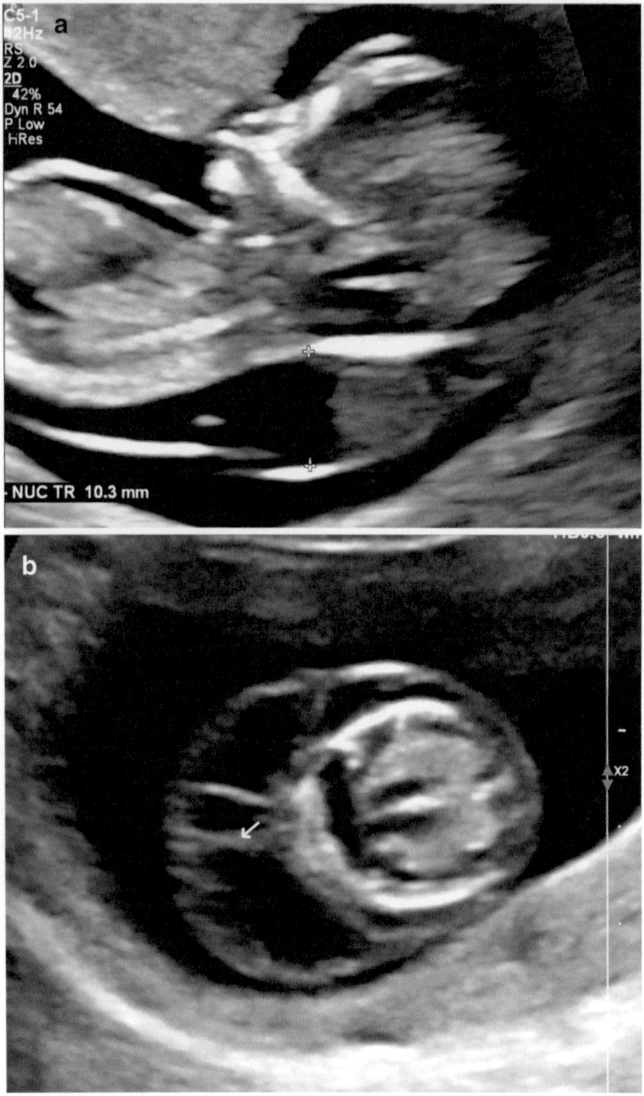

Fig. 2.10 Cystic hygromas in a fetus with Turner syndrome. (**a**) Raised nuchal translucency of 10.3 mm. (**b**) Cystic hygroma with the nuchal ligament (*arrow*) separating the lymphatic sacs on either side of the midline. (**c**) Coronal view of the head and neck showing bilateral enlarged lymphatic sacs (*arrows*). (**d**) Bilateral axillary cystic hygromas (*arrows*)

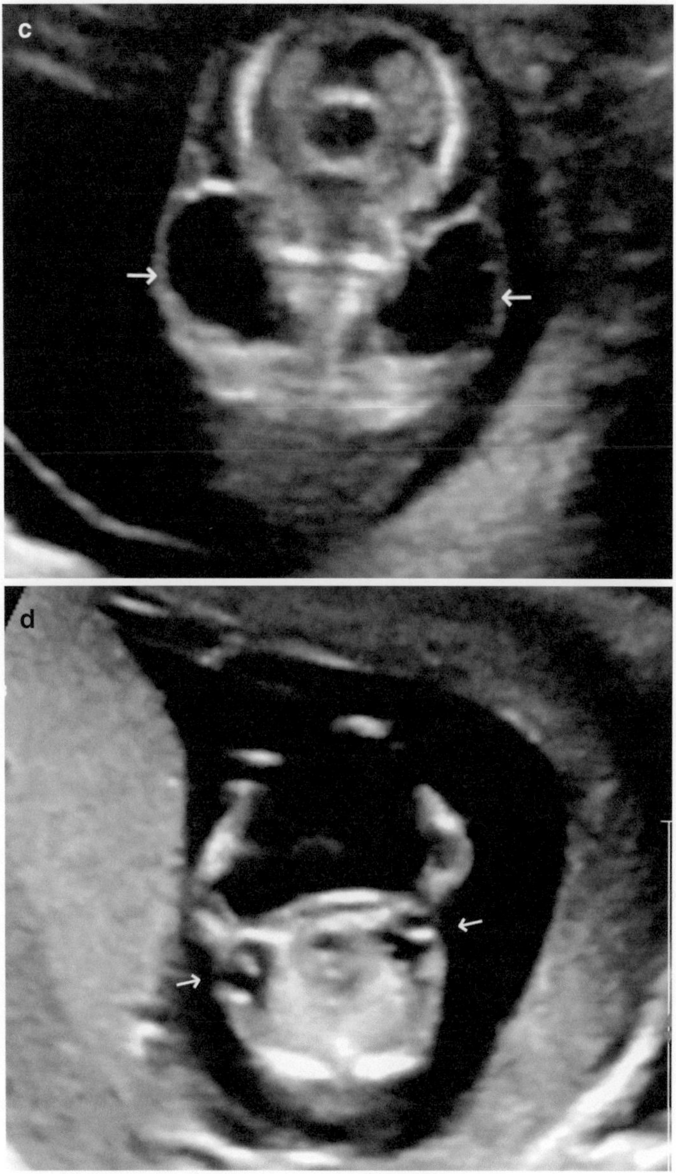

Fig. 2.10 (continued)

was nearly 80% when aneuploidy, associated malformations, and hydrops were excluded [21].

2.7.2 Megacystis

Fetal megacystis ('large bladder') is diagnosed when the fetal bladder measures more than 7 mm longitudinally at the 11–13 + 6 weeks scan (Fig. 2.11a, b). The etiology of megacystis includes chromosomal abnormalities, bladder outlet obstruction, and rarely, syndromes like prune belly syndrome and megacystis-microcolon-intestinal hypoperistalsis syndrome (MMIHS).

The incidence of aneuploidy (mostly trisomies 13, 18, and 21) is 23% when the longitudinal bladder diameter is 7–15 mm, and only 11% when the diameter is >15 mm. Conversely, overall outcomes are better in euploid fetuses with smaller bladders, with 90% of fetuses having spontaneous resolution when the bladder size is <15 mm. Fetuses with large megacystis usually progress to significant lower urinary tract obstruction [22].

2.7.3 Open Neural Tube Defect

Open neural tube defects (ONTDs) are caused by an incomplete closure of the neural tube, leading to exposure of the brain or spinal cord (Fig. 2.12). As most cases are multifactorial in origin and have a uniformly poor outcome, invasive testing has a limited role. However, invasive testing can establish the causality and help in counseling about the recurrence risk in future pregnancies. It is also mandatory in women considering in utero repair of ONTD. Aneuploidy is detected in approximately 10% of cases, with trisomy 18 being the commonest, followed by trisomy 13 [23]. Chapter 15 provides a detailed discussion on ONTDs.

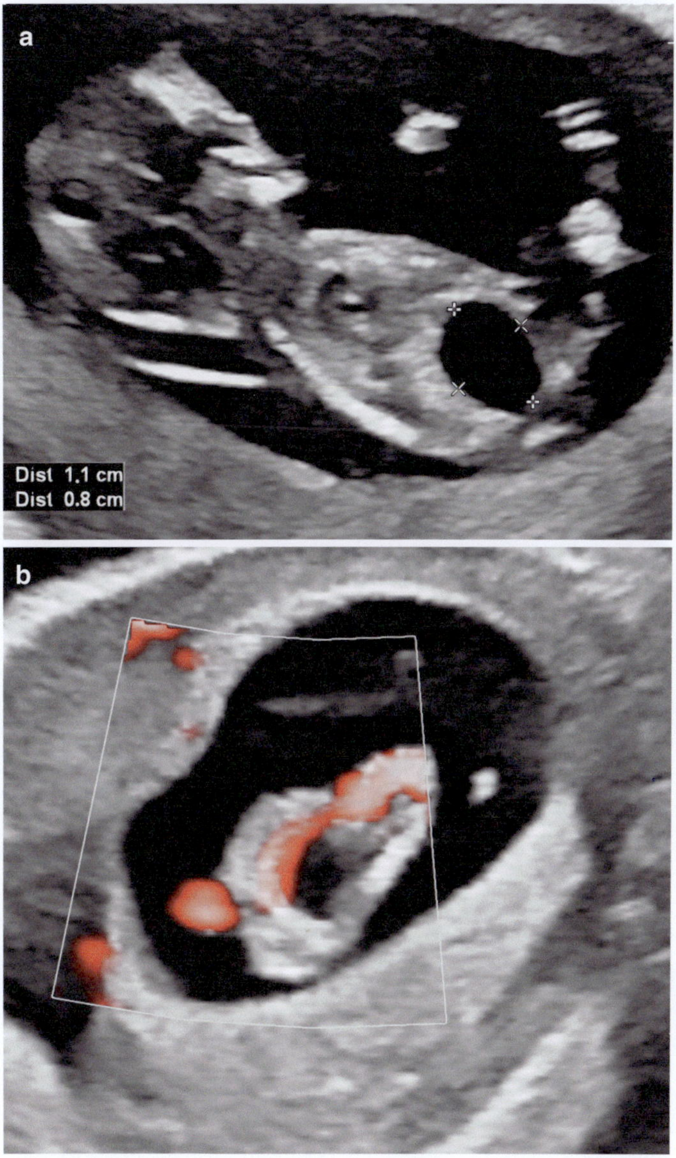

Fig. 2.11 (**a**) Sagittal view of a 12-week fetus with trisomy 21 showing megacystis. The longitudinal diameter of fetal bladder is 11 mm. Note that the NT is also raised. (**b**) Axial view with color Doppler insonation confirms the cystic structure to be the bladder, and has identified a single umbilical artery

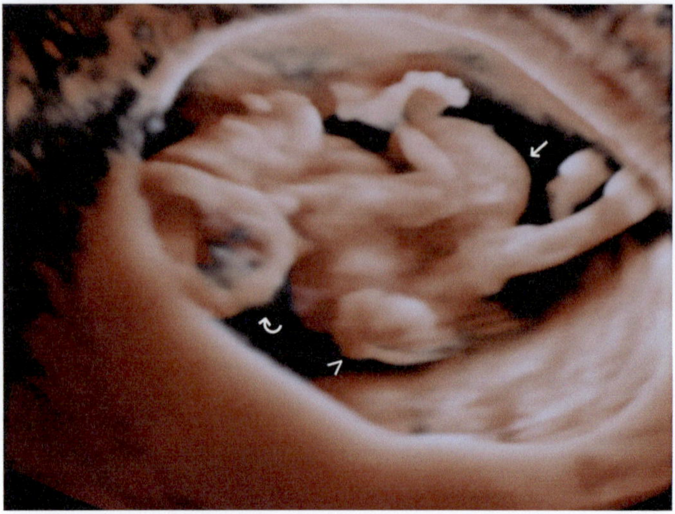

Fig. 2.12 Three-dimensional ultrasound in surface mode in a 13-week fetus with trisomy 18 showing severe malformations: iniencephaly (*curved arrow*), open spina bifida (*arrowhead*), and omphalocele (*straight arrow*)

2.7.4 Omphalocele

Physiological herniation of bowel into the base of the umbilical cord occurs between 6 and 11 weeks of gestation due to lack of space in the abdominal cavity. Omphalocele can be differentiated from physiological gut herniation when it is seen after 12 weeks. In addition, a size of >7 mm and presence of the liver within the sac are considered pathological. Omphalocele appears as a bulge in the lower abdomen which is covered by a membrane, with the umbilical cord inserted at its apex (Fig. 2.12).

Omphaloceles in the first trimester are associated with chromosomal abnormalities in 40% of cases, the commonest being trisomy 18 followed by trisomy 13 [24]. In isolated omphaloceles with a normal karyotype, the possibility of genetic conditions like Beckwith-Wiedemann syndrome should be kept in mind as the other features may be difficult to demonstrate in the first trimester.

2.7.5 Holoprosencephaly

Holoprosencephaly is a condition in which the forebrain (prosencephalon) fails to divide into two hemispheres. Depending on the degree of fusion, it can be classified as alobar, semilobar, lobar, and the middle interhemispheric variant.

In alobar holoprosencephaly, the fetal intracranial anatomy appears distinctly abnormal with the absence of midline falx (Fig. 2.13a). The two lateral ventricles are replaced by an anterior crescentic monoventricle. The thalami are completely fused in the midline. In addition, there can be associated abnormalities of the face, like cyclopia, proboscis, or facial cleft (Fig. 2.13b). The semilobar, lobar, and interhemispheric variants are difficult to diagnose in the first trimester.

2.7.6 Limb Defects

First-trimester limb defects associated with aneuploidy include limb reduction defects, polydactyly (Fig. 2.14), and abnormalities of the upper limbs (club hand, cleft hand, or clenched hand), or lower limbs (rocker-bottom foot).

2.8 Safety of Ultrasound in the First Trimester

Ultrasound is a form of energy which has the potential to produce thermal and mechanical effects on biological tissue. The following points should be noted regarding its use in the first trimester:

1. The potential of ultrasound to cause tissue damage is measured in the form of 'thermal index.' The higher the thermal index, the more the risk to the fetus. Thermal index is lowest when using the B-mode or the M-mode and rises progressively with the use of color Doppler, power Doppler, and pulsed wave Doppler. Modern ultrasound systems have in-built first-trimester presets which maintain the thermal index within the permissible limit of 1.0.

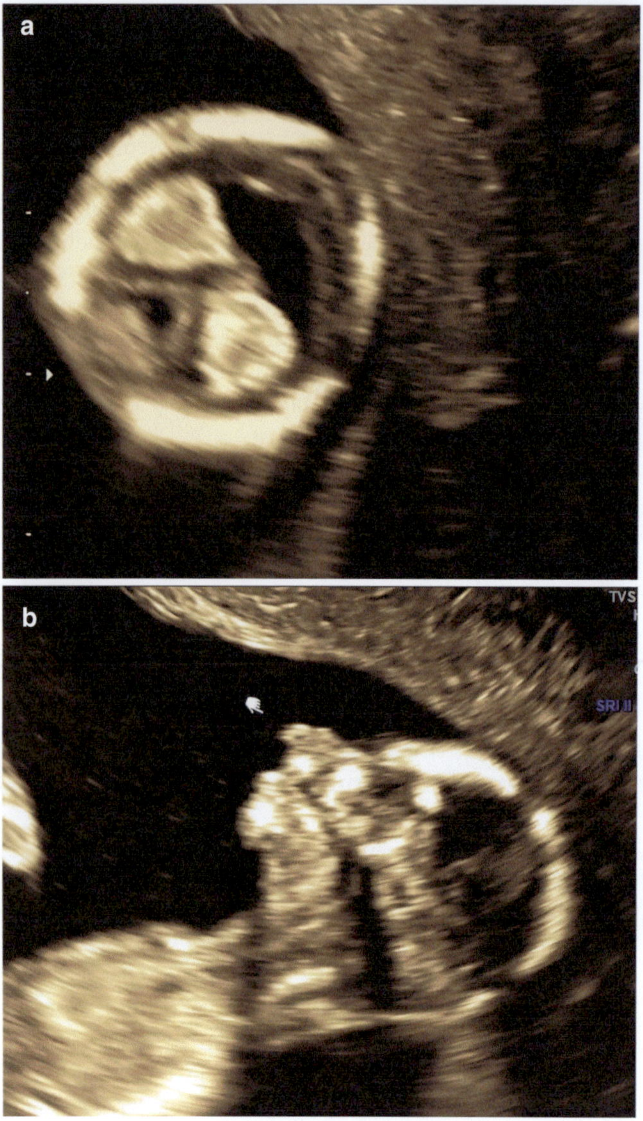

Fig. 2.13 (**a**) Transvaginal ultrasound of the fetal head at 12 weeks of gestation showing alobar holoprosencephaly. (**b**) Sagittal view of the face in the same fetus showing an abnormal facial profile (*hand icon*)

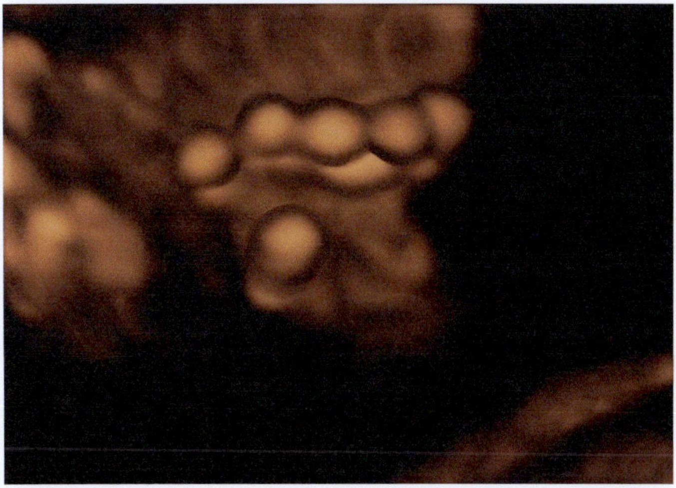

Fig. 2.14 Three-dimensional ultrasound in surface mode showing polydactyly in a 13-week fetus with trisomy 13. Additional findings included a raised NT of 6.7 mm, absent NB, and TR

2. The embryonic period of gestation lasts until the tenth menstrual week. During this phase, there is rapid cell division, organogenesis, and the establishment of fetal circulation. Only B-mode or M-mode should be used during this time.
3. After 11 weeks, it is safe to use Doppler ultrasound modalities when specifically indicated, e.g., for cardiac evaluation and aneuploidy screening, provided the exposure time is restricted to a maximum of 5–10 min [13].
4. Uterine artery Doppler does not expose the fetus to the ultrasound waves.
5. In all cases, the ALARA principle should be followed to avoid undue exposure for the fetus (ALARA—As Low As Reasonably Achievable).

2.9 Key Messages

1. Standardized technique should be strictly followed while evaluating NT, NB, DV, and tricuspid flow.
2. NB, DV, and tricuspid flow are technically difficult to evaluate and highly prone for errors in interpretation. Incorrect assessment can reduce the efficacy of screening, rather than enhance it.
3. Women with fetal NT >3 mm or structural malformations should directly be offered invasive testing along with DNA storage.
4. In the first trimester, NB length should not be reported. NB should be mentioned as present or absent, and used only as a part of combined FTS.
5. Color Doppler, power Doppler, and pulsed wave Doppler should be avoided before 11 weeks of gestation.

References

1. Nicolaides KH, Azar G, Byrne D, Mansur C, Marks K. Fetal nuchal translucency: ultrasound screening for chromosomal defects in first trimester of pregnancy. BMJ. 1992;304(6831):867–9.
2. Nicolaides KH. Screening for fetal aneuploidies at 11 to 13 weeks. Prenat Diagn. 2011;31(1):7–15.
3. Nicolaides KH. The 11–13 weeks scan [Online course]. The Fetal Medicine Foundation. https://fetalmedicine.org/education/the-11-13-weeks-scan. Accessed 2 May 2023.
4. Petersen OB, Smith E, Van Opstal D, Polak M, Knapen MFCM, Diderich KEM, et al. Nuchal translucency of 3.0-3.4 mm an indication for NIPT or microarray? Cohort analysis and literature review. Acta Obstet Gynecol Scand. 2020;99(6):765–74.
5. Souka AP, Von Kaisenberg CS, Hyett JA, Sonek JD, Nicolaides KH. Increased nuchal translucency with normal karyotype. Am J Obstet Gynecol. 2005;192(4):1005–21.
6. Souka AP, Krampl E, Bakalis S, Heath V, Nicolaides KH. Outcome of pregnancy in chromosomally normal fetuses with increased nuchal

translucency in the first trimester. Ultrasound Obstet Gynecol. 2001;18(1):9–17.

7. Sotiriadis A, Papatheodorou S, Makrydimas G. Neurodevelopmental outcome of fetuses with increased nuchal translucency and apparently normal prenatal and/or postnatal assessment: a systematic review. Ultrasound Obstet Gynecol. 2012;39(1):10–9.
8. Äyräs O, Eronen M, Tikkanen M, Rahkola-Soisalo P, Paavonen J, Stefanovic V. Long-term outcome in apparently healthy children with increased nuchal translucency in the first trimester screening. Acta Obstet Gynecol Scand. 2016;95(5):541–6.
9. Ali MM, Chasen ST, Norton ME. Testing for Noonan syndrome after increased nuchal translucency. Prenat Diagn. 2017;37(8):750–3.
10. Sandikcioglu M, Mølsted K, Kjaer I. The prenatal development of the human nasal and vomeral bones. J Craniofac Genet Dev Biol. 1994;14(2):124–34.
11. Cicero S, Curcio P, Papageorghiou A, Sonek J, Nicolaides K. Absence of nasal bone in fetuses with trisomy 21 at 11–14 weeks of gestation: an observational study. Lancet. 2001;358(9294):1665–7.
12. Moreno-Cid M, Rubio-Lorente A, Rodríguez MJ, Bueno-Pacheco G, Tenías JM, Román-Ortiz C, Arias Á. Systematic review and meta-analysis of performance of second-trimester nasal bone assessment in detection of fetuses with Down syndrome. Ultrasound Obstet Gynecol. 2014;43(3):247–53.
13. International Society of Ultrasound in Obstetrics and Gynecology, Bilardo CM, Chaoui R, Hyett JA, Kagan KO, Karim JN, Papageorghiou AT, Poon LC, Salomon LJ, Syngelaki A, Nicolaides KH. ISUOG Practice Guidelines (updated): performance of 11–14-week ultrasound scan. Ultrasound Obstet Gynecol. 2023;61(1):127–43.
14. Geipel A, Willruth A, Vieten J, Gembruch U, Berg C. Nuchal fold thickness, nasal bone absence or hypoplasia, ductus venosus reversed flow and tricuspid valve regurgitation in screening for trisomies 21, 18 and 13 in the early second trimester. Ultrasound Obstet Gynecol. 2010;35(5):535–9.
15. Maiz N, Valencia C, Kagan KO, Wright D, Nicolaides KH. Ductus venosus Doppler in screening for trisomies 21, 18 and 13 and Turner syndrome at 11–13 weeks of gestation. Ultrasound Obstet Gynecol. 2009;33(5):512–7.
16. Timmerman E, Oude Rengerink K, Pajkrt E, Opmeer BC, van der Post JAM, Bilardo CM. Ductus venosus pulsatility index measurement reduces the false-positive rate in first-trimester screening. Ultrasound Obstet Gynecol. 2010;36(6):661–7.
17. Falcon O, Faiola S, Huggon I, Allan L, Nicolaides KH. Fetal tricuspid regurgitation at the 11 + 0 to 13 + 6-week scan: association with chromosomal defects and reproducibility of the method. Ultrasound Obstet Gynecol. 2006;27(6):609–12.

18. Scala C, Morlando M, Familiari A, Leone Roberti Maggiore U, Ferrero S, D'Antonio F, Khalil A. Fetal tricuspid regurgitation in the first trimester as a screening marker for congenital heart defects: systematic review and meta-analysis. Fetal Diagn Ther. 2017;42(1):1–8.
19. Liao AW, Snijders R, Geerts L, Spencer K, Nicolaides KH. Fetal heart rate in chromosomally abnormal fetuses. Ultrasound Obstet Gynecol. 2000;16(7):610–3.
20. Graesslin O, Derniaux E, Alanio E, Gaillard D, Vitry F, Quéreux C, Ducarme G. Characteristics and outcome of fetal cystic hygroma diagnosed in the first trimester. Acta Obstet Gynecol Scand. 2007;86(12):1442–6.
21. Malone CM, Mullers S, Kelliher N, Dalrymple J, O'Beirnes J, Flood K, Malone F. Euploid first-trimester cystic hygroma: a more benign entity than previously thought? Fetal Diagn Ther. 2021;48(9):667–71.
22. Liao AW, Sebire NJ, Geerts L, Cicero S, Nicolaides KH. Megacystis at 10–14 weeks of gestation: chromosomal defects and outcome according to bladder length. Ultrasound Obstet Gynecol. 2003;21(4):338–41.
23. Sepulveda W, Corral E, Ayala C, Be C, Gutierrez J, Vasquez P. Chromosomal abnormalities in fetuses with open neural tube defects: prenatal identification with ultrasound. Ultrasound Obstet Gynecol. 2004;23(4):352–6.
24. Syngelaki A, Guerra L, Ceccacci I, Efeturk T, Nicolaides KH. Impact of holoprosencephaly, exomphalos, megacystis and increased nuchal translucency on first-trimester screening for chromosomal abnormalities. Ultrasound Obstet Gynecol. 2017;50(1):45–8.

Serum Markers Used for Screening

3

3.1 Introduction

Maternal serum markers in combination with maternal age and nuchal translucency form a powerful tool to screen for the common trisomies. In this chapter, the focus is on the individual serum markers and their importance in first- and second-trimester screening. The chapter delves into the concept of multiples of median (MoM), alterations in marker levels seen in the common aneuploidies, and the factors that impact screening performance. Additionally, it addresses newer markers such as placental growth factor and hyperglycosylated hCG.

3.2 Beta Subunit of Human Chorionic Gonadotropin (β-hCG)

Human chorionic gonadotropin (hCG) is a glycoprotein, largely produced by the syncytiotrophoblast cells and found abundantly in the blood and urine of pregnant women. It comprises two subunits, α and β, of which the α subunit is coded by chromosome 6, and is common to follicle-stimulating hormone, luteinizing hormone, and thyroid-stimulating hormone. The β subunit comprises 145 amino acids coded by chromosome 19 and is unique to hCG. Levels of β-hCG peak at 8–10 weeks and then remain steady

© The Author(s), under exclusive license to Springer Nature Singapore Pte Ltd. 2023
A. Kamat, *Down Syndrome Screening*,
https://doi.org/10.1007/978-981-99-7758-1_3

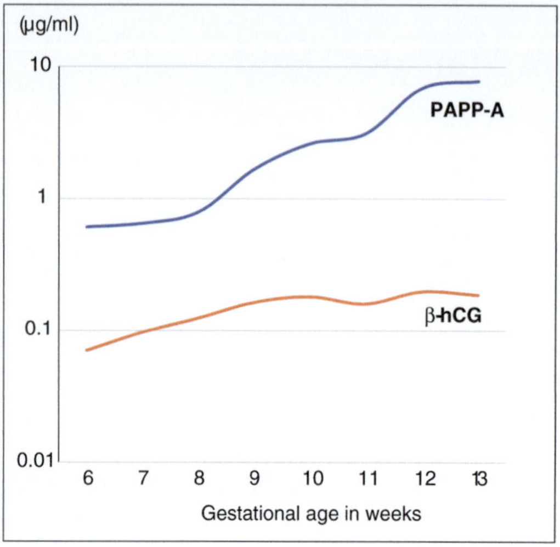

Fig. 3.1 Mean maternal serum concentration of β-hCG and PAPP-A in the first trimester. (Data from Bischof et al. [2])

until 18–20 weeks [1]. Figure 3.1 shows the changes in β-hCG levels during the first trimester.

There are at least four types of hCG molecules [3]:

Native hCG is the intact hCG molecule. Since the α subunit is common to several hormones, its measurement is of no significance. The β subunit being unique to hCG, its measurement is used as a surrogate for the total hCG. In practice, both the terms 'hCG' and 'β-hCG' are used interchangeably.

Hyperglycosylated hCG is a sugar variant with much larger N- and O-linked oligosaccharides. It has autocrine functions within the cytotrophoblast, and promotes cell division, implantation, and invasion into the endometrium.

Free β-hCG refers to a hyperglycosylated β subunit of hCG that is not bound to the α subunit. Free β-hCG makes up less than 4% of the total circulating hCG and originates from either direct placental production of the β subunit or separation of α and β subunits. Free β-hCG level rises rapidly in whole blood at room temperature, because of its liberation from intact hyperglycosylated hCG.

Pituitary hCG is the fourth variant which functions in an LH-like manner in the brain.

Human chorionic gonadotropin acts on the LH receptors present in the corpus luteum, the decidua, the cytotrophoblast, the myometrial vessels, fetal and umbilical cord cells, and the maternal brain. It promotes progesterone secretion by luteal cells, and stimulates uterine growth, angiogenesis, and muscle relaxation. It helps mitosis and differentiation of cytotrophoblast and syncytiotrophoblast cells. It also prevents immune rejection of the fetus and positively influences its growth. The hCG/LH receptor in the maternal brain plays a role in hyperemesis gravidarum.

First-trimester screening tests use the *free β-hCG* value, while the quadruple test may use either *free* β-hCG or *total* β-hCG value, depending on the testing laboratory.

Maternal serum levels of hCG are elevated when the fetus has Down syndrome (Table 3.1). This results from a marked increase in placental synthesis of β-hCG as evidenced by an increased β-hCG mRNA expression in trophoblasts. The increase in secretion of α-hCG is more modest [1]. Falsely raised β-hCG levels in

Table 3.1 NT, PAPP-A, and β-hCG MoM values in the first trimester seen in various aneuploidies. Arrows indicate an increase (↑), decrease (↓), or no significant change (↔). (Data from Eiben et al. [4], and Spencer et al. [5–7])

Aneuploidy	NT (MoM)	PAPP-A (MoM)	Free β-hCG (MoM)
Trisomy 21	2.67 ↑	0.51 ↓	2.15 ↑
Trisomy 13	2.87 ↑	0.25 ↓↓	0.51 ↓
Trisomy 18	3.27 ↑↑	0.18 ↓↓	0.28 ↓↓
Turner's syndrome (45, X)	4.76 ↑↑	0.49 ↓	1.11 ↔
47XXX, XXY, XYY	2.07 ↑	0.88 ↔	1.07 ↔
Triploidy	1.89 ↑	3.13 ↑↑	4.59 ↑↑

euploid pregnancies may be caused by a delay in shipping the sample, recent hCG injection, or a vanishing twin. Far rarer causes include partial moles and hCG-secreting tumors.

3.3 Pregnancy-Associated Plasma Protein A (PAPP-A)

Pregnancy-associated plasma protein A (PAPP-A) is a metalloproteinase found in the plasma of pregnant women, encoded by a gene on chromosome 9. Circulating PAPP-A is largely synthesized by the syncytiotrophoblast and by the decidua. Ninety-nine percent of PAPP-A is bound to the proform of eosinophil major basic protein (proMBP). This complex cannot bind to the cell surface, hence nearly all the synthesized PAPP-A/proMBP is released into maternal circulation [8].

Within the placenta, PAPP-A increases the levels of insulin-like growth factor (IGF), which stimulates cell division and inhibits apoptosis. Thus, PAPP-A plays a crucial role in trophoblast formation and invasion. It is also synthesized by non-placental tissues such as the ovary, fibroblasts, osteoblasts, and smooth muscle cells in blood vessels, where it may play an autocrine role [8].

PAPP-A in pregnant women can be detected shortly after implantation, and it increases throughout the pregnancy till term, doubling every 3–4 days in the first trimester (Fig. 3.1). Due to this exponential increase, PAPP-A levels are very specific to gestational age. Hence, PAPP-A is reported as multiples of the median (MoM) value for a particular gestation. Using MoM instead of absolute concentration makes the value independent of gestational age. The difference in PAPP-A levels between euploid and aneuploid pregnancies is more at 11 weeks compared to 13 weeks. This difference is also greater than the difference in free β-hCG levels. Combined and biochemical screening is therefore more sensitive at 11 weeks [1].

Circulating PAPP-A levels closely correlate with placental function. Low PAPP-A levels are not specific to trisomy 21, and are also seen in other aneuploidies. In Down syndrome, the maternal serum levels of PAPP-A are significantly low, despite only a mild reduction in placental synthesis (Table 3.1). Possibly, the low serum levels result either from an altered release or a reduced stability of the molecule in these fetuses.

In euploid pregnancies, gestational age and placental function are the major factors influencing PAPP-A levels. Other factors include multiple pregnancy and smoking (which influence placental size), and maternal weight (which affects the serum concentration and distribution of PAPP-A). Parity, race, and assisted reproduction also cause a change in PAPP-A levels, though the exact mechanisms are not clear. Low PAPP-A levels in euploid pregnancies are linked with adverse pregnancy outcomes (see Chap. 4). The significance of elevated PAPP-A levels in the first trimester is not clear.

3.4 Alpha-Fetoprotein

Alpha-fetoprotein (AFP) is a glycoprotein encoded by the AFP gene on Chromosome 4, and is secreted by the yolk sac and the fetal liver. It is the predominant protein in fetal plasma akin to albumin in post-natal life [9]. Fetal serum levels of AFP are a hundred times higher than amniotic fluid, though its exact role in the fetus has not yet been elucidated. One of its possible functions may be to prevent the virilization of the female fetal brain by androgens derived from maternal estrogen.

Maternal serum alpha-fetoprotein (MSAFP) starts rising toward the end of the first trimester and remains elevated till approximately 32 weeks [9]. When prenatal Down syndrome screening was first introduced, MSAFP was the only serum marker used. Since there is a significant overlap in MSAFP values in women carrying aneuploid fetuses and those with euploid fetuses it has poor sensitivity and specificity as a standalone marker for aneuploidy. Conversely, MSAFP significantly increases when the fetus has an open neural tube defect (ONTD), making it a useful marker (Table 3.2).

Diabetic mothers have lower levels of MSAFP, though the risk of ONTDs is higher, and therefore this correction is very important. Other conditions which raise MSAFP include multiple preg-

Table 3.2 Levels of second-trimester serum markers in common trisomies. Values are in multiples of median (MoM). Arrows indicate an increase (↑), decrease (↓), or no significant change (↔). MSAFP: maternal serum alpha-fetoprotein; uE3: unconjugated estriol; hCG: human chorionic gonadotropin; inh A: inhibin A. Data from Wald et al. [10] (SURUSS), and Bestwick et al. [11]

Aneuploidy	MSAFP	uE3	hCG	inh A
Trisomy 21	0.74 ↓	0.70 ↓	2.05 ↑	2.54 ↑
Trisomy 13	1.17 ↔	0.95 ↔	1.15 ↔	1.61 ↑
Trisomy 18	0.72 ↓	0.47 ↓	0.25 ↓↓	1.11 ↔
Open neural tube defects	>2.5			

nancy, fetal demise, placental abnormalities, and oligohydramnios. Apart from ONTDs, other fetal anomalies associated with raised MSAFP are abdominal wall defects, polycystic kidneys, esophageal atresia, duodenal atresia, teratoma, cystic hygroma, and hydrops [9].

Congenital fetal AFP deficiency is a rare condition associated with abnormally low levels of MSAFP. This condition is not known to have any adverse effect on pregnancy outcome [12].

3.5 Unconjugated Estriol

Estriol is the dominant estrogen during pregnancy which is secreted by the fetoplacental unit. It has a lower potency compared to estradiol. Dehydroepiandrosterone sulfate (DHEAS) produced in fetal adrenals undergoes aromatization in the syncytiotrophoblasts to form estriol. Estriol levels continue to increase throughout pregnancy till term. Nearly all the placental estriol enters maternal circulation and reaches maternal liver, where it is conjugated to form a glucuronide conjugate. Because of a short half-life of 30 min, and rapid conjugation by maternal liver, unconjugated estriol (uE3) forms only 10–15% of the total circulating estriol in maternal plasma [13].

Unconjugated estriol levels are low in both Down syndrome and trisomy 18 because of placental dysfunction and/or immaturity of fetal adrenals or liver. Used as a single marker, uE3 has a poor predictive value, but increases the sensitivity and specificity when added to other markers in the triple and quadruple marker tests (Table 3.2).

Unconjugated estriol levels can also be low in fetal adrenal insufficiency, Smith-Lemli-Opitz syndrome, X-linked ichthyosis, and aromatase deficiency. High levels of uE3 are associated with fetal congenital adrenal hyperplasia and impending preterm birth [13].

3.6 Inhibin A

Inhibins and activins belong to the family of transforming growth factor β, named because of their earliest identified function of suppression and stimulation of follicle-stimulating hormone, respectively. Though they were first isolated from the gonads, they have been subsequently detected in other tissues as well. Inhibin A is an α-βA dimer and inhibin B is α-βB dimer. In non-pregnant women, inhibin A is secreted by the dominant follicle and the subsequently formed corpus luteum, and inhibin B by the small antral follicles [14].

In pregnant women, large amounts of inhibin A are produced by the placenta and released into maternal circulation. Inhibin A levels rise from 5 weeks of gestation, peaking at 8–9 weeks and then decline, remaining low throughout the second trimester. The levels rise again in the third trimester, with a second peak close to term [15].

The exact function of inhibin A in pregnancy is unknown. It likely has paracrine and autocrine functions, including regulation of secretion of other placental hormones and suppression of maternal ovarian folliculogenesis. The rise during the third trimester suggests the possibility of an additional role in late gestation.

In Down syndrome, maternal serum levels of inhibin A remain unaltered until the 11th week of gestation, but are significantly elevated at 15–18 weeks because of increased placental synthesis [15]. Inhibin A is raised in trisomy 13, but not in trisomy 18 (see Table 3.2). The quadruple test does not screen for trisomy 13, as the other markers are not significantly different from unaffected pregnancies.

3.7 Maternal Characteristics Affecting Screening

Several maternal characteristics and pregnancy-related factors alter the levels of serum markers. These details need to be entered correctly on the requisition form for every patient undergoing screening. Correcting for these variables results in an increase in detection rate and/or a lower false-positive rate (FPR).

3.7.1 Gestational Age

The accurate estimation of gestational age on the day of screening cannot be overstated. All markers are expressed in MoM values adjusted for gestational age, and incorrect dating leads to erroneous screening results. Menstrual dates are often incorrect, and ultrasound dating is mandatory.

For first-trimester screening, the crown-rump length should be measured on the same day as nuchal translucency. Aneuploidy itself can cause growth restriction. Therefore, for the quadruple test, gestational age should be calculated from the earliest scan available, rather than the measurements taken on the day of the test. Finally, the scan date should be clearly mentioned in the requisition form.

3.7.2 Ethnicity

Maternal ethnicity causes slight variations in levels of serum markers. Correcting for ethnicity equalizes the FPR in all populations. Some variations noted for different ethnic groups (compared to Caucasian women) are as follows [14, 16, 17]:

- Asians: Higher β-hCG and PAPP-A.
- Blacks: Higher β-hCG, PAPP-A, and AFP, and lower inhibin A.
- Aboriginals: Higher uE3.

3.7.3 Maternal Weight

Overweight women have lower levels of serum markers as compared to thin women, likely because of the dilution caused by an increased blood volume. Maternal weight has the greatest effect on PAPP-A levels. Adjusting for maternal weight increases the detection rate of Down syndrome by 1%. As maternal weight distribution varies with ethnicity, correction should be based on weight percentiles specific to the local population.

3.7.4 Assisted Reproductive Technology (ART)

An analysis of 962 pregnancies in the multicenter FASTER trial showed that pregnancies achieved by in vitro fertilization (IVF) were associated with altered second-trimester serum markers, resulting in a higher screen-positive rate. Specifically, inhibin A and hCG levels were increased, and estriol levels were reduced. Inexplicably, MSAFP levels were only elevated in donor egg IVF patients [18].

The effect of ART on first-trimester markers is less pronounced. PAPP-A levels are slightly lower in pregnancies resulting from IVF and intrauterine insemination following ovarian stimulation [18]. Chapter 11 explains the nuances of assisted reproduction and Down syndrome screening.

3.7.5 Multiple Pregnancies

In twin pregnancies, the median β-hCG levels are at 2.023 MoM compared to singletons. Levels of PAPP-A differ according to chorionicity. The MoM correction factor is 1.788 in MC twins and 2.192 in DC twins [19].

Compared to singleton pregnancies, the MoM values for alpha fetoprotein, hCG, unconjugated estriol, and inhibin A are 1.6, 1.84, 1.99, and 2.13, respectively [20]. Despite making the necessary adjustments, second-trimester screening does not perform as well in twin pregnancies.

3.7.6 Diabetes Mellitus

Insulin-dependent diabetes mellitus reduces uE3 levels, but the effect is not substantial enough to alter screening results. As explained earlier, diabetes is associated with lower MSAFP levels. Therefore, this factor correction is vital in order to maintain the detection rate for open neural tube defects [9]. Other markers are not affected.

3.7.7 Human Chorionic Gonadotropin Injections

Women with a history of recurrent miscarriages may receive hCG injections to support their pregnancy. Since hCG takes approximately 10 days to clear from maternal blood, serum screening should be avoided for 2 weeks following the last hCG injection.

3.7.8 Vaginal Bleeding

Vaginal bleeding at any time prior to screening causes subtle alterations in maternal serum markers, but does not affect screening performance in pregnancies that ultimately continue till term. A history of vaginal bleeding does not require a correction in MoM values for any marker.

3.7.9 Smoking

Smokers have altered levels of serum markers in the first and second trimesters. Levels of hCG, PAPP-A, and uE3 are lower, while MSAFP and inhibin A levels are raised. Aneuploidy screening in smokers has similar sensitivity compared to non-smokers, but higher false-positive rates (FPR). Correcting for smoking status significantly lowers the FPR (and therefore, invasive procedures) in these women [21].

3.8 Newer Serum Markers

Newer markers have been proposed to either supplement or replace one of the existing markers in the screening tests. As serum screening (using β-hCG and PAPP-A alone) without NT has poor sensitivity for the detection of Down syndrome, additional markers can be potentially added to improve screening performance, particularly in centers that do not have trained sonographers. At present, these newer markers should only be used in clinical trials as there is limited data about their efficacy for Down syndrome screening.

3.8.1 Placental Growth Factor

Placental growth factor (PlGF) is a protein belonging to the vascular endothelial growth factor (VEGF) family, and is synthesized by trophoblasts. Any condition causing placental dysfunction alters PlGF levels. Its levels are significantly reduced in Down syndrome, with the median level in affected cases being 0.67 MoM. Addition of PlGF along with AFP in the first-trimester screening protocol modestly improves the detection rate of trisomy 21 by 1.4–3.3% depending on the FPR [22]. An advantage of including it in first-trimester screening is the ability to screen for both Down syndrome and preeclampsia simultaneously (see Chap. 14). Disadvantages include an increase in the cost of screening, and, as mentioned earlier, lack of sufficient data showing the benefit of this approach.

3.8.2 Hyperglycosylated hCG

Hyperglycosylated hCG (H-hCG), also known as invasive trophoblast antigen, is a structurally complex high-carbohydrate hCG variant. In Down syndrome, besides the twofold increase in hCG secretion, there is a threefold increase in its glycosylation. This causes H-hCG levels to be elevated even more than levels of free β-hCG.

While the initial research on H-hCG was encouraging, more recent studies have reported less promising results. Despite serum H-hCG being significantly raised in mothers carrying trisomy 21 fetuses, there is a significant overlap between normal and affected pregnancies. This offsets the benefit of its high median value in affected pregnancies, and brings down its efficacy to that of free β-hCG [23].

Maternal urinary H-hCG levels are also raised in trisomy 21 pregnancies compared to normal. This is seldom used in clinical practice because of the requirement of a urine sample in addition to the serum sample, and the lack of validation by large-scale randomized trials [24].

3.8.3 A Disintegrin and Metalloprotease-12 (ADAM12)

A disintegrin and metalloprotease-12 is a placental glycoprotein with proteolytic activity against insulin-like growth factor binding proteins, which regulates the bioavailability of IGF-I and IGF-II. Maternal serum levels of ADAM 12 are reduced in Down syndrome, being most significant between 8 and 10 weeks of gestation [25].

Maternal serum ADAM12 is unlikely to be added to the 11–13 weeks combined screening test for several reasons [26]. First, ADAM12 levels are not significantly different in Down syndrome fetuses compared to euploid fetuses between 11 and 13 weeks. Second, ADAM12 levels are affected by PAPP-A and β-hCG levels. Third, using an additional marker increases the cost of screening without improving sensitivity or FPR. A serum test consisting of ADAM12 and PAPP-A, with or without additional markers, may prove useful in the future for aneuploidy screening before 11 weeks [25].

References

1. Shiefa S, Amargandhi M, Bhupendra J, Moulali S, Kristine T. First trimester maternal serum screening using biochemical markers PAPP-A and free β-hCG for Down syndrome, Patau syndrome and Edward syndrome. Indian J Clin Biochem. 2013;28(1):3–12.
2. Bischof P, DuBerg S, Herrmann W, Sizonenko PC. Pregnancy-associated plasma protein-A (PAPP-A) and hCG in early pregnancy. Br J Obstet Gynaecol. 1981;88(10):973–5.
3. Cole LA. Biological functions of hCG and hCG-related molecules. Reprod Biol Endocrinol. 2010;8:102.
4. Eiben B, Glaubitz R. First-trimester screening: an overview. J Histochem Cytochem. 2005;53(3):281–3.
5. Spencer K, Ong C, Skentou H, Liao AW, Nicolaides KH. Screening for trisomy 13 by fetal nuchal translucency and maternal serum free beta-hCG and PAPP-A at 10-14 weeks of gestation. Prenat Diagn. 2000;20(5):411–6.
6. Spencer K, Tul N, Nicolaides KH. Maternal serum free beta-hCG and PAPP-A in fetal sex chromosome defects in the first trimester. Prenat Diagn. 2000;20(5):390–4.
7. Spencer K, Liao AW, Skentou H, Cicero S, Nicolaides KH. Screening for triploidy by fetal nuchal translucency and maternal serum free beta-hCG and PAPP-A at 10-14 weeks of gestation. Prenat Diagn. 2000;20(6):495–9.
8. Kirkegaard I, Uldbjerg N, Oxvig C. Biology of pregnancy-associated plasma protein-A in relation to prenatal diagnostics: an overview. Acta Obstet Gynecol Scand. 2010;89(9):1118–25.
9. Adigun OO, Yarrarapu SNS, Khetarpal S. Alpha fetoprotein. In: StatPearls. Treasure Island, FL: StatPearls Publishing; 2020. http://www.ncbi.nlm.nih.gov/books/NBK430750. Accessed 22 May 2023.
10. Wald NJ, Rodeck C, Hackshaw AK, Walters J, Chitty L, Mackinson AM. First and second trimester antenatal screening for Down's syndrome: the results of the Serum, Urine and Ultrasound Screening Study (SURUSS). J Med Screen. 2003;10(2):56–104.
11. Bestwick JP, Huttly WJ, Wald NJ. Detection of trisomy 18 and trisomy 13 using first and second trimester Down's syndrome screening markers. J Med Screen. 2013;20(2):57–65.
12. Muller F, Dreux S, Sault C, Galland A, Puissant H, Couplet G, et al. Very low alpha-fetoprotein in Down syndrome maternal serum screening. Prenat Diagn. 2003;23(7):584–7.
13. Falah N, Torday J, Quinney S, Haas D. Estriol review: clinical applications and potential biomedical importance. Clin Res Trials. 2015;1(2):29–33.

14. Benn PA. Advances in prenatal screening for Down syndrome: I. General principles and second trimester testing. Clin Chim Acta. 2002;323(1–2):1–16.
15. Aitken DA, Wallace EM, Crossley JA, Swanston IA, van Pareren Y, van Maarle M, et al. Dimeric inhibin A as a marker for Down's syndrome in early pregnancy. N Engl J Med. 1996;334(19):1231–6.
16. O'Brien JE, Dvorin E, Drugan A, Johnson MP, Yaron Y, Evans MI. Race-ethnicity-specific variation in multiple-marker biochemical screening: alpha-fetoprotein, hCG, and estriol. Obstet Gynecol. 1997;89(3):355–8.
17. Spencer K, Ong CY, Liao AW, Nicolaides KH. The influence of ethnic origin on first trimester biochemical markers of chromosomal abnormalities. Prenat Diagn. 2000;20(6):491–4.
18. Lambert-Messerlian G, Dugoff L, Vidaver J, Canick JA, Malone FD, Ball RH, et al. First- and second-trimester Down syndrome screening markers in pregnancies achieved through assisted reproductive technologies (ART): a FASTER trial study. Prenat Diagn. 2006;26(8):672–8.
19. Spencer K, Kagan KO, Nicolaides KH. Screening for trisomy 21 in twin pregnancies in the first trimester: an update of the impact of chorionicity on maternal serum markers. Prenat Diagn. 2008;28(1):49–52.
20. Bender W, Dugoff L. Screening for aneuploidy in multiple gestations: the challenges and options. Obstet Gynecol Clin North Am. 2018;45(1):41–53.
21. Zhang J, Lambert-Messerlian G, Palomaki GE, Canick JA. Impact of smoking on maternal serum markers and prenatal screening in the first and second trimesters. Prenat Diagn. 2011;31(6):583–8.
22. Badeghiesh A, Volodarsky-Perel A, Lasry A, Hemmings R, Gil Y, Balayla J. Use of placental growth factor for trisomy 21 screening in pregnancy: a systematic review. AJP Rep. 2020;10(3):e234–40.
23. Palomaki GE, Neveux LM, Haddow JE, Wyatt P. Hyperglycosylated-hCG (h-hCG) and Down syndrome screening in the first and second trimesters of pregnancy. Prenat Diagn. 2007;27(9):808–13.
24. Weinans MJN, Butler SA, Mantingh A, Cole LA. Urinary hyperglycosylated hCG in first trimester screening for chromosomal abnormalities. Prenat Diagn. 2000;20(12):976–8.
25. Tørring N, Ball S, Wright D, Sarkissian G, Guitton M, Darbouret B. First trimester screening for trisomy 21 in gestational week 8-10 by ADAM12-S as a maternal serum marker. Reprod Biol Endocrinol. 2010;8:129.
26. Poon LC, Chelemen T, Minekawa R, Frisova V, Nicolaides KH. Maternal serum ADAM12 (A disintegrin and metalloprotease) in chromosomally abnormal pregnancy at 11-13 weeks. Am J Obstet Gynecol. 2009;200(5):508.e1–6.

Maternal Serum Screening and Counselling

4

4.1 Introduction

Chromosomal abnormalities are one of the leading causes of intellectual disability in children. Early detection allows women to make an informed choice regarding continuation or termination of pregnancy.

This chapter focuses primarily on Down syndrome for several reasons. First, Down syndrome is the commonest aneuploidy. Second, most fetuses having trisomy 13 or trisomy 18 typically have severe malformations detected on prenatal ultrasound, while those with Down syndrome may not. Third, infants with trisomy 18 and trisomy 13 die within hours or days after birth; individuals with Down syndrome can have a long lifespan plagued by physical and intellectual disabilities. Detection of trisomy 21, therefore, assumes great significance during the antenatal period. Chapter 13 provides an in-depth discussion on trisomy 13 and trisomy 18.

4.2 General Considerations

4.2.1 Maternal Age

The risk of having a baby with trisomy 21 increases with the mother's advancing age. This risk remains relatively constant in

© The Author(s), under exclusive license to Springer Nature Singapore Pte Ltd. 2023

A. Kamat, *Down Syndrome Screening*,
https://doi.org/10.1007/978-981-99-7758-1_4

Table 4.1 Maternal age and risk of trisomy 21 at term [1]. Note that the reported risks vary slightly depending on the study and the population sampled

Age at term	Risk of trisomy 21	Age at term	Risk of trisomy 21
18	1:1500	32	1:690
19	1:1490	33	1:570
20	1:1470	34	1:460
21	1:1460	35	1:350
22	1:1450	36	1:270
23	1:1410	37	1:200
24	1:1390	38	1:150
25	1:1330	39	1:110
26	1:1280	40	1:85
27	1:1220	41	1:70
28	1:1130	42	1:55
29	1:1040	43	1:45
30	1:930	44	1:40
31	1:820	45	1:35

younger women, being approximately 1 in 1300 at 25 years. It rises steadily till the age of 35, and rapidly thereafter [1]. Approximately 40% of Down syndrome fetuses die in utero. The risk is therefore higher at 12 weeks compared to mid-trimester, and lowest at term [2]. Most screening tests calculate the risk at term, which roughly translates to the actual possibility of giving birth to an affected baby. Table 4.1 shows the risk of trisomy 21 at term with increasing maternal age.

Despite being the single most important demographic factor determining the risk of trisomy 21, maternal age serves as a poor screening test when used alone. Because of a disproportionately high fecundity, a significant number of Down syndrome babies are born to young women despite their individual risk being low. When obstetricians first started screening for Down syndrome, they used a simple protocol of performing amniocentesis in all women older than 35 years. Understandably, this approach had a poor detection rate and resulted in numerous women being unnecessarily subjected to invasive procedures.

Such a crude approach has no role in present-day practice. With the availability of nuchal translucency (NT) and maternal serum screening, invasive testing should not be offered based on maternal age alone. All pregnant women, irrespective of their age, should be counseled and offered the screening test as an option. It should be the patient's decision whether to do the screening test. For example, a 20-year-old woman may opt for screening, while a 42-year-old woman may decline it. Both these decisions are clinically and legally valid, and should be respected.

4.2.2 Cutoffs for Screening Tests

Every screening test, such as the combined first-trimester screening test (FTS) or the quadruple test has a fixed cutoff to decide whether the patient should be referred for further testing like amniocentesis. When the calculated risk is greater than this cutoff, the patient gets a 'high-risk' or 'screen-positive' result. If the calculated risk is lower, a 'low-risk' or 'screen-negative' result is obtained. The patient 'risk' calculated in any screening test does not indicate her actual chance of having an affected baby (see the explanation below). It is simply a statistical value that helps us to place her in the low-risk or high-risk group.

This cutoff was originally fixed at 1:250, an arbitrary value based on the probability of a 35-year-old woman giving birth to a baby with Down syndrome. The rationale was to achieve the same sensitivity as that obtained by performing amniocentesis in all women older than 35 years [3]. This approach lacks scientific reason. The cutoff risk value should ideally be fixed such that an intended 5% false-positive rate (FPR) is achieved, while maximizing the detection rate. In two-step screening techniques, the cutoff should be lower, as there is an intermediate risk group which will be subjected to further screening before being advised amniocentesis or CVS.

Recommended cutoff values for screen-positive results vary widely between different countries and screening programs. The National Health Service (UK) recommends a cutoff value of

1:150 for trisomy 13, 18, and 21 [4]. In Australia, women who get a risk of >1:300 for either of the trisomies are recommended for further testing [5]. In India, the cutoff value used is 1:250 for Down syndrome, and 1:100 for Edward syndrome and Patau syndrome [6]. Clinicians should follow the recommendations of professional organizations in their own country.

4.2.3 Interpretation of Serum Screening Result

In this book, we consider a risk threshold of 1 in 250 as the cutoff value for combined first-trimester screening. When the screening test shows the patient risk to be higher than 1:250 (e.g., 1:50, 1:100, 1:230), further evaluation by either invasive testing or non-invasive prenatal testing (NIPT) should be offered. If the patient's calculated risk is lower than 1:250 (e.g., 1:260, 1:2000, 1:8000), no further testing is required.

If a contingent screening approach is used, three risk groups are defined: high-risk (>1:250), intermediate-risk (1:250–1:1000), and low-risk (<1:1000). Patients in the high-risk group are offered invasive testing, while those in the low-risk group are reassured and advised no further testing. Those in the intermediate-risk group undergo further screening to refine their intermediate risk into either high risk or low risk. Contingent screening is explained in Chap. 9.

4.2.4 Age Risk, Biochemical Risk, and NT Risk

Screening test reports typically mention the patient's age-related risk (a priori risk) and her risk after the screening test (posterior risk). Some labs report multiple risk calculations for the same patient, such as biochemical risk, NT risk, and combined risk. This practice causes confusion for both, pregnant women and their obstetricians, and should be avoided. Once a patient undergoes combined FTS, only her final risk calculated from Maternal Age + NT + PAPP-A + free β-hCG should be considered.

Example: Consider a 37-year-old woman with a normal ultrasound whose age-related risk is 1:90, biochemical risk is 1:200, and combined FTS risk is 1:1200. This woman should be considered as low risk based on her combined FTS risk, and no further testing is required.

4.2.5 Calculated Risk Versus Real Risk

The actual chance that a high-risk patient is carrying a Down syndrome fetus does not depend on her 'risk' calculated in the screening test. The 'risk' mentioned in the screening test report is just a statistical calculation used to divide patients into high-risk and low-risk groups. Once a woman receives a high-risk report, the actual risk depends on her age (Table 4.2).

Let us consider a few examples:

- **Example 1:** A 20-year-old woman who screens positive with a calculated risk of 1:80—Actual probability of a trisomy 21 result at amniocentesis is 1:33.
- **Example 2:** A 40-year-old woman who screens positive with a calculated risk of 1:80—Actual probability of a trisomy 21 result at amniocentesis is 1:17.
- **Example 3:** A 40-year-old woman who screens positive with a calculated risk of 1:200—Actual probability of a trisomy 21 result at amniocentesis is 1:17.

Table 4.2 Actual chance of having a Down syndrome fetus after testing screen positive [7]

Maternal age (years)	Chance that invasive testing will confirm trisomy 21
20	1:33
25	1:32
30	1:29
35	1:25
40	1:17
45	1:9

In conclusion, we should not falsely reassure a patient with a calculated risk of 1:200 that her chance of having an aneuploid baby is 1 in 200. All patients with a calculated risk above the cut-off value should be offered further evaluation, either by invasive testing or NIPT.

4.2.6 Minimum Standard for Screening

Other than invasive testing, no test can diagnose Down syndrome with certainty. To maintain a high detection rate (DR) and avoid unnecessary invasive procedures, only the screening tests which follow a minimum standard should be used. For a first-trimester screening test, the minimum standard is defined as a detection rate of at least 75% for a 3% FPR. For the second-trimester screening, a 75% detection rate for a 5% FPR is acceptable. Among the single-step maternal serum screening tests, only the combined FTS (using NT, PAPP-A, and β-hCG) and quadruple test meet the minimum standard for screening [8].

4.2.7 Fixing the Protocol and Documentation

Since the maternal serum tests are not diagnostic tests, it is possible that they may occasionally be wrong. Coherent pre-test and post-test counseling can go a long way in helping the clinician deal with upset parents. When establishing a screening program, the following measures need to be adopted to reduce the risk of litigation and be able to defend oneself successfully if called to do so:

- The screening protocol that the center follows must be fixed and documented. (Chapter 10 describes a sample protocol you can follow.)
- The same protocol should be followed in all patients.
- Any deviation from the standard protocol should be documented in patient notes with reason.

- In case the center changes the screening protocol, these changes must be documented and dated.
- It is ideal to provide patients with printed information or brochures explaining the screening process in a simplified manner.

4.3 Combined First-Trimester Screening

Combined first-trimester screening (FTS) involves risk calculation by a combination of maternal age, nuchal translucency (NT), serum pregnancy-associated plasma protein A (PAPP-A), and free beta human chorionic gonadotropin (free β-hCG). It is the only first-trimester screening test which meets the minimum screening standard. Nasal bone (NB) may be included, provided a sonographer trained in NB assessment is available.

4.3.1 Components of Combined First-Trimester Screening

Maternal Age Maternal age is the most important variable which determines the risk of having an aneuploid fetus. The convention is to consider the maternal age at childbirth (40 weeks) calculated from the mother's date of birth.

With assisted reproduction, maternal age calculation is slightly complex (see Chap. 11). If the embryo transfer (ET) does not occur in the same cycle, the date of ovum pickup (OPU) is used to calculate the maternal age. With donor egg or donor embryo cycle, the age of the donor on the day of OPU is considered. In pregnancies resulting from donor egg IVF, a false-positive result is extremely likely if we enter the patient's own age in the maternal age column of the requisition form, since these women are significantly older than the egg donors.

Nuchal Translucency (NT) The nuchal translucency is the subcutaneous layer of fluid in the fetal neck. Chapter 2 explains the correct technique for measuring the NT as described by the Fetal Medicine Foundation [9]. In brief, NT is measured at a gestation of 11–13 + 6 weeks. The fetus is imaged in a strict mid-sagittal plane, with the fetal neck in a neutral position. Image magnification is used such that only the fetal head, face, neck, and thorax are visible. The calipers are placed exactly on the inner borders of the two lines defining the retro-nuchal fluid collection, and the largest such measurement is considered. If the NT measurement is over 3 mm, it is wiser to proceed directly for invasive testing.

Pregnancy-associated Plasma Protein A (PAPP-A) This is a maternal plasma glycoprotein which is first detected shortly after implantation and continues to rise throughout pregnancy. Because of its rapid rise, it is expressed in multiples of median (MoM) for a particular gestation. The use of MoM values allows each of the components of the FTS to be measured on different dates and still be combined meaningfully. Values of PAPP-A are significantly reduced when the fetus has either trisomy 21, trisomy 13, or trisomy 18 (Table 3.1).

Free Beta Chorionic Gonadotropin (Free β-hCG) Free β-hCG is a hyperglycosylated β subunit of hCG. Free β-hCG is increased in pregnancies with a Down syndrome fetus, while lower than normal values are associated with trisomy 13 and 18 (Table 3.1). Some laboratories test for total hCG (or β-hCG) instead of free β-hCG, which has a slightly lower sensitivity but is more stable at room temperatures compared to free β-hCG.

4.3.2 Effect of Gestational Age on Test Results

The difference in free β-hCG between normal and aneuploid pregnancies is greater at 13 + 6 weeks compared to 11 weeks. For PAPP-A, it is exactly the opposite. PAPP-A can be measured as early as 9 weeks to improve the sensitivity of combined FTS; however, it is seldom done, because of the logistic difficulties of taking multiple blood samples for a single test.

In clinical practice, both PAPP-A and free β-hCG are measured from a single blood sample taken at a gestational age of 11–13 + 6 weeks, usually on the same day as the NT scan.

4.3.3 Screening Methodology

- A trained operator performs the 11–13 weeks scan and takes the NT measurement. If the gestational age is less than 11 weeks, the patient is called after 11 completed weeks. If the gestational age is 14 + 0 weeks or more, combined FTS cannot be performed.
- In case a significant anomaly is detected, or the NT value is >3 mm, invasive testing is offered.
- The patient is counseled about aneuploidy screening. The woman's partner, if present, should also be included in the counseling session.
- If the patient refuses screening, the same should be documented in her notes. No further aneuploidy screening or testing is performed.
- If the patient accepts screening, a blood sample is taken on the same day. Serum is separated and dispatched to the testing laboratory after filling in all the details in the test requisition form. The patient is informed regarding the expected turnaround time (TAT) and a post-test counseling date is fixed.
- The test should never be repeated in the same or another lab, as this can generate contradictory results.
- Women with screen-positive or high-risk results should be referred for invasive testing or NIPT.

4.3.4 Sensitivity and False-Positive Rate

Combined FTS for detection of Down syndrome has a sensitivity of 83–90% for a 5% FPR or 78% for a 3% FPR [10, 11]. This sensitivity is not a constant, but depends on the maternal age, the predetermined cutoff value and the FPR chosen. The detection rates for trisomy 18 and 13 are 97% and 92% respectively, with a risk cutoff of 1:100 and a 4% FPR [12].

4.3.5 Screening with Maternal Age + NT Alone

Using maternal age and NT without serum markers reduces the sensitivity of first-trimester screening for Down syndrome to 75% for a 5% FPR [11]. It is an acceptable screening option in twins and in singleton pregnancies with a vanishing twin. In higher order multiples, it is the only screening option available.

4.3.6 Nasal Bone in Combined First-Trimester Screening

Successful integration of NB into the combined first-trimester screening program increases the detection rate for Down syndrome. A contingent screening model with nasal bone as the second step has been suggested. In this model, the initial screening is done with NT and serum markers, and patients with an intermediate risk are referred to a specialized fetal medicine unit for nasal bone assessment. This model reduces the number of invasive procedures by half without affecting screening goals for the whole population [13]. Chapter 2 explains the methodology for the assessment of NB, while Chap. 9 discusses contingent screening with ultrasound markers. Assessment of NB is difficult, and prone to errors. Incorrect assessment reduces the screening performance. Sonographers performing NB assessment must undergo formal certification and regular audit.

4.3.7 Ductus Venosus Flow and Tricuspid Regurgitation

Ductus venosus (DV) and tricuspid valve Doppler can increase the accuracy of combined FTS. Down syndrome fetuses have a greater prevalence of reversed 'a' wave in the DV. Ductus venosus pulsatility index for vein (DV-PIV), which is an auto-traced measurement by the ultrasound machine, is more sensitive than 'a' wave reversal. Tricuspid regurgitation (TR) is also more frequent in aneuploid fetuses.

However, DV and tricuspid valve flow are technically difficult to assess and require specific and intensive training (see Chap. 2). Routine reporting of these parameters by untrained sonographers frequently results in false-positive reports and unnecessary referral for invasive procedures. Even more unfortunate is the fact that numerous women opt for pregnancy termination based on these findings alone, without confirmatory testing.

Routine assessment, reporting, and use of DV flow or TR in Down syndrome screening are not recommended. Few specialized fetal medicine units may employ these markers for the contingent screening model or for research. Even in such units, regular training of ultrasound operators and frequent audits are mandatory.

4.3.8 Patient Selection

Patient selection for combined FTS is important to optimize the efficacy of the test and to avoid getting into difficult situations. Not all patients should be coerced to undergo screening. Maternal age of 35 years should not be used as a cutoff to offer screening.

Some patients who may *not* be ideal candidates for combined FTS are:

1. Those in whom the screening test should not be performed.

    - Women not willing to undergo screening.
    - Those who have not undergone NT scan and pre-test counseling.
    - Those not willing to undergo further testing if a screen-positive result is obtained.

2. Those in whom serum biochemistry is not reliable (ultrasound alone may be used to assess risk).

    - Vanishing twin where fetal pole/placenta are visible.
    - Higher order multiple pregnancies.
    - History or receiving hCG injection in the past 2 weeks.

3. Those who should be considered directly for invasive testing.

    - NT value >3.0 mm, cystic hygroma.
    - Those with a structural malformation identified on ultrasound.
    - Previous baby with translocation Down syndrome.

4. Those needing invasive procedures to test for other genetic disorders, e.g., if both parents have beta-thalassemia trait, fetal karyotyping can be performed on the same CVS sample used to test for beta-thalassemia mutations.

4.4 The Quadruple Marker Test (Quad Screen)

Combined FTS is the preferred screening test when (a) the woman presents before 14 weeks of gestation, and (b) a trained sonographer for assessment of NT is available. In other cases, the quadruple marker test (quad screen) performed between 15 and 22 weeks is the next best option. This test screens for trisomy 21, trisomy 18, and open neural tube defects. It excludes trisomy 13 as this condition does not significantly alter the second-trimester markers.

The quad screen includes maternal serum alpha-fetoprotein (MSAFP), human chorionic gonadotropin (β-hCG or free β-hCG), unconjugated estriol, and inhibin A. Fetal biometry is performed on the day of the test to reconfirm the gestational age.

4.4.1 Components of the Quadruple Marker Test

Maternal Age Maternal age at term is used to calculate the baseline risk of Down syndrome for a fetus. With IVF conception,

OPU and ET date and donor's date of birth (in donor IVF) should be noted.

Maternal Serum Alpha-Fetoprotein (MSAFP) Maternal serum alpha-fetoprotein is a useful marker for both aneuploidy and open neural tube defects. Levels of MSAFP are reduced in both trisomy 21 and trisomy 18, while they are increased in open neural tube defects. To estimate the risk for Down syndrome and trisomy 18, the reporting software uses a statistical calculation with maternal age and MoM values of all four markers. For calculating the risk of open neural tube defects, only the MSAFP value is considered, with a fixed cutoff screen positive value of >2.5 MoM.

Human Chorionic Gonadotropin (β-hCG or Free β-hCG) In the second trimester, β-hCG levels are twice as high in trisomy 21 fetuses, while they are 75% lower than normal in trisomy 18 fetuses. Laboratories may use either β-hCG or free β-hCG in the quadruple marker test as per the availability of testing machines (Table 3.2).

Unconjugated Estriol (uE3) While uE3 alone is a poor screening tool for aneuploidy, it is useful in conjunction with MSAFP and inhibin A. Estriol levels are abnormally low in trisomy 21 as well as trisomy 18.

Inhibin A Inhibin A is a dimeric glycoprotein belonging to the inhibin family of alpha-beta subunit glycoproteins, known for their selective inhibition of follicle stimulation hormone from the anterior pituitary. Addition of inhibin A as a fourth marker has dramatically improved the efficiency of second-trimester screening for Down syndrome, and made the triple marker test obsolete. The results of two large studies, SURUSS from the United Kingdom and FASTER conducted in the United States, have shown an incremental gain of 6–11% in Down syndrome detection rate when inhibin A is added to the triple test [10, 14].

4.4.2 Methodology

- An ultrasound scan should be performed before the quadruple test. In case of a significant abnormality, the patient should be offered genetic testing by amniocentesis. In case of a lethal abnormality, termination of pregnancy may be offered.
- Fetal measurements are taken to confirm the gestational age and include biparietal diameter (BPD), head circumference (HC), abdominal circumference (AC), and femur length (FL). Aneuploidy itself causes growth restriction, leading to incorrect estimation of gestational age. *Hence, if gestational age has been already fixed by an earlier scan, the same should be retained.*
- The patient is counseled about aneuploidy screening. If the patient refuses screening, no further aneuploidy screening or testing is performed.
- A blood sample is taken, serum is separated and dispatched to the testing laboratory after filling in all the details in the test requisition form. The patient is informed regarding the expected turnaround time (TAT) and the post-test counseling date is fixed.
- The test should never be repeated. Women getting a screen-positive result for aneuploidy should be referred for invasive testing (or NIPS, as per policy). If only MSAFP is raised, a targeted anomaly scan is indicated to look for open neural tube defects and abdominal wall defects.

4.4.3 Sensitivity and False-Positive Rate

The quad screen has a sensitivity of 81–83% for an FPR of 5% [10, 14]. Optimal performance of this test is between 16 and 18 weeks of gestation.

4.5 Details to Be Filled in the Requisition Form

Table 4.3 provides a list of details that need to be entered in the requisition form for combined FTS or quad screen. Incomplete or erroneous filling of the requisition form can introduce significant errors in the screening result.

Table 4.3 Details to be filled on the requisition form for combined FTS and Quad screen

1. Patient details • Name, address, and ID of the patient • Date of birth • Ethnicity • Weight • Last menstrual period • Number of pregnancies and number of live births • History of Down syndrome in previous pregnancy • Family history of Down syndrome • Diabetic status • Smoking status
2. Pregnancy details • Type of conception • Bleeding in the last 2 weeks • Last date of hCG injection (if applicable) • Date of OPU and ET, and egg source (for IVF conceptions) • Donor's date of birth (for donor IVF conceptions)
3. Fetus details (for combined FTS) • Date of ultrasound scan • Singleton or twin pregnancy • Chorionicity in twins • Crown rump length • Nuchal translucency • Nasal bone presence or absence (if included) • Fetal heart rate
4. Fetus details (for quad screen, singleton pregnancy only) • Date of ultrasound scan • BPD, HC, AC, and FL

4.6 Sample Collection and Transport

Whether combined FTS or second-trimester screening is being done, the sample should be meticulously collected and transported. Otherwise, the serum marker levels in the sample get altered, affecting the performance of the screening test.

A blood sample volume of 2–4 mL is sufficient for the analysis of PAPP-A and β-hCG levels. For whole blood, levels of PAPP-A and free β-hCG remain stable for 7 days at a constant temperature of 4 °C, for 2 days at 20 °C and 2 h at 30 °C. When whole blood is being transported, it should be sent within 24 h of collection with ice packs to maintain a cold chain. A delay in shipping the sample can cause free β-hCG levels to rise, as it is liberated from hyperglycosylated hCG at room temperature.

If serum is being transported, it should be separated within 4 h of blood collection to maintain the serum analyte levels. Separated serum samples maintain stability for 2 days at 20 °C and hence, should still be shipped with ice packs. If a longer duration is expected between blood collection and analysis, the serum sample should be frozen. Frozen serum samples show no significant change in either free β-hCG or PAPP-A levels for at least a week, even after the partial freeze-thaw cycles that naturally occur during storage, transport, and testing.

Likewise, whole blood levels of MSAFP, uE3, and inhibin A change at room temperatures, leading to erroneous results. When sending a sample for second-trimester screening, the serum should be separated within 4 h, stored in the refrigerator, and shipped within 24 h along with ice packs.

4.7 First-Trimester Versus Second-Trimester Screening

Women who present for antenatal booking prior to 14 weeks of gestation should be offered combined FTS. In case additional screening for open neural tube defects is required and skilled sonographers are not available, only MSAFP, rather than the quadruple test, should be done in the second trimester. Women who present for the first time between 15 and 22 weeks should be offered a quadruple test (ideally performed between 16 and 18 weeks).

4.7.1 Advantages of Combined FTS over Quad Screen

1. The combined FTS is more sensitive and specific.
2. First-trimester screening allows for adequate time for subsequent testing if needed.
3. It is the only serum screening test which fulfills the minimum standard for screening in twins.
4. Serum screening for trisomy 13 is possible only in the first trimester.
5. Low PAPP-A level detected during combined FTS is a marker for subsequent placental dysfunction.
6. Preeclampsia screening can be integrated into combined FTS.

4.7.2 Advantages of Quad Screen over Combined FTS

1. The quadruple test permits screening of women who get booked after 14 weeks.
2. It provides additional screening for open neural tube defects.
3. It can be used in centers where trained NT operators are not available.
4. It can be performed in case of a vanishing twin (provided the second fetus and placenta are no longer visible).
5. It is useful for patients receiving hCG injections in the first trimester.

4.8 Double Marker, Triple Marker, and Penta Marker Tests

Among the single-step screening tests, only the combined FTS and the quadruple test meet the minimum standard for screening. Screening tests offering fewer markers have a reduced detection rate or a high FPR. Single-step screening tests with more than four markers have not conclusively shown greater efficacy for the increased cost they demand.

4.8.1 Double Marker Test

The double marker test uses a combination of maternal age with β-hCG and PAPP-A without including nuchal translucency. It detects only 60–70% of cases of Down syndrome for a 5% FPR and does not meet the minimum standard for screening [11]. *It is an obsolete test which should be abandoned.* Instead, women who opt for screening between 11 and 13 + 6 weeks should be offered the combined FTS (which includes NT). In case a skilled NT operator is not available, it is better to wait till 15–16 weeks and do the quadruple test.

4.8.2 Triple Marker Test

The triple marker test combines maternal age with three serum markers, namely MSAFP, hCG, and unconjugated estriol. It has a trisomy 21 detection rate of only 69% for a 5% FPR [14]. *It is considerably inferior to the quadruple test, does not meet the minimum standard, and, like the double marker test, has no role in contemporary practice.*

4.8.3 Single-Step Penta Marker Tests

Several single-step penta marker tests have been proposed for aneuploidy screening. They involve the addition of placental growth factor (PlGF) and MSAFP to the combined FTS, or PAPP-A, αhCG, or hyperglycosylated hCG to the quad screen. None of them have been validated in prospective trials or shown to be more efficient or cost-effective than the combined FTS [15, 16]. While it is possible that these multiple marker tests may be validated in the future, it is even more likely that NIPT will eventually replace maternal serum screening altogether. Contingent and integrated (two-step) screening strategies using first-trimester and second-trimester markers improve the detection rate; these are elaborated in Chap. 9. The use of PlGF in screening for pre-eclampsia is discussed in Chap. 14.

4.9 Choosing a Screening Test

Table 4.4 provides a summary of the various single-step screening tests. Among all the tests, only the combined FTS and the quadruple test are recommended in singleton pregnancies.

Table 4.4 Recommendations for selecting an appropriate single-step screening test [10, 11, 14–16]

Screening test	Sensitivity for a 5% FPR	Current recommendation
Maternal age	30%	Not recommended
Maternal age + NT	75%	*Recommended only for vanishing twin and higher order multiple pregnancies*
Double marker (PAPP-A + β-hCG)	60–70%	Not recommended
Combined FTS (NT + PAPP-A + β-hCG)	83–90%	*Recommended in first trimester for singleton and twin pregnancies*
Triple test (AFP + β-hCG + uE3)	69%	Not recommended
Quadruple test (AFP + β-hCG + uE3 + inhibin A)	81–83%	*Recommended in second trimester for singleton pregnancies*
Penta marker tests	84–90%	Not recommended at present

4.10 False-Positive Results and Pregnancy Outcome

Maternal serum markers are produced by the placenta. Abnormal marker profiles seen in aneuploidy reflect the pattern of placental dysfunction in these pregnancies. Any condition which causes significant placental dysfunction can alter the ratio of the serum markers, giving rise to a false-positive screening result. Euploid fetuses with an increased NT or altered serum marker levels are at risk for pregnancy complications (miscarriage, preterm birth, growth restriction) and adverse perinatal outcomes.

4.10.1 Increased NT

An increased NT is associated with structural malformations, especially cardiac anomalies and congenital diaphragmatic hernia. All fetuses with significant nuchal edema should be evaluated with a targeted anomaly scan and echocardiography at 19–20 weeks, followed by serial growth scans in the third trimester. Fetuses with enlarged NT who have a normal karyotype, no anomalies, and no growth restriction usually have good perinatal outcomes. Discordance in NT among monochorionic twins is a marker for twin-to-twin transfusion syndrome [17].

4.10.2 Low PAPP-A

Pregnancy-associated plasma protein-A level in the first trimester is the most significant predictor of adverse pregnancy outcomes. A PAPP-A level of *less than 0.4 MoM* is associated with an increased risk of miscarriage, fetal growth restriction, oligohydramnios, preeclampsia, preterm deliveries, and stillbirths [18]. Women who have had low first-trimester PAPP-A levels should undergo increased surveillance during pregnancy. Induction of labor may be considered in those who do not deliver by 40 weeks. A recent study by Fruscalzo and coworkers has linked low

PAPP-A levels in the first trimester of pregnancy to short stature in the offspring and de novo development of maternal diabetes mellitus in later life [19].

4.10.3 Other Markers

Women with an increased MSAFP, inhibin-A or β-hCG level, and a genetically normal fetus are also at an increased risk of placental dysfunction. This is particularly seen when two or more markers are elevated. The elevation of these serum markers may result from placental hypoxia in early pregnancy or an attempt by the placenta to secrete more proteins as a compensatory mechanism in the face of an inadequate blood supply and impaired placental growth.

Low levels of estradiol (uE3) also increase the risk of adverse pregnancy outcomes. In addition, low uE3 levels are seen in X-linked ichthyosis, Smith-Lemli-Opitz syndrome, and congenital adrenal hypoplasia [20]. Extremely low (or undetectable) levels of MSAFP may be because of the congenital AFP deficiency, a rare condition which surprisingly has no effect on the fetus and neonate [21]. Isolated low levels of β-hCG or inhibin A do not seem to have a significant effect on the fetus.

4.11 Pre-test Counseling

The pre-test counseling session is a time for expectant parents to receive information about Down syndrome and the screening process, and to ask any questions they may have. The counseling should include information about the different screening tests available, including their accuracy and the potential risks and benefits of each test. Parents should also be informed about the potential implications of a positive or negative screening result.

Aneuploidy screening is stressful for the couple, and not without reason. The mere introduction of aneuploidy screening changes the couple's perception of their unborn child from normal to potentially abnormal. Care must be taken to devote time for pre-test counseling in order to ease as much of this stress as possible until the test results arrive.

Before discussing aneuploidy screening, the pregnant woman should undergo an ultrasonography to assess the fetal number, size, and viability, and rule out lethal malformations as far as possible.

Screening for Down syndrome and other aneuploidies is every woman's choice, and it must not be enforced. The counseling should be non-directive irrespective of patient's age. Both partners must be counseled together. Depending on the literacy level of the couple, the complexity of information may need to be dialed down for better understanding. While documenting the counseling session in patient notes, however, the use of correct medical terms is mandatory.

The conditions being screened for should be outlined in brief. Using terms like 'intellectual disability' and 'learning difficulty' is strongly recommended over 'mental retardation.' Caution must be exercised while counseling couples with a previous abnormal child. The risk of giving birth to a Down syndrome child should be explained depending upon maternal age. At 18 years, the risk is approximately 1:1500. At 30 years, it is 1:900 and triples every 5 years thereafter, being approximately 1:300 at 35 years, 1:100 at 40 years, and 1:35 at 45 years.

Many couples have difficulty in understanding the difference between a screening test and a diagnostic test. They may assume that genetic testing rules out all problems in the baby, and that a screen-negative result implies that the baby would be born perfectly normal. It is important to clarify that this test only screens for three specific genetic conditions (trisomy 13, trisomy 18, and trisomy 21). Other conditions causing intellectual disability (e.g., autism) are not detected.

Both screen-positive and screen-negative outcomes must be discussed. Subsequent tests (CVS, amniocentesis, or NIPT) with their costs and risks should be explained. We rarely mention intermediate risk at this stage, as it makes the process far too complicated for most patients to understand. In case the screening test reports an intermediate risk, it can be further evaluated within the ambit of the tests already explained.

Finally, it is important to drive home the point that genetic conditions are uncommon in the general population, and even if the couple refuses screening altogether, there is a strong likelihood that the baby is normal.

4.11.1 Example of Pre-test Counseling

The following is an example of a brief pre-test counseling session for a combined first-trimester screening test after a normal 11–13 + 6 weeks scan. The patient's age is assumed to be 30 years:

Counselor: *"Good morning. I am here to provide you with pre-test counseling for the genetic screening test you will be undergoing today. This counseling session helps you understand the purpose, benefits, and potential risks associated with the test. If you have questions, feel free to interrupt me."*

Counselor: *"At the outset, your 11–14 weeks scan is normal. This means that the parts which should be visible on ultrasound by 3 months are all formed well. Occasionally, there are certain genetic conditions in the baby that may not always be detected on ultrasound. These are called Down syndrome, Edward syndrome and Patau syndrome. The commonest among these is Down syndrome, which affects 1 in 900 babies born to women of your age."*

Patient: *"Doctor, will you not be able to detect it at the anomaly scan?"*

Counselor: *"Edward syndrome and Patau syndrome can usually be detected on ultrasound. Down syndrome may not always be detected, as physical parts can be normal in these babies."*

Patient: *"How do we detect these conditions?"*

Counselor: *"To detect these conditions with certainty, we must remove a tiny sample from the placenta or a small amount of amniotic fluid with a needle, and send it for testing. We cannot do that in all patients, as it is associated with 1% risk of miscarriage. Therefore, we offer a blood test to all expecting mothers called the 'screening test.' This is not a hundred per-*

cent guaranteed test, but it tells us whether you are at high risk or low risk for having an affected child. Most pregnant women get a low-risk or screen-negative result, which means their babies are unlikely to have these problems. A few women (about 5%) get a high-risk or screen-positive result. These few women need to undergo further testing with NIPT or invasive testing."

Patient: *"What is an NIPT?"*

Counselor: *"After 10 weeks, the baby's placenta keeps releasing bits of DNA into the mother's bloodstream. NIPT is a blood test which analyzes this DNA in your blood. It can detect over 99% babies with Down syndrome. It is still a screening test, but its high detection rate makes it less likely to get a false-positive result. NIPT is expensive, and can be done as a second-tier test if your combined FTS shows a high risk. A few women prefer to do it as the first-step test."*

Patient: *"What are my options if Down syndrome is confirmed in my baby?"*

Counselor: *"In case of a confirmed diagnosis on CVS or amniocentesis, you will have the option to either terminate or continue the affected pregnancy. In either case, we will completely respect your decision. You will be referred to a counselor who will guide you and support you."*

Patient: *"Doctor, are screening tests mandatory?"*

Counselor: *"No. This test is entirely voluntary, and you may refuse it completely or stop the process at any point."*

4.12 Post-test Counseling and Follow Up

Unless aneuploidy screening is done at a one-step clinic (where the 11–13 + 6 weeks scan, serum biochemistry, and consequent risk reporting are done together), it is likely that screening report will take a few days. Even if the screening test shows a low risk, it is prudent to have a brief discussion with the woman and her partner, and document it in her notes.

4.12.1 Screen-Positive (High-Risk) Result

Post-test counseling following a screen-positive result demands ample time as it is crucial to address the concerns and emotions of the expectant mother, who is likely to experience distress and anxiety. Handling the counseling session with utmost care and patience is of paramount importance.

A screen-positive result for trisomy 21 indicates that the patient has an increased risk of giving birth to a child with trisomy 21 compared to other women of her age. However, most patients with screen-positive results have normal babies. Depending on the institutional policy, patients with screen-positive results should be offered either definitive testing by CVS or amniocentesis, or cell-free DNA (NIPT) as an intermediate step. In case the woman refuses any further testing, her choice should be respected (and documented clearly). Under no circumstances should a pregnancy be terminated without confirmation of aneuploidy by CVS or amniocentesis.

Once a screening test shows an increased risk, the same test must never be repeated. Statistically, if any test is repeated several times, its values tend to regress to the mean. Since the levels of serum markers in pregnancies with a euploid fetus and an aneuploid fetus fall on different sides of the cutoff, repeat values in both cases are statistically likely to move toward each other. Additionally, there is a possibility of ending up with two reports, one screen-negative and one screen-positive, for the same patient. In such a case, NIPT or invasive testing would still be required.

Comprehensive ultrasound evaluation of the fetus should be performed following a screen positive test and the findings should be incorporated into clinical decision-making. In case a structural abnormality is detected, invasive testing should be offered rather than NIPT.

4.12.2 Screen-Negative (Low-Risk) Result

A screen-negative result indicates that the present pregnancy is unlikely to result in a baby with trisomy 13, 18, or 21. The patient should be reassured that no further testing is required. It must be emphasized that this test is not diagnostic. In case a structural abnormality is noted at a subsequent scan, a patient who has tested screen negative on maternal serum screening would still need referral for amniocentesis.

4.12.3 Intermediate Risk Result

Some labs report an intermediate risk as well. An intermediate risk for Down syndrome is defined as a first-trimester screening risk in between the cutoff (e.g., 1:250) and 1:1000. Patients with an intermediate-risk result should be offered additional tests for the refinement of risk.

Two approaches are available when dealing with this group of patients. One option is to offer a cfDNA test (NIPT). The other option is to repeat the maternal serum test at 16 weeks, and generate a combined risk result after taking into consideration the risk generated by the first-trimester test (contingent screening). This option is available in the risk calculation software used by most laboratories. Contingent screening is discussed in greater detail in Chap. 9. As mentioned earlier, one should never do an independent quadruple test in such cases, as it is likely to generate a different risk than that generated by the combined FTS. Risk modification using second-trimester soft markers is no longer recommended (See Chap. 9).

In either case, if the second test shows a screen-positive result, invasive testing should be offered. If cfDNA screening returns a low fetal fraction or test failure, invasive testing should still be offered, as low fetal fraction itself is associated with aneuploidy. Finally, if the woman herself requests a confirmatory invasive test, her request must not be denied.

4.13 Key Messages

1. When combined FTS is performed, only the final combined risk should be considered.

2. For a woman who screens positive, the chance that invasive testing will confirm trisomy 21 depends on her age and not on the risk value calculated by the test.
3. Only a trained and certified ultrasound operator should measure NT.
4. Nasal bone evaluation is technically difficult, but improves sensitivity of combined FTS. Evaluation of DV and TR is not routinely recommended.
5. Double marker test (without NT) and triple marker test have poor sensitivity, and should be abandoned.
6. Maternal serum screening should be performed at least 2 weeks after the last hCG injection.
7. A low-risk result on combined FTS or quadruple test does not rule out Down syndrome with certainty. Pre-test and post-test counseling are extremely important.
8. Pregnancies with raised serum markers and a euploid fetus should be monitored for placental dysfunction.

References

1. Morris JK, Wald NJ, Mutton DE, Alberman E. Comparison of models of maternal age-specific risk for Down syndrome live births. Prenat Diagn. 2003;23(3):252–8.
2. Morris JK, Wald NJ, Watt HC. Fetal loss in Down syndrome pregnancies. Prenat Diagn. 1999;19(2):142–5.
3. Nicolaides KH. Screening for fetal chromosomal abnormalities: need to change the rules. Ultrasound Obstet Gynecol. 1994;4(5):353–4.
4. National Health Service (NHS) England. Service specification no.16: NHS Fetal Anomaly Screening Programme (Trisomy Screening). July 2019 [cited 2023 May 13]. https://www.england.nhs.uk/wp-content/uploads/2017/04/Service-Specification-No.16-NHS_FASP_Trisomy_Screening.pdf.
5. Maxwell S, James I, Dickinson JE, O'Leary P. First trimester screening cut-offs for noninvasive prenatal testing as a contingent screen: balancing detection and screen-positive rates for trisomy 21. Aust N Z J Obstet Gynaecol. 2016;56(1):29–35.
6. Manikandan K, Seshadri S. Down syndrome screening in India: are we there yet? J Obstet Gynaecol India. 2017;67(6):393–9.
7. Spencer K. Age related detection and false positive rates when screening for Down's syndrome in the first trimester using fetal nuchal translucency

and maternal serum free betahCG and PAPP-A. BJOG. 2001;108(10):1043–6.
8. Chitayat D, Langlois S, Wilson RD. No. 261-prenatal screening for fetal aneuploidy in singleton pregnancies. J Obstet Gynaecol Can. 2017;39(9):e380–94.
9. Nicolaides KH. The 11–13 weeks scan [Online course]. The Fetal Medicine Foundation https://fetalmedicine.org/education/the-11-13-weeks-scan. Accessed 2 May 2023.
10. Wald NJ, Hackshaw AK, Walters J, Mackinson AM, Rodeck C, Chitty L. First and second trimester antenatal screening for Down's syndrome: the results of the serum, urine and ultrasound screening study (SURUSS). J Med Screen. 2003;10(2):56–104.
11. Nicolaides KH. Screening for fetal aneuploidies at 11 to 13 weeks. Prenat Diagn. 2011;31(1):7–15.
12. Santorum M, Wright D, Syngelaki A, Karagioti N, Nicolaides KH. Accuracy of first-trimester combined test in screening for trisomies 21, 18 and 13. Ultrasound Obstet Gynecol. 2017;49(6):714–20.
13. Cicero S, Avgidou K, Rembouskos G, Kagan KO, Nicolaides KH. Nasal bone in first-trimester screening for trisomy 21. Am J Obstet Gynecol. 2006;195(1):109–14.
14. Malone FD, Canick JA, Ball RH, Nyberg DA, Comstock CH, Bukowski R, Berkowitz RL, Gross SJ, Dugoff L, Craigo SD, Timor-Tritsch IE, Carr SR, Wolfe HM, Dukes K, Bianchi DW, Rudnicka AR, Hackshaw AK, Lambert-Messerlian G, Wald NJ, D'Alton ME, First- and Second-Trimester Evaluation of Risk (FASTER) Research Consortium. First-trimester or second-trimester screening, or both, for Down's syndrome. N Engl J Med. 2005;353(19):2001–11.
15. Huang T, Dennis A, Meschino WS, Rashid S, Mak-Tam E, Cuckle H. First trimester screening for Down syndrome using nuchal translucency, maternal serum pregnancy-associated plasma protein A, free-β human chorionic gonadotrophin, placental growth factor, and α-fetoprotein. Prenat Diagn. 2015;35(7):709–16.
16. Alldred SK, Deeks JJ, Guo B, Neilson JP, Alfirevic Z. Second trimester serum tests for Down's syndrome screening. Cochrane Database Syst Rev. 2012;2012(6):CD009925.
17. Souka AP, Von Kaisenberg CS, Hyett JA, Sonek JD, Nicolaides KH. Increased nuchal translucency with normal karyotype. Am J Obstet Gynecol. 2005;192(4):1005–21.
18. Livrinova V, Petrov I, Samardziski I, Jovanovska V, Simeonova-Krstevska S, Todorovska I, Atanasova-Boshku A, Gjeorgjievska M. Obstetric outcome in pregnant patients with low level of pregnancy-associated plasma

protein A in first trimester. Open Access Maced J Med Sci. 2018;6(6):1028–31.
19. Fruscalzo A, Cividino A, Rossetti E, Maurigh A, Londero AP, Driul L. First trimester PAPP-A serum levels and long-term metabolic outcome of mothers and their offspring. Sci Rep. 2020;10(1):5131.
20. Falah N, Torday J, Quinney S, Haas D. Estriol review: clinical applications and potential biomedical importance. Clin Res Trials. 2015;1(2):29.
21. Muller F, Dreux S, Sault C, Galland A, Puissant H, Couplet G, et al. Very low alpha-fetoprotein in Down syndrome maternal serum screening. Prenat Diagn. 2003;23(7):584–7.

Noninvasive Prenatal Testing (NIPT)

5

5.1 Introduction

Noninvasive prenatal testing (NIPT) has emerged as a groundbreaking approach that offers expectant parents a safe and accurate means of evaluating fetal genetic abnormalities, based on the study of fetal cell-free DNA (cfDNA) in the mother's bloodstream. Noninvasive prenatal screening (NIPS) is synonymous with NIPT and illustrates the true nature of the test.

This chapter delves into the fundamentals of NIPT, including the sequencing technologies, interpretation of results, and efficacy in screening for common aneuploidies and sex chromosome abnormalities. In addition, it thoroughly examines the advantages and limitations of NIPT in comparison to conventional screening methods, while also elucidating its implementation in clinical practice.

5.2 Origin of Cell-Free DNA

5.2.1 Fetal Cells in Maternal Blood

During pregnancy, a small number of fetal cells cross the placenta and enter the maternal bloodstream. These were first identified in maternal blood by direct staining of the Y chromosome originat-

© The Author(s), under exclusive license to Springer Nature Singapore Pte Ltd. 2023
A. Kamat, *Down Syndrome Screening*,
https://doi.org/10.1007/978-981-99-7758-1_5

ing from male fetuses [1]. Fetal cells are scarce in maternal blood, making their detection and isolation difficult.

5.2.2 Cell-Free DNA in Maternal Blood

Cell-free DNA (cfDNA) refers to degraded DNA fragments present in maternal plasma, which are formed as a result of several destructive processes like apoptosis, necrosis, and autophagy. Whenever apoptosis or programmed cell death occurs, intracellular enzymes degrade the cellular contents. Within the nucleus of the cell, DNA exists in the form of 'nucleosomes,' which are coils of DNA wrapped around protein cores. This DNA is highly resistant to enzymatic destruction and gets released as cfDNA. Maternal plasma contains abundant cfDNA originating from various maternal tissues and cells, particularly the leucocytes. Cell-free DNA is rapidly cleared by macrophages through the process of phagocytosis [2].

The fetal fraction of cfDNA does not originate from the fetus, the name itself being a misnomer. As DNA fragments are large molecules, the transplacental transfer of fetal DNA is poor. Whatever little fetal DNA that crosses the placenta is swiftly engulfed by maternal macrophages, resulting in a remarkably short half-life. The so-called 'fetal' fraction of cfDNA originates from the apoptosis of villous cytotrophoblast cells (Fig. 5.1). Therefore, it more accurately reflects the genetic constitution of the placenta rather than that of the fetus [3, 4].

At 10 weeks of gestation, 90% of the total cfDNA in plasma is of maternal origin and only 10% is of fetal origin. Fetal cfDNA increases by 0.1% per week between 10 weeks and 20 weeks, and 0.6% per week thereafter. The fetal fraction is significantly lower in obese women, likely because of a high adipocyte turnover causing an increase in maternal cfDNA concentration [5]. It is completely cleared from maternal circulation within 24 h of delivery. Aneuploidy itself alters the levels of fetal cfDNA. The median fetal fraction is increased in Down syndrome, while reduced levels are seen in trisomy 13, trisomy 18, triploidy and monosomy X. Pregnancies with mosaic fetuses (mixture of normal and aneu-

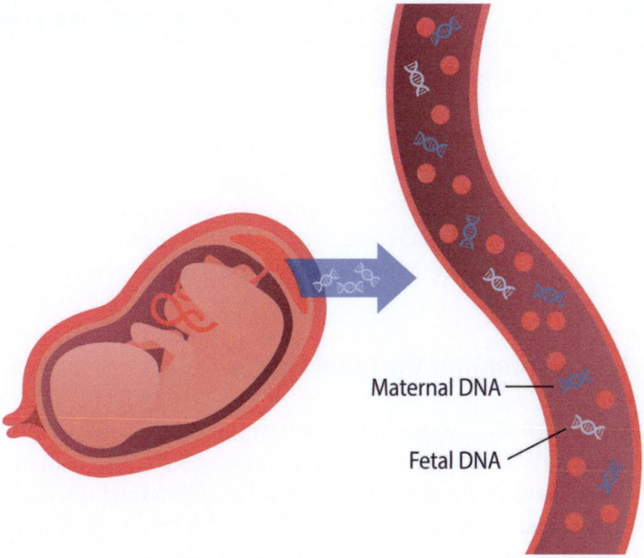

Fig. 5.1 The cfDNA analyzed by NIPT is a mixture of maternal and fetal fraction. The 'fetal' fraction of cfDNA originates from the placenta

ploid cells) have fetal cfDNA fractions not significantly different from euploid pregnancies [6].

5.3 Testing Methodology

Isolation and differentiation of fetal cfDNA from maternal cfDNA is difficult due to its low concentration in maternal plasma. Moreover, the fetus shares half of its genetic constitution with its mother, leading to a considerable similarity in DNA segments.

5.3.1 Sample Collection and Transport

NIPT can be performed at any time after 9 weeks of gestation. The possibility of test failure due to low fetal fraction is higher for samples drawn before 13 weeks. Approximately 8–10 cc maternal venous blood is collected in special K3EDTA stabilized tubes such as the Strek Cell-Free DNA BCT® or the Roche Cell-Free DNA Collection Tube®. The preservative agent stabilizes maternal blood cells and prevents the release of maternal cfDNA during transport. The tube should be inverted completely for approximately ten times for proper mixing and then sealed carefully before shipping. The sample should not be frozen. Cell-free DNA remains very stable and can be transported at room temperature (ideally 18–25 °C). Total duration from blood sample withdrawal to processing should not exceed 7 days.

5.3.2 Estimating the Fetal Fraction

Even though the separation of fetal cfDNA from the pool of maternal cfDNA is not a strict requirement of NIPT, the fetal fraction still needs to be estimated. This is because a fetal fraction of <4% can lead to inaccurate results. The fetal fraction can either be derived from the sequencing data itself or estimated using a separate test. Fetal cfDNA fragments are shorter than maternal fragments, and this difference in size can be used to calculate the fetal fraction. Additional techniques, such as differential DNA methylation and single nucleotide polymorphisms (SNP), can also be used [7]. In case the fetal fraction is low, a repeat blood sample is required. If the repeat sample also shows the same, invasive testing is indicated, as aneuploidy itself can lead to low fetal cfDNA levels in maternal blood [6].

5.3.3 Extraction of Cell-Free DNA

Maternal blood is centrifuged to separate the plasma from the buffy coat and the RBCs. Maternal plasma is subjected to DNA extraction techniques to separate the cfDNA.

5.3.4 Amplification

The amount of total cfDNA present in plasma is itself quite low, out of which only a small proportion is of fetal origin. Even if the

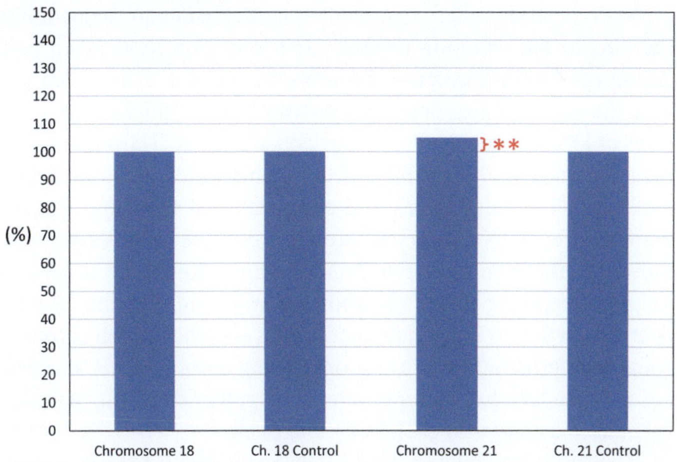

Fig. 5.2 Illustrative graph showing the minuscule increase (**) in chromosome 21 cfDNA in maternal blood when the fetus has trisomy 21

fetal fraction is 10% and the fetus has Down syndrome, the relative increase in chromosome 21 DNA fragments in maternal blood is as low as 5% [8]. It is indeed remarkable that modern technology can detect such small differences to reach meaningful conclusions (Fig. 5.2). Understandably, millions of sequence reads are needed to ensure that the detected change in DNA content is real, and not merely by chance. Therefore, polymerase chain reaction (PCR) is used to increase the DNA content of the sample before sequencing.

5.3.5 Sequencing

DNA sequencing involves determination of the precise order of nucleotides (adenine, cytosine, guanine, and thymine) in DNA. The commonest method used for sequencing of DNA is called the *next-generation sequencing* (NGS), and is explained below [6, 8]. Other techniques are briefly described at the end of the chapter.

NGS is also called massively parallel shotgun sequencing (MPSS) or the counting method, as it relies on sequencing and counting of all informative chromosome regions. This technique uses fluorescent bases and DNA polymerases to quickly turn millions of DNA molecules into color-coded images. The sequencing data obtained is then subjected to sophisticated bioinformatics analysis, where algorithms and computational tools are used to compare the cfDNA with the reference genome to look for chromosomal abnormalities. For detecting aneuploidy, the reads are mapped according to the chromosome of origin. The increase or decrease in the expected number of reads specific to each chromosome is interpreted as an extra or missing chromosome. To keep costs down, labs run multiple samples together by adding patient-specific 'bar-codes' to each DNA fragment.

NGS does not analyze fetal cfDNA separately from maternal cfDNA, but processes all the cfDNA together. In case a genetic abnormality is detected, its source cannot be ascertained. In such a scenario, the analyzer software presumes that the mother is genetically normal, and gives a screen-positive result for the fetus. This technical limitation can lead to a false-positive result in any situation where maternal cfDNA pattern is abnormal. Similarly, triploidy cannot be detected due to a proportionate increase in the entire fetal genome. In twins, it is not possible to identify which of the two fetuses is the affected one.

Targeted MPSS (t-MPSS) is a modification of the above technique, involving sequencing of cfDNA corresponding to selected regions on a few chromosomes of interest. This technique requires 20 times fewer reads compared to whole-genome sequencing in NGS, making it time and cost-efficient. The result can be further refined by statistically combining it with maternal age, previous history of aneuploidy, or the risk calculated in maternal serum screening [8].

5.4 Interpretation of NIPT Result

Even at the cost of repetition, one point needs to be re-emphasized. The commonly used NGS technique bases its results on the analysis of the entire (maternal + fetal) cfDNA content to arrive at a reasonably accurate 'best guess.' Unlike karyotyping or FISH, it does not actually image the fetal chromosomes.

5.4.1 Screen-Positive Result

Laboratories usually report NIPT results as a *z*-score. Depending on the lab, the *z*-score may be converted into a patient-specific risk, or reported as screen-positive or screen-negative. The former has the advantage of clarifying that the test is not diagnostic. Few laboratories report the positive predictive value, an often-overlooked statistic signifying how likely is it that the baby is actually affected. All patients with an abnormal or screen-positive NIPT result should be offered CVS or amniocentesis. *Decision regarding termination of pregnancy should never be taken based on the NIPT report alone.*

5.4.2 Screen-Negative Result

A screen-negative NIPT result is highly reassuring and requires no further testing. The fact that NIPT is not a 100% diagnostic test should be explained to the patient. Ideally, this discussion should happen prior to testing. If a subsequent ultrasound reveals a structural abnormality known to be associated with aneuploidy (e.g., duodenal atresia), amniocentesis should still be performed.

5.4.3 Low Fetal Fraction or No-Call Result

A no-call result is possible either when the sequencing shows too much noise in the data obtained or when the blood sample shows a low fetal fraction. To provide a meaningful result, NIPT requires the fetal fraction to be at least 4% of the total cfDNA in maternal blood. Low fetal fraction occurs in 1–8% of women [9], and can be due to:

- Gestational age: being more common at 9–10 weeks.
- Blood sample volume <10 mL.
- Obese women.
- Fetal aneuploidy (trisomy 13, 18, monosomy X, and triploidy).

In such cases, a repeat sample should be sent. The woman should be informed that there is a 25% chance of a repeat test failure. In case of a repeat no-call result, invasive testing should be offered. No-call results add to the false-positive rate of cfDNA screening.

5.5 Screening Performance for Common Aneuploidies (Singleton Pregnancies)

Noninvasive prenatal testing is a highly efficient screening test for the detection of common autosomal trisomies. It is particularly suitable in women who are at high risk of having a child with a trisomy, but without structural abnormalities on ultrasound. In the presence of a specific anomaly detected on ultrasound, invasive testing is recommended.

5.5.1 Sensitivity for Common Trisomies

Table 5.1 shows the estimated detection rate (DR) and false-positive rate (FPR) for trisomy 13,18, and 21

Table 5.1 Screening performance of NIPT in the general population [8, 10, 11]

Aneuploidy	Review	DR in % (95% CI)	FPR in % (95% CI)
Trisomy 21	Benn et al. [8]	99.3 (98.2–99.8)	0.16 (0.08–0.31)
	Gil et al. [10]	99.2 (98.5–99.6)	0.09 (0.05–0.13)
	Rose et al. [11]	98.80 (97.81–99.34)	0.04 (0.02–0.08)
Trisomy 18	Benn et al. [8]	97.4 (93.7–99.0)	0.15 (0.07–0.31)
	Gil et al. [10]	96.3 (94.3–97.9)	0.12 (0.08–0.17)
	Rose et al. [11]	98.83 (95.45–99.71)	0.07 (0.03–0.17)
Trisomy 13	Benn et al. [8]	78.9 (65.9–91.9)	0.41 (0.22–0.61)
	Gil et al. [10]	91.7 (86.9–95.5)	0.11 (0.06–0.16)
	Rose et al. [11]	100 (0–100)	0.04 (0.02–0.08)

As is clear from Table 5.1, NIPT has a very high DR for all the three autosomal trisomies despite its statistical approach. The slightly lower DR for chromosome 13 is attributed to a relatively lower proportion of guanine (G) and cytosine (C) nucleotides (as enrichment during PCR and sequencing depends on the GC content) [12]. Despite the low FPR, a significant number of false positives occur (see the section on 'limitations of NIPT'). With NIPT being marketed as a highly accurate test, the general impression conveyed to both healthcare providers and patients is that it is an infallible test. An unfortunate result of this is the termination of many normal fetuses when false-positive results occur. Therefore, every high-risk NIPT report must be confirmed by invasive testing before taking a decision to terminate pregnancy.

5.5.2 Sex Chromosome Aneuploidies (SCAs)

In a systematic review by Gil and coworkers, the sensitivity of NIPT for monosomy X (Turner syndrome) was found to be 90.3% for an FPR of 0.23%. For other SCAs, the DR was 93.0% for a 0.14% FPR [10]. Several mechanisms could account for the lower detection rate observed with SCAs [8]:

- Almost one-third of fetuses with SCAs are mosaics, with a mixture of euploid and aneuploid cell lines.
- The Y chromosome is small and shares some homologous sequences with the X chromosome.
- The pregnant woman herself can have mosaicism for Turner syndrome, and this can influence the test results (see Sect. 5.6.5).
- Normal women show an age-related loss of an X chromosome in some cells, leading to an increase in 45,X cells. Few women also demonstrate cells which have gained an extra X chromosome.
- While each trisomy is a genetically specific condition, SCAs collectively refer to several conditions with variable ratio of X and Y chromosome-derived cfDNA.

5.6 Limitations of NIPT and Other Concerns

Despite being a highly sensitive test, NIPT faces challenges related to accuracy, interpretation, and ethical considerations. In this section, the current limitations of NIPT are discussed.

5.6.1 False-Positive Rate (FPR) and Positive Predictive Value (PPV)

False-positive rate refers to the percentage of the tested population who get an abnormal result, but are normal. It is important to understand that a false-positive rate applies to the entire population being tested, not only to the cases detected. Positive predictive value (PPV) refers to the chance that a fetus, which is labeled as abnormal, is, in reality, abnormal.

Example 1: Down syndrome (Age risk 1:1000 at 29 years)
Let us consider 1,00,000 low-risk women who are 29 years old undergoing NIPT for Down syndrome screening (See Fig. 5.3). Assuming an FPR as low as 0.05%, the number of women getting a false-positive result will be 50 (0.05% of 1,00,000). The total number of women who are carrying Down syndrome fetuses in this cohort will be 100 (age risk 1:1000), out of which 99 would be detected (DR of 99%). Hence, out of 149 screen-positive NIPT reports, only two-thirds would be correct, and one-third would be incorrect. Many of these normal babies would unfortunately be aborted if confirmatory invasive testing is not done.

Example 2: Prader–Willi syndrome (risk: 1 in 20,000)
We repeat the above calculations for a rare condition, Prader–Willi syndrome which has a birth incidence of 1 in 20,000. As seen from Fig. 5.4, only 5 women out of 55 who screen positive for this syndrome will be carrying an affected fetus (positive predictive value = 9%). The remaining 50 women will have a normal fetus. This means that 91% of NIPT screen-positive results for Prader–Willi syndrome will be wrong!

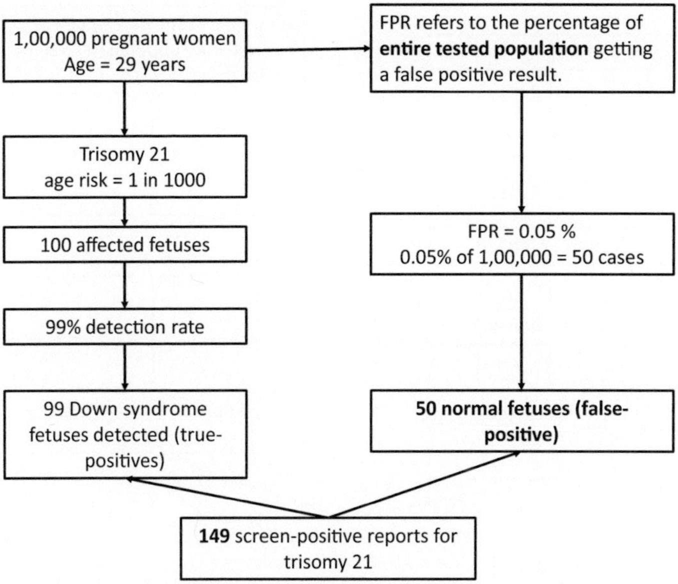

Fig. 5.3 Screening performance of NIPT for Down syndrome in 1,00,000 women aged 29 years, assuming a sensitivity of 99% and a specificity of 99.95%. Note that one-third of screen-positive results are wrong (false-positive)

As seen from the above examples, the PPV for any condition depends on its prevalence in the tested population. In Example 1 above, which considers universal screening in a low-risk population, the PPV is 66% (two-thirds of positive NIPT results are correct). In high-risk populations, such as older women, and those with screen-positive quadruple test results, the prevalence is higher, and so is the PPV. As the women undergoing NIPT for Down syndrome screening tend to be older, the PPV is typically much higher than that calculated in Example 1.

In a systematic evidence review in 2022, Rose and coworkers showed the PPV to be 91% for Down syndrome, 65% for Edward syndrome, and only 37% for Patau syndrome [11]. Importantly, the PPV for sex chromosome aneuploidies was <50%, implying that over half of the screen-positive results were incorrect.

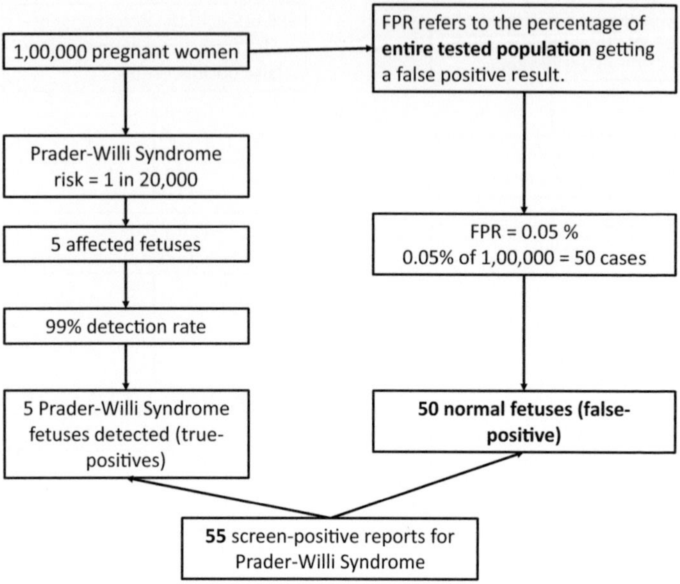

Fig. 5.4 Screening performance of NIPT for Prader–Willi in 1,00,000 women assuming a sensitivity of 99% and a specificity of 99.95%. Note that 91% of screen-positive results are wrong (false-positive)

5.6.2 Microdeletions and Rare Autosomal Trisomies (RATs)

Several laboratories now offer NIPT for microdeletion syndromes and autosomal trisomies other than 13, 18, and 21 (expanded NIPT). There are several reasons why expanded NIPT should not be routinely offered:

- Microdeletions are submicroscopic gene deletions which are associated with minuscule changes in cfDNA levels. This change is often too small to be accurately interpreted.
- Positive predictive value of NIPT depends on the prevalence of a condition in the population. Because of a low prevalence, NIPT has a poor PPV for these rare disorders.

- Some chromosomal abnormalities, like complete trisomy 1, have never been reported in humans and are incompatible with a live fetus. In case the NIPT report shows the possibility of these conditions in the setting of a normal NT scan, counseling patients regarding unnecessary invasive testing is difficult.

In a study of 712 women, the PPV was only 21% for DiGeorge syndrome (22q11.2 deletion), and 0% for Cri-du-Chat syndrome and Prader-Willi/Angelman syndrome using the counting method [13]. Similarly, Chen and coworkers reported a 0% PPV for genetic abnormalities involving chromosomes 8, 9, and 10 [14].

5.6.3 Mosaicism

Mosaicism is a condition in which an individual has two different cell lines. For example, a baby with mosaicism for Down syndrome has some cells in the body with trisomy 21, while other cells are completely normal. Fetal mosaicism poses a unique challenge for NIPT. As cfDNA testing platforms use placental cfDNA as a proxy for fetal genotype, the results of NIPT will depend on which of the two cell lines predominate within the placenta.

In rare cases (1%), only the placenta may have an abnormal genetic constitution, referred to as confined placental mosaicism (CPM). Two genetic mechanisms can cause CPM. One of them is postmitotic nondisjunction, in which case a few cells destined to form the placenta separate from those destined to form the embryo. If these extraembryonic cells undergo nondisjunction after this event, only the placenta can be aneuploid. The second mechanism is aneuploidy rescue. In aneuploidy rescue, the fertilized ovum has a trisomy. As it divides, a few of the cells expel out the extra chromosome in an attempt to become euploid. These normal cells then form the embryo, while the trisomic cells are segregated together to form the placenta. In CPM, there is an increased risk of miscarriage, fetal growth restriction, and fetal death because of placental dysfunction. (In most cases, however, it is associated with a normal fetal outcome.)

CPM was first reported while testing CVS samples. In CVS, the placental villi are cultured and tested using two methods: (1) short-term culture and (2) long-term culture. Short-term culture involves the culture of the outer layer of the chorionic villi (comprising cytotrophoblasts) for 24–48 h for a rapid analysis. Long-term culture involves culturing the mesodermal core of the chorionic villi, which is expected to be concordant with fetal genotype. Rarely, different results arise between the two, leading to suspicion of CPM [15].

When the placenta and the fetus differ genetically, it is the placenta that is almost always abnormal, leading to false-positive results on NIPT and CVS. If CVS is performed following a positive NIPT, it is important that both cell lines are evaluated. Uncultured CVS tissue can be evaluated by FISH or after the short-term culture, and this should be followed by long-term culture. In case the CVS tissue sample also reveals mosaicism, repeat fetal sampling by amniocentesis is mandatory before taking a decision to terminate the pregnancy. If the NIPT shows a screen-positive result, and the gestational age is close to 14 weeks, it is better to wait and do an amniocentesis. Amniocentesis gives a direct confirmation of the fetal genotype and is not affected by CPM.

5.6.4 Multiple Pregnancy

Noninvasive prenatal testing in multiple pregnancies is marred by several challenges and shortcomings. The intricacies of screening multiple pregnancies with NIPT are elaborated in Chap. 8. Some concerns specific to multiple pregnancies are:

- If NIPT returns a screen-positive result, it is not possible to know which fetus is affected.
- Zygosity, not chorionicity, determines whether the fetuses will be genetically identical. It may not always be possible to detect zygosity on ultrasound. In monozygotic twins, screening performance of NIPT is as good as singleton pregnancy, with a higher fetal fraction.

- As aneuploidy can be associated with a low cfDNA production, the cfDNA from the normal twin can mask that produced by the aneuploid twin.
- A vanishing twin can lead to confounding results because of the inconsistent release of cfDNA from the dead twin's placenta.
- Postzygotic nondisjunction is an event whereby one of the monochorionic (MC) fetuses undergoes a genetic alteration after the splitting of the zygote, leading to nonidentical fetuses.
- In higher order gestations, NIPT is not possible.

The use of SNP analysis (discussed later in the chapter) has been shown to improve screening performance in twins. Data from the Fetal Medicine Foundation using the Harmony® prenatal test showed a DR of 95%, 90%, and 50% for trisomy 21, 18, and 13 respectively [16].

5.6.5 Maternal Chromosomal Abnormalities

A woman may have subtle genetic abnormalities like low-level mosaicism for Turner syndrome with no clinical consequences. During cfDNA screening, it may have two effects. Abnormal levels of sex chromosomal cfDNA may be interpreted as fetal sex chromosomal abnormalities, especially if NGS is used. If the SNP approach is used, the SCA is likely to be correctly attributed to the mother, leading to a negative psychological impact.

Another source of confusion can be maternal copy number variations (CNVs). These refer to the varying number of copies of a particular gene from individual to individual due to a gain or loss of genetic material. While maternal copy number variations may have no clinical effects, they may be misinterpreted as fetal microdeletions or microduplications by NIPT platforms.

5.6.6 Malignancies and Other Conditions Affecting Maternal cfDNA

Maternal cancers can affect NIPT results, as dying cancer cells release large amounts of cfDNA into maternal circulation. Neoplastic cells often exhibit a combination of several genetic abnormalities. A suspicion of maternal malignancy may be raised by an NIPT report showing multiple aneuploidies in the same fetus. Maternal malignancies reported to affect NIPT results include neuroendocrine carcinoma, non-Hodgkin lymphoma, leukemia, and colorectal cancer. As these cases are far and few, there is very little data to recommend specific guidelines for the workup of such women.

Similarly, NIPT is not recommended for women who have had a blood transfusion within the past 3 months. It is also not suitable in recipients of transplants, stem cell therapy, or immunotherapy.

5.6.7 Donor Oocyte IVF

The fetal fraction of cfDNA comprises DNA fragments which partly resemble paternal and maternal genomes. In donor oocyte IVF, a third source of genetic material is introduced, which can be misinterpreted by the MPSS technique. If NIPT is to be performed in women conceived through donor oocyte programs, the blood sample needs to be sent to a laboratory having (a) a high fetal fraction accuracy and (b) using the SNP technique of NIPT.

IVF pregnancies are also associated with a lower fetal fraction, higher test failure rate, and lower PPV for trisomies 13, 18, and SCAs [17]. The ensuing increase in the false-positive rate, along with hesitancy of these women to undergo invasive testing, creates difficult situations for clinicians. A thorough pre-test counseling should include a discussion about the possible need for an invasive procedure.

5.6.8 Fetuses with Structural Malformations

Invasive testing is recommended over NIPT in anomalous fetuses because of several reasons [18]:

1. NIPT is a screening test, and not a diagnostic test.
2. Structural malformations are typically detected at mid-pregnancy and using NIPT as an intermediate test increases time taken to reach a specific diagnosis.
3. Sensitivity of NIPT is validated only for the common trisomies. Fetal anomalies can be associated with rare aneuploidies and submicroscopic abnormalities.

5.6.9 Increased Cost of Screening

Noninvasive screening is a highly sensitive, cost-effective tool when used in high-risk populations, such as women with high-risk result on maternal serum screening. In low-risk populations, it is difficult to justify the cost of using NIPT as a first-line screening test, considering that aneuploidy itself is a relatively uncommon condition.

A cross-sectional survey to quantify willingness-to-pay among 192 pregnant women in Singapore showed that most women preferred maternal serum screening over NIPT [19]. Acceptance as a first-line screening test is likely to vary across different countries and health systems depending on beliefs of women and their obstetricians, and financial implications. Contingent screening with NIPT is the most cost-effective strategy for cfDNA testing. In this strategy, NIPT is used as a second-tier test in women who screen positive on maternal serum screening.

Contingent *serum* screening is a method wherein women with an intermediate risk result in the first-trimester serum screening are screened again in the second trimester. Contingent serum screening has a sensitivity of 95% and is a cost-effective alternative to NIPT.

5.6.10 Other Concerns Regarding NIPT

Several other concerns remain regarding the widespread use of NIPT. These are briefly discussed below.

Social Inequality As NIPT is an expensive test which is not covered by most insurance providers and health schemes, individuals from lower socioeconomic strata may face financial barriers that prevent them from seeking or affording genetic testing. This results in the diagnosis of genetic abnormalities being skewed according to the economic status.

Genetic Discrimination There is no such thing as a genetically perfect human being. As cfDNA testing expands to include whole genome sequencing, there is every possibility of discovering subtle genetic abnormalities in many individuals. Identification of abnormalities with mild phenotypic expression, variants of unknown significance, and genes which make an individual susceptible to a particular disease can cause lifelong anxiety to individuals and their families. Furthermore, it will lead to many individuals being unnecessarily labeled as abnormal. Some would prefer not to procreate, fearing inheritance of these abnormalities.

Misuse for Sex-selective Abortions NIPT can be done as early as 9 weeks and is diagnostic for fetal sex. In most countries, it is not regulated as strictly as ultrasound and invasive testing. Therefore, NIPT has the possibility of being misused for sex determination and sex-selective abortions.

Training in Invasive Procedures As NIPT gradually replaces maternal serum screening, it will reduce the number of invasive procedures, making training of new operators difficult. As fetal loss rates are inversely proportional to the number of procedures performed in any unit, this can slightly offset the risk reduction provided by NIPT.

Commercialization and Rapid Deployment NIPT has been commercially available since 2011. The aggressive promotion of NIPT by laboratories, especially for uncommon genetic conditions, raises concerns about the ethical and clinical implications of its widespread adoption.

Conflict of Interest Among Researchers A worrisome trend pertains to financial conflicts of interest among authors of journal papers and guidelines, potentially influencing the impartiality of research outcomes. To ensure responsible use of NIPT and optimize patient outcomes, it is crucial to prioritize evidence-based practice, collaborative research, and transparent reporting.

5.7 Implementation in Clinical Practice

Noninvasive prenatal screening is a double-edged sword. While it reduces the invasive procedures for diagnosing common trisomies, using it without due caution can cause anxiety and uncertainty, sometimes resulting in an unwarranted pregnancy termination.

5.7.1 Current Recommendations for Use of NIPT

Screening using NIPT is presently recommended in the following situations:

1. High-risk or intermediate-risk result on maternal serum screening: In these women, NIPT helps in reducing the number of invasive procedures. This is probably the most important indication.

2. As a first-line screening test instead of serum screening: NIPT exhibits high performance and cost-effectiveness in older women. Younger women may also opt for NIPT, if cost is not a concern.
3. Previous child with Down syndrome: When the woman has a previous baby with free trisomy 21 or mosaicism, the risk of recurrence is approximately 1%, and NIPT may be offered instead of serum screening in subsequent pregnancies. In case of previous *translocation* Down syndrome, invasive testing should be offered as the first step.
4. Insignificant soft marker on ultrasound: When an isolated soft marker such as choroid plexus cyst or echogenic intracardiac focus is noted, and the patient wants a sensitive screening test, NIPT is a good option.
5. Detecting fetal Rhesus D (RhD) genotype and fetal sex: RhD-positive genotype and fetal gender (either male or female) have a high prevalence in the general population (Correlate with Fig. 5.3). As a result, NIPT is considered a diagnostic test for these two indications. *Sex determination is not permitted in some countries like India, China, and Taiwan.*

Numerous laboratories offer cfDNA testing for rare genetic conditions, in many instances, without providing validation data. Rare conditions diagnosed by NIPT have a poor positive predictive value, meaning most patients who test positive are carrying a normal fetus.

NIPT is not recommended in the following situations:

1. Presence of a structural abnormality.
2. Nuchal translucency ≥3.0 mm (some consider 3.5 mm as cut-off).
3. Testing for rare autosomal trisomies.
4. Testing for microdeletions, microduplications, or single-gene disorders.
5. Previous baby with translocation Down syndrome.
6. Higher order multiple pregnancies.
7. Vanishing twin or after selective fetal reduction.
8. Donor egg IVF.

9. Blood transfusion within the last 12 months.
10. Bone marrow transplantation or stem cell therapy.
11. Maternal cancer or known genetic mosaicism.

In many of these scenarios, labs may still offer to do NIPT. In such cases, if the woman requests cfDNA screening rather than an invasive procedure, a detailed pre-test counseling is mandatory. Reduced sensitivity, high false-positive rates, probability of needing subsequent invasive testing, and a resultant delay in diagnosis must be discussed and documented. Overall, it is best to avoid NIPT altogether, and proceed directly to CVS or amniocentesis.

The above list reflects the shortcomings of NGS-based NIPT, which is the method employed by most labs at present. Although SNP-based cfDNA tests claim high accuracy in cases such as vanishing twin or maternal mosaicism, there is insufficient data for their universal recommendation.

5.7.2 NIPT as a First-Line Screening Test

Barring the high cost, NIPT is superior to maternal serum screening for detection of trisomy 13, 18, and 21. Over time, as this cost gap narrows down, it is likely that maternal serum screening will become obsolete. Nevertheless, careful consideration of its limitations, and potential consequences of false-positive and false-negative results would be crucial when deciding whether to implement cfDNA as a first-line screening test.

The American College of Medical Genetics and Genomics (ACMG) published a clinical guideline in 2022 strongly recommending NIPT as a first-line screening test in all singleton and twin pregnancies for trisomies 13, 18, and 21, SCAs, and 22q11.2 deletion syndrome. This guideline largely ignored the economic considerations, boldly stating, 'The utility and value of NIPS to pregnant individuals extends beyond the price of the test' [20].

Contrarily, most guidelines, including those by the International Society of Ultrasound in Obstetrics and Gynecology (ISUOG) and the National Health Service (UK) recommend NIPT as a second-tier test. Still, they allow women to make an informed choice to opt for it as the primary screening test (though it may not be publicly funded or covered by insurance in many countries) [21, 22].

5.8 Nuchal Translucency Scan in the Era of cfDNA

While NIPT has revolutionized the screening for common aneuploidies, it is unlikely it will ever replace the 11–13 + 6 weeks scan for several reasons:

1. The 11–14 weeks scan provides a comprehensive assessment of the fetus, including structural malformations.
2. Crucial details can be documented in multiple pregnancies (such as chorionicity and vanishing fetus).
3. Uterine artery Doppler is a predictor of future placental dysfunction.
4. It permits the assessment of the placenta and the cervix and pathologies of the uterus and adnexa.
5. This scan is performed relatively early in the pregnancy, allowing for early detection of potential issues. Early detection gives parents more time to decide, consult with experts, and act if needed.
6. The results of the 11–14 weeks scan are typically available immediately or shortly after the examination. This immediate feedback can ease anxiety and provide timely information for the parents.
7. 11–13 + 6 weeks scan may be more accessible and covered by insurance plans.

5.9 Single Nucleotide Polymorphism (SNP)-Based NIPT

Single nucleotide polymorphisms (SNPs) are individual variations in the sequence of the nucleotides adenine (A), cytosine (C), guanine (G), and thymine (T) which give a unique genetic identity to each individual. Sequencing of SNPs allows the differentiation of fetal and maternal cfDNA using paternal blood sample as a reference. If paternal blood is not available, a reference map of the human genome can be used as a substitute [23].

5.9.1 Technique

- After centrifugation of maternal blood, three layers are formed: the RBC layer at the bottom, the buffy coat in the middle, and the plasma at the top. The buffy coat comprises the leucocytes and platelets, and contains only maternal DNA. The supernatant plasma contains a mixture of maternal and fetal cfDNA.
- The SNP-based approach employs PCR amplification of both layers separately, followed by sequencing of nearly 20,000 SNPs.
- For each chromosome, the analyzer considers three hypotheses: monosomy, disomy (normal), or trisomy. Using data from the Human Genome Project, several million sub-hypotheses are considered for crossovers.
- Based on the number and position of SNPs, the fetal/maternal cfDNA pattern is compared to each of the hypotheses to find the closest match. As a result, the statistical probability of the fetus being normal or abnormal is calculated.

5.9.2 Advantages [23]

1. The SNP-based approach has high sensitivity for trisomies 13, 18, and 21, Turner syndrome, and triploidy, with a 90.9% PPV for trisomy 21 [24, 25].
2. It is less dependent on the fetal fraction. In case the fetal fraction is <4%, the SNP-based method returns a no-call result rather than providing erroneous results.
3. The SNP-based method is less prone to GC amplification bias, and therefore, retains a high detection rate for trisomy 13, and monosomy X.

4. This technique can detect triploidy, uniparental disomy, zygosity in twins, and maternal mosaicism for SCAs.
5. SNP-based NIPT can identify a vanishing twin by detecting an additional haplotype.

Despite the claimed advantages, the SNP-based method has false positives (and rarely, false negatives). Therefore, every screen-positive result must be confirmed by invasive testing before terminating the pregnancy.

5.10 Experimental Approaches and Techniques

Emerging approaches in fetal cell-free DNA testing can potentially lead to a significant advancement in prenatal diagnostics. Researchers are continuously exploring new avenues within this field to widen its scope, reduce the cost, or both. As these approaches continue to evolve and improve, they hold the promise of providing a precise and cost-effective diagnosis, allowing for early decision-making during pregnancy.

5.10.1 DNA Methylation-Based Assay

The fetal genome differs from the maternal genome in its methylation pattern, with some sites being relatively hypomethylated or hypermethylated. These sites are called as differentially methylated regions (DMRs). Methylated DNA immunoprecipitation is a technique that uses antibodies to selectively extract and enhance methylated fetal DNA fragments from maternal plasma by targeting specific DMRs. Presently, low cfDNA yield remains the major limitation of this technique. If this limitation is addressed, the DMR-based approach could be a sensitive and cost-effective alternative to present methods [26].

5.10.2 Long Chimeric Reads

Long chimeric reads refer to DNA sequencing reads that span multiple distinct regions or genomic segments. These reads are generated by sequencing technologies that can produce long fragments of DNA by joining several cfDNA fragments. Using this technique, Belova and coworkers showed it was possible to get a larger amount of useful diagnostic information from each read compared to the currently used techniques. They also reported a shorter turnaround time and a 40% reduction in cost [27].

5.10.3 NIPT for Single-Gene Disorders (NIPT-SGD)

Single-gene disorders (SGDs), also known as monogenic disorders, are genetic disorders caused by mutations or alterations in a single gene. These disorders are typically inherited in a Mendelian pattern, meaning they are passed down from parents to their children in a predictable manner. Examples of SGDs are skeletal disorders (osteogenesis imperfecta, Ehlers-Danlos syndrome, achondroplasia, thanatophoric dysplasia), craniosynostosis syndromes (Crouzon syndrome, Apert syndrome), Noonan spectrum disorders, and multi-system disorders (Cornelia de Lange syndrome, tuberous sclerosis, Sotos syndrome). Single-gene disorders are extremely rare, being present in <0.5% fetuses with normal ultrasounds. Prenatal diagnosis of SGDs is uncommon and often happens in a subsequent pregnancy following the birth of an affected child. Diagnosis usually requires sequencing the entire exome or specific gene panels.

Mohan and coworkers reported their clinical experience using the Vistara NIPT-SGD test® which analyzes fetal cfDNA by NGS to look for pathogenic or likely pathogenic variants implicated in 25 dominant conditions. They reported a high sensitivity in cases with a known paternal mutation or fetal anomalies strongly suggestive of SGD [28].

Limitations of NIPT-SGD include an inability to detect copy-number variations and structural rearrangements. It has a very low PPV in low-risk populations, and cannot detect maternally inherited disorders. NIPT-SGD is in its earliest stages of development and is currently unsuitable for routine screening.

5.10.4 Free Fetal RNA in Maternal Plasma

Like cfDNA, maternal plasma also contains fetal cell-free RNA originating from the placenta. Using SNP-based techniques, it is possible to quantify and sequence this RNA. Unfortunately, it has not yet been possible to use this research to develop a clinically useful test. This approach also requires maternal plasma to be processed within 12 h of sample collection, posing significant logistic difficulties [6].

5.10.5 Fetal Cells in Maternal Blood

As mentioned earlier, fetal cells were isolated from maternal blood several decades before cfDNA. Fetal cells are extremely sparse (estimated to be one per ten million maternal cells), which makes it difficult to extract sufficient data or get conclusive results from their analysis.

In 2014, Hatt and colleagues published a study on fetal cell identification in 78 maternal blood samples using the marker-set CD105 and CD141 for fetal cell enrichment. They were successful in detecting fetal cells in 91% of the samples and identifying fetal gender (using FISH for chromosomes X and Y) in 85% of the samples [29]. Research is ongoing to improve techniques for isolating and analyzing these rare fetal cells in maternal blood.

5.10.6 Endocervical Fetal Trophoblasts

Cells originating from the extravillous trophoblast can be sampled from maternal endocervix using a cytobrush. Using a platform called trophoblast retrieval and isolation from the cervix (TRIC), Kadam and coworkers were able to isolate these cells as early as 5 weeks of gestation with >90% purity [30]. If validated, this technique could provide greater insight into the fetal genome, and possibly help in predicting placental dysfunction.

5.11 Key Messages

1. The fetal fraction of cfDNA originates from the placenta, not the fetus. This is usually <10% of the total cfDNA found in maternal blood.
2. Most labs use the NGS method, which cannot differentiate between fetal and maternal cfDNA. It generates a statistical result based on the total increase in cfDNA specific to a chromosome.
3. NIPT is a highly sensitive screening test for common trisomies, with over 99% DR for trisomy 21.
4. The most important role of NIPT is to reduce the number of invasive procedures in women who screen positive on the combined FTS or the quadruple test, or those with an isolated minor soft marker.
5. No pregnancy should be terminated based on a screen-positive result without invasive testing.
6. Low fetal fraction or no-call results are more common in aneuploid fetuses. Invasive testing is recommended.
7. Women whose fetuses have an NT >3 mm or structural malformations should be offered invasive testing as the first step rather than cfDNA screening.
8. NIPT has a poor PPV for rare autosomal trisomies, microdeletions, and single-gene disorders.
9. Maternal mosaicism and malignancies can interfere with NIPT results.
10. NIPT can be performed in twins, but with caution, and having understood its limitations.

References

1. Herzenberg LA, Bianchi DW, Schröder J, Cann HM, Iverson GM. Fetal cells in the blood of pregnant women: detection and enrichment by fluorescence-activated cell sorting. Proc Natl Acad Sci U S A. 1979;76(3):1453–5.
2. Grabuschnig S, Bronkhorst AJ, Holdenrieder S, Rosales Rodriguez I, Schliep KP, Schwendenwein D, Ungerer V, Sensen CW. Putative origins of cell-free DNA in humans: a review of active and passive nucleic acid release mechanisms. Int J Mol Sci. 2020;21(21):8062.
3. Lo YM, Chan KC, Sun H, Chen EZ, Jiang P, Lun FM, Zheng YW, Leung TY, Lau TK, Cantor CR, Chiu RW. Maternal plasma DNA sequencing reveals the genome-wide genetic and mutational profile of the fetus. Sci Transl Med. 2010;2(61):61ra91.
4. Hochstenbach R, Nikkels PG, Elferink MG, Oudijk MA, van Oppen C, van Zon P, van Harssel J, Schuring-Blom H, Page-Christiaens GC. Cell-free fetal DNA in the maternal circulation originates from the cytotrophoblast: proof from an unique case. Clin Case Rep. 2015;3:489–91.
5. Ashoor G, Syngelaki A, Poon LC, Rezende JC, Nicolaides KH. Fetal fraction in maternal plasma cell-free DNA at 11–13 weeks' gestation: relation to maternal and fetal characteristics. Ultrasound Obstet Gynecol. 2013;41(1):26–32.
6. Dar P, Shani H, Evans MI. Cell-free DNA: comparison of technologies. Clin Lab Med. 2016;36(2):199–211.
7. Straver R, Oudejans CB, Sistermans EA, Reinders MJ. Calculating the fetal fraction for noninvasive prenatal testing based on genome-wide nucleosome profiles. Prenat Diagn. 2016;36(7):614–21.
8. Benn P, Cuckle H, Pergament E. Non-invasive prenatal testing for aneuploidy: current status and future prospects. Ultrasound Obstet Gynecol. 2013;42(1):15–33.
9. Grace MR, Hardisty E, Dotters-Katz SK, Vora NL, Kuller JA. Cell-free DNA screening: complexities and challenges of clinical implementation. Obstet Gynecol Surv. 2016;71(8):477–87.
10. Gil MM, Quezada MS, Revello R, Akolekar R, Nicolaides KH. Analysis of cell-free DNA in maternal blood in screening for fetal aneuploidies: updated meta-analysis. Ultrasound Obstet Gynecol. 2015;45(3):249–66.
11. Rose NC, Barrie ES, Malinowski J, Jenkins GP, McClain MR, LaGrave D, Leung ML, ACMG Professional Practice and Guidelines Committee. Electronic address: documents@acmg.net. Systematic evidence-based review: the application of noninvasive prenatal screening using cell-free DNA in general-risk pregnancies. Genet Med. 2022;24(7):1379–91.
12. Hu H, Wang L, Wu J, Zhou P, Fu J, Sun J, Cai W, Liu H, Yang Y. Noninvasive prenatal testing for chromosome aneuploidies and sub-

chromosomal microdeletions/microduplications in a cohort of 8141 single pregnancies. Hum Genomics. 2019;13(1):14.
13. Petersen AK, Cheung SW, Smith JL, Bi W, Ward PA, Peacock S, Braxton A, Van Den Veyver IB, Breman AM. Positive predictive value estimates for cell-free noninvasive prenatal screening from data of a large referral genetic diagnostic laboratory. Am J Obstet Gynecol. 2017;217(6):691.e1–6.
14. Chen Y, Yu Q, Mao X, Lei W, He M, Lu W. Noninvasive prenatal testing for chromosome aneuploidies and subchromosomal microdeletions/microduplications in a cohort of 42,910 single pregnancies with different clinical features. Hum Genomics. 2019;13(1):60.
15. Eggenhuizen GM, Go A, Koster MPH, Baart EB, Galjaard RJ. Confined placental mosaicism and the association with pregnancy outcome and fetal growth: a review of the literature. Hum Reprod Update. 2021;27(5):885–903.
16. Judah H, Gil MM, Syngelaki A, Galeva S, Jani J, Akolekar R, Nicolaides KH. Cell-free DNA testing of maternal blood in screening for trisomies in twin pregnancy: updated cohort study at 10–14 weeks and meta-analysis. Ultrasound Obstet Gynecol. 2021;58(2):178–89.
17. Lee TJ, Rolnik DL, Menezes MA, McLennan AC, da Silva CF. Cell-free fetal DNA testing in singleton IVF conceptions. Hum Reprod. 2018;33(4):572–8.
18. Beulen L, Faas BHW, Feenstra I, van Vugt JMG, Bekker MN. Clinical utility of non-invasive prenatal testing in pregnancies with ultrasound anomalies. Ultrasound Obstet Gynecol. 2017;49(6):721–8.
19. Sim WS, Yeo SH, Choi C, Yeo TW, Lee JJ, Huynh VA, Finkelstein EA, Ozdemir S. Preferences for a non-invasive prenatal test as first-line screening for Down Syndrome: a discrete choice experiment. Prenat Diagn. 2022;42(11):1368–76.
20. Dungan JS, Klugman S, Darilek S, Malinowski J, Akkari YMN, Monaghan KG, Erwin A, Best RG; ACMG Board of Directors. Electronic address: documents@acmg.net. Noninvasive prenatal screening (NIPS) for fetal chromosome abnormalities in a general-risk population: an evidence-based clinical guideline of the American College of Medical Genetics and Genomics (ACMG). Genet Med. 2023;25(2):100336.
21. International Society of Ultrasound in Obstetrics and Gynecology, Bilardo CM, Chaoui R, Hyett JA, Kagan KO, Karim JN, Papageorghiou AT, Poon LC, Salomon LJ, Syngelaki A, Nicolaides KH. ISUOG Practice Guidelines (updated): performance of 11–14-week ultrasound scan. Ultrasound Obstet Gynecol. 2023;61(1):127–43.
22. Bowden B, de Souza S, Puchades A, Williams K, Morgan S, Anderson S, Tucker D, Hillier S. Implementation of non-invasive prenatal testing within a national UK antenatal screening programme: impact on women's choices. Prenat Diagn. 2022;42(5):549–56.

23. Kim K. Advantages of the single nucleotide polymorphism-based noninvasive prenatal test. J Gene Med. 2015;12:66–71.
24. Nicolaides KH, Syngelaki A, Gil M, Atanasova V, Markova D. Validation of targeted sequencing of single-nucleotide polymorphisms for non-invasive prenatal detection of aneuploidy of chromosomes 13, 18, 21, X, and Y. Prenat Diagn. 2013;33(6):575–9.
25. Dar P, Curnow KJ, Gross SJ, Hall MP, Stosic M, Demko Z, Zimmermann B, Hill M, Sigurjonsson S, Ryan A, Banjevic M, Kolacki PL, Koch SW, Strom CM, Rabinowitz M, Benn P. Clinical experience and follow-up with large scale single-nucleotide polymorphism-based noninvasive prenatal aneuploidy testing. Am J Obstet Gynecol. 2014;211(5):527.e1–17.
26. Akbariqomi M, Heidari R, Gargari SS, Omrani MD, Rigi G, Sanikhani NS, Kooshki H, Mahmoudian F, Mazlomi MA, Tavoosidana G. Evaluation and statistical optimization of a method for methylated cell-free fetal DNA extraction from maternal plasma. J Assist Reprod Genet. 2019;36(5):1029–38.
27. Belova V, Plakhina D, Evfratov S, Tsukanov K, Khvorykh G, Rakitko A, Konoplyannikov A, Ilinsky V, Rebrikov D, Korostin D. NIPT technique based on the use of long chimeric DNA reads. Genes (Basel). 2020;11(6):590.
28. Mohan P, Lemoine J, Trotter C, Rakova I, Billings P, Peacock S, Kao CY, Wang Y, Xia F, Eng CM, Benn P. Clinical experience with non-invasive prenatal screening for single-gene disorders. Ultrasound Obstet Gynecol. 2022;59(1):33–9.
29. Hatt L, Brinch M, Singh R, Møller K, Lauridsen RH, Schlütter JM, Uldbjerg N, Christensen B, Kølvraa S. A new marker set that identifies fetal cells in maternal circulation with high specificity. Prenat Diagn. 2014;34(11):1066–72.
30. Kadam L, Jain C, Kohan-Ghadr HR, Krawetz SA, Drewlo S, Armant DR. Endocervical trophoblast for interrogating the fetal genome and assessing pregnancy health at five weeks. Eur J Med Genet. 2019;62(8):103690.

Second-Trimester Soft Markers Associated with Aneuploidy

6

6.1 Introduction

No pregnancy should be terminated solely because of the presence of fetal soft markers. While this chapter could have begun in several ways, no sentence in this entire chapter is as important as the preceding one.

Soft markers are variations in normal fetal anatomy, which are occasionally found at the time of the second-trimester anomaly scan. As the name suggests, soft markers themselves do not reflect significant structural abnormalities. Presence of a soft marker increases the risk of Down syndrome and other aneuploidies. The risk of aneuploidy rises sharply when there are multiple soft markers present.

Soft markers are also seen in normal fetuses and their presence is not diagnostic of aneuploidy. Most fetuses with isolated soft markers are genetically normal. Conversely, only one-third of fetuses with Down syndrome have any abnormal finding on ultrasound. Soft markers on their own cannot reliably diagnose nor exclude any condition, including Down syndrome.

Chapter 9 explains why aneuploidy risk modification using soft marker likelihood ratios (LRs) is no longer recommended. In this chapter, therefore, we shall consider each soft marker separately.

© The Author(s), under exclusive license to Springer Nature Singapore Pte Ltd. 2023

A. Kamat, *Down Syndrome Screening*,
https://doi.org/10.1007/978-981-99-7758-1_6

6.2 Aberrant Right Subclavian Artery

The right subclavian artery (RSA) normally arises from the brachiocephalic artery, which is the first branch of the aortic arch. In about 1.5% of individuals, this artery directly arises as the fourth branch from the descending portion of the aortic arch, and is called an aberrant right subclavian artery (ARSA). An ARSA is noted in 29%, 18%, and 8% of fetuses with Down syndrome, Edwards syndrome, and other aneuploidies respectively. One in six fetuses with ARSA has an associated cardiac anomaly [1]. When present along with additional soft markers or structural malformations, ARSA is associated with a significant risk of aneuploidy and pathogenic or likely pathogenic copy number variations (CNVs) [2].

While ARSA has the potential to play a role in refining the risk of aneuploidy, robust data in low-risk populations is presently lacking. Many fetal medicine units include ARSA as a part of fetal echocardiography.

6.2.1 Diagnosis and Management

- Identification of ARSA is not considered a part of a routine screening ultrasound, and presently, its use as a soft marker should be limited to units specialized in fetal medicine or in research.
- The normal RSA is imaged in the horizontal view of the upper thorax. Normally, it arises from the aortic arch and courses horizontally in front of the trachea to reach the right arm, with the right subclavian vein next to it (Fig. 6.1). ARSA arises inferiorly and posteriorly and crosses the thorax posterior to the trachea. The vein retains its normal horizontal anterior position and appears separated from the ARSA, forming an angle (Fig. 6.2).

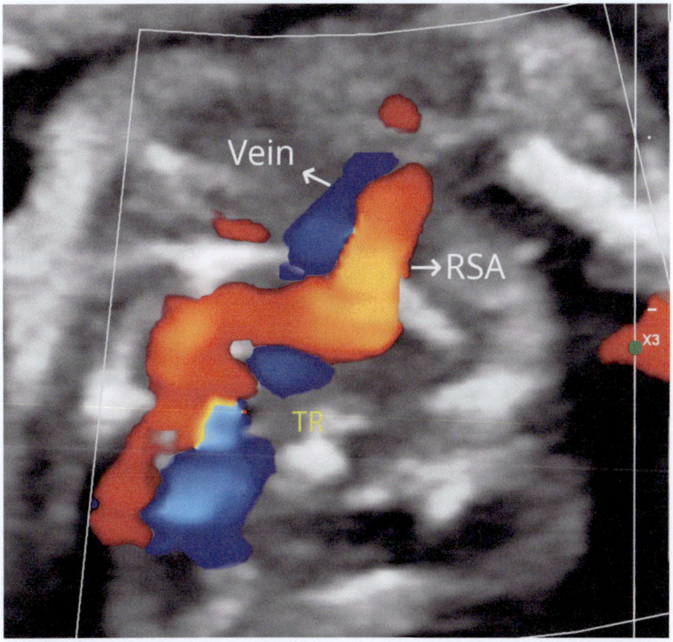

Fig. 6.1 Axial section of the thorax showing normal course of the RSA. Note that the artery accompanies the vein and lies anterior to the trachea (*TR*)

- If an isolated ARSA is detected during fetal echocardiography, the women should be given an option of either NIPT or amniocentesis with karyotyping. When additional findings are present, karyotyping and testing for 22q11.2 microdeletion are recommended. Chromosomal microarray (CMA) may also be considered in these cases [2, 3].

6.2.2 Outcome and Postnatal Follow-Up

Isolated ARSA is considered as a normal variant. No specific follow-up is required. Very rare instances of neonatal respiratory distress or dysphagia have been reported [2].

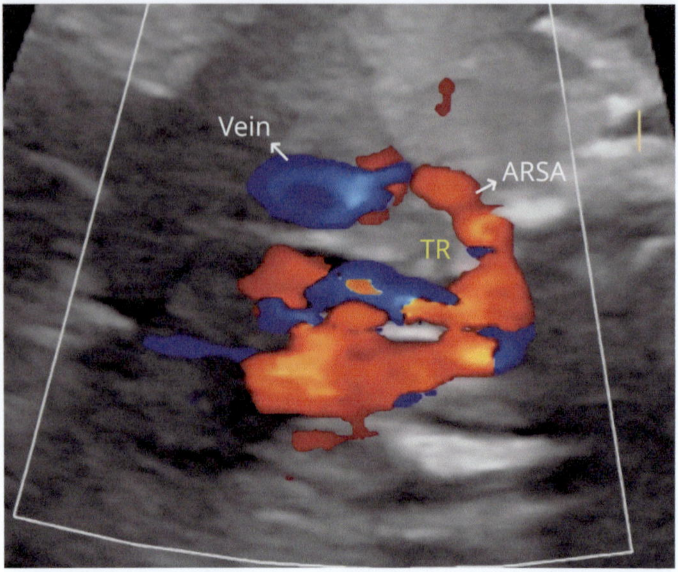

Fig. 6.2 Slightly inferior section showing the course of ARSA. Note the separation between the artery and the right subclavian vein and the relative position of the trachea (*TR*)

6.3 Absent or Hypoplastic Nasal Bone

Absent or hypoplastic nasal bone (NB) is considered an important soft marker for Down syndrome. Rarely, it may be associated with other genetic abnormalities like trisomy 18, trisomy 13, sex chromosomal abnormalities, and other aneuploidies. Approximately 60% of fetuses with Down syndrome have an absent or hypoplastic NB compared to 0.8% of normal fetuses [4].

Ultrasound evaluation of NB in the first trimester has been described in Chap. 2.

6.3.1 Diagnosis and Management (Second Trimester)

- Nasal bone is imaged in the midsagittal section perpendicular to the longitudinal axis of the nose (Fig. 6.3). When NB is not visualized, it is labeled as an absent NB (Fig. 6.4a, b).
- Hypoplastic NB is defined either as a ratio against the BPD (BPD-to-NB ratio >10), by length (<2.5 mm), by gestational age-based percentiles (<2.5th percentile), or by multiples of the median (≤0.7 MoM) [4].
- Nasal bone length varies among different populations, and population-specific charts should be used whenever possible. Hypoplastic NB correlates less well with the risk of aneuploidy compared to absent NB, and therefore must be interpreted with caution.

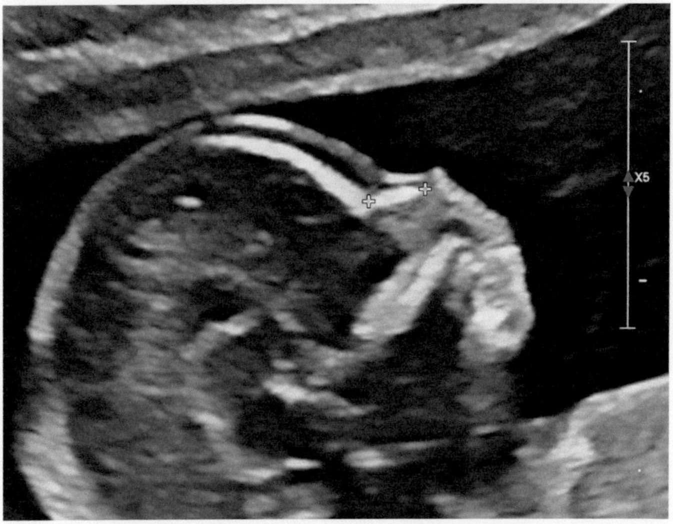

Fig. 6.3 Midsagittal section of the fetal face at a gestational age of 18 weeks demonstrating a normal NB (*calipers*)

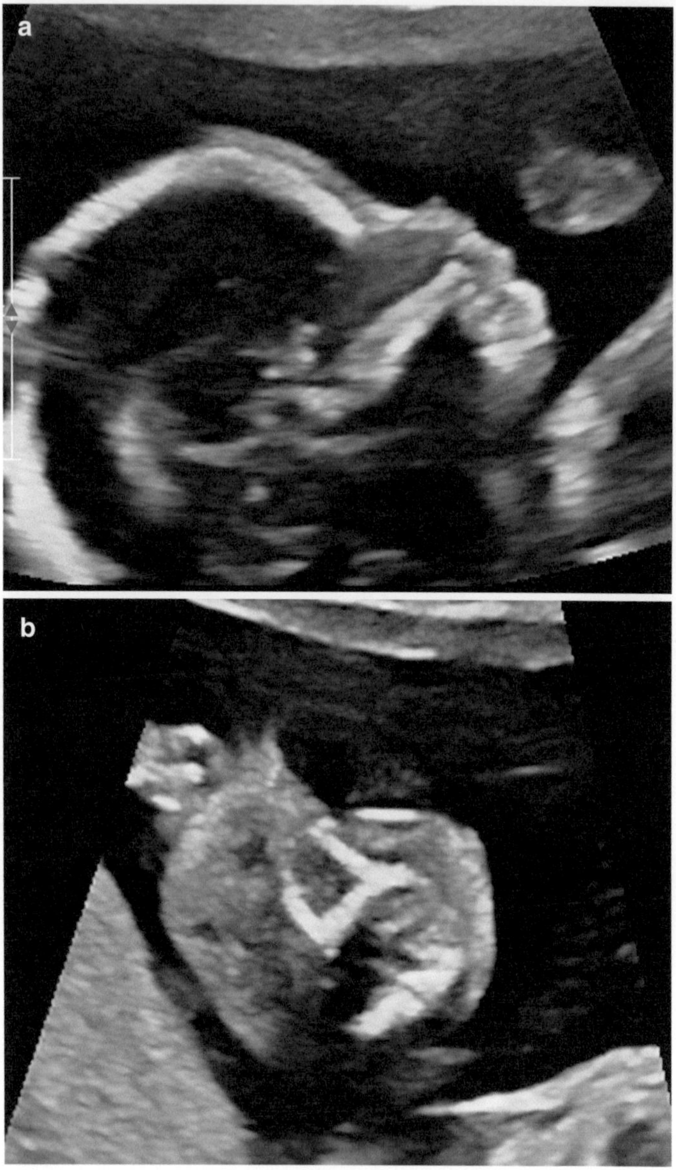

Fig. 6.4 (**a**) Midsagittal section of the fetal face at a gestational age of 19 weeks demonstrating an absent NB (compare with Fig. 6.3). (**b**) Coronal section of the face in the same fetus demonstrating an incomplete retronasal triangle

- If an absent or hypoplastic NB is detected, a comprehensive ultrasound scan is mandatory to look for structural anomalies and other soft markers.
- If this is an isolated finding, genetic counseling should be done and the woman should be offered either amniocentesis or NIPT. NIPT has a high sensitivity for the common trisomies associated with an absent NB, but it is still a screening test.
- In the presence of a negative cfDNA screening result or a normal fetal karyotype, no further evaluation is necessary [5]. *Absent or hypoplastic NB in euploid fetuses is a normal variation which does not produce any cosmetic defect.*

6.3.2 Outcome and Postnatal Follow-Up

Isolated absent or hypoplastic NB is considered a normal variant and requires no follow-up. The parents should be counseled that it does not cause any cosmetic defect in the baby.

6.4 Choroid Plexus Cysts

Choroid plexus cysts (CPCs) are cystic areas >2 mm in diameter in the choroid plexus of the lateral ventricles seen between 14 and 24 weeks of gestation. Choroid plexus cysts are present in 1% of all fetuses and are usually identified during the anomaly scan. CPCs are not associated with Down syndrome. While CPCs are associated with trisomy 18, the risk is extremely low in the absence of multiple structural abnormalities [5].

6.4.1 Diagnosis and Management

- CPCs are visible in the trans-ventricular plane of the fetal brain (Fig. 6.5).
- The number, size, and laterality of CPCs are irrelevant.
- Identification of CPCs should prompt referral to a fetal medicine unit for comprehensive evaluation of the fetus.

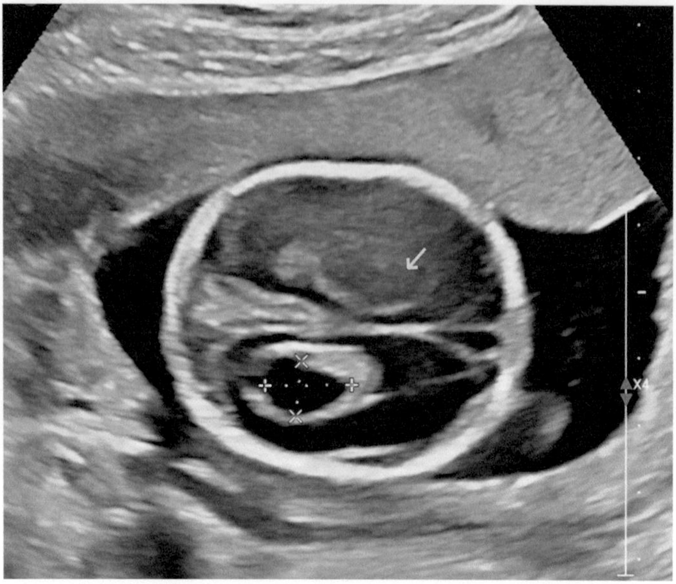

Fig. 6.5 Axial section of the fetal head at 19 weeks of gestation showing bilateral CPCs. Note that the cyst in the near-field choroid plexus is difficult to visualize (*arrow*) due to acoustic shadowing by the overlying bone

- If CPCs are an isolated finding, maternal serum screening or NIPT should be offered. If the screening result is negative, amniocentesis is not required [5].
- In the presence of associated anomalies or soft markers, genetic counseling and amniocentesis with karyotyping should be offered.
- Very large persisting CPCs warrant a follow-up neurosonography to differentiate them from ganglionic eminence cavitations and to assess the possible association with cortical malformations [6].

6.4.2 Outcome and Postnatal Follow Up

Isolated CPCs have no effect on neurological outcome and are considered as a benign finding. The pregnant woman should be reassured. No specific follow-up is required and nearly all disappear by the third trimester.

6.5 Echogenic Bowel

Echogenic bowel is a nonspecific finding in which portions of the small bowel are seen to have a signal brightness equal to or greater than that of fetal bone (Fig. 6.6). The adjacent fetal iliac bone is used for comparison. Fetal bowel can be graded according to the degree of echogenicity into three grades [7].

- Grade 1: Echogenicity increased, but less than bone.
- Grade 2: Echogenicity equal to bone.
- Grade 3: Echogenicity greater than bone.

Grade 1 echogenicity is a highly subjective finding, and likely to be benign. Fetal bowel is labeled as echogenic bowel if it is at least as bright as bone. *Note that the grade of echogenicity should not be reported.*

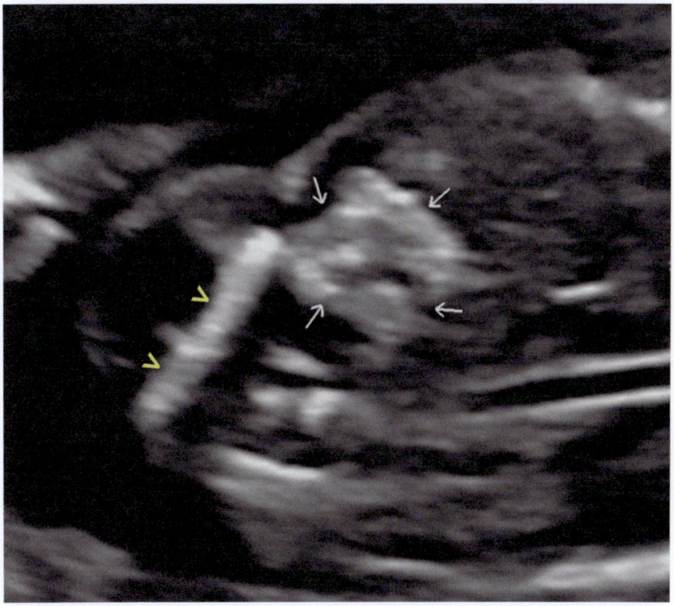

Fig. 6.6 Echogenic bowel (*arrows*) in a fetus with trisomy 21. Note that the echogenicity is equal to that of the adjacent iliac bone (*arrowheads*). Also note that the image gain has been reduced

6.5.1 Etiology and Pathophysiology

Echogenic bowel can be seen in various conditions enumerated below [5, 8]:

1. Aneuploidy (the commonest being trisomy 21).
2. TORCH and parvovirus infections.
3. IUGR.
4. Bowel abnormalities.
5. Cystic fibrosis.
6. Intra-amniotic hemorrhage.
7. Physiological finding (0.5% of fetuses).

The possible mechanisms responsible for the echogenic appearance include:

- Reduced fluid content (Down syndrome).
- Hypoperistalsis (cystic fibrosis).
- Gut ischemia (IUGR).
- Direct damage, perforation, or minimal ascites (infections).
- Swallowed blood (intra-amniotic bleeding).

6.5.2 Recommended Ultrasound Settings

- Route: transabdominal.
- Transducer frequency: low.
- Harmonic imaging: off.
- Compound imaging: off.
- Gain: reduced, just enough to identify fetal bowel and iliac bone (Fig. 6.6).

6.5.3 Diagnosis and Management

- If the small bowel appears at least as bright as bone after using the above settings, the bowel is labeled as echogenic.
- Following the diagnosis of echogenic bowel, a detailed evaluation in a fetal medicine unit is recommended to look for coexisting abnormalities.

- Aneuploidy testing by amniocentesis should be offered even in isolated cases. Cell-free DNA screening (NIPT) may be offered to patients not willing for invasive testing, but its limitations should be explained.
- Maternal TORCH testing should be done. If maternal testing reveals presence of IgM antibodies or IgG antibodies with low avidity, amniotic fluid PCR for fetal TORCH should be considered.
- In populations where cystic fibrosis is prevalent, testing both parents for cystic fibrosis transmembrane conductance regulator (CFTR) gene mutations is indicated. If either parent tests positive, fetal testing should be performed.
- Monitoring for fetal growth restriction and placental dysfunction should be initiated with uterine artery Doppler and serial scans for interval growth, placental appearance, and liquor.
- Follow-up scans in the third trimester should be performed to look for evolving bowel malformations.
- High-frequency transducers can produce false-positive results due to enhanced delineation of the bowel wall and its contents.
- Echogenic bowel should not be reported in the first trimester.

6.5.4 Outcome and Postnatal Follow-Up

Following a second-trimester diagnosis of echogenic bowel, 60% of fetuses are normal at birth, with the rest having either growth restriction or one of the other abnormalities mentioned above [8]. Second-trimester ultrasound findings of early growth restriction, oligohydramnios, thick placenta, and abnormal uterine artery Doppler are associated with a poor outcome, including late second-trimester fetal demise. In the absence of fetal aneuploidy or infection, bowel problems in the neonatal period are unlikely if the bowel appears normal on a late third-trimester ultrasound scan.

6.6 Echogenic Intracardiac Focus

An echogenic intracardiac focus (EIF) is defined as an echogenic spot measuring <6 mm in one or both ventricles, appearing at least as bright as fetal bone, and seen in at least 2 planes (Fig. 6.7).

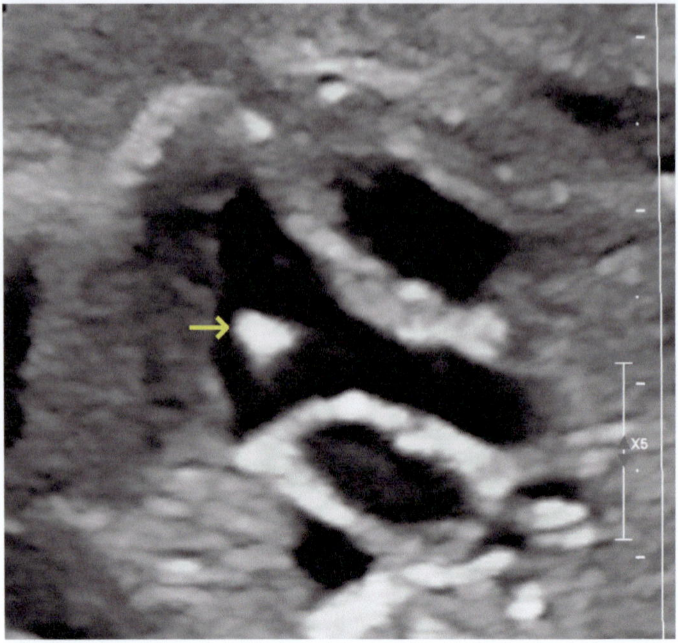

Fig. 6.7 Left ventricular outflow tract view of the heart showing an EIF in the left ventricle (*arrow*)

An EIF is thought to reflect a mineral deposit on one of the papillary muscles, with no effect on cardiac function. It is observed in 3–4% of normal fetuses, with left ventricle being the commonest site. Though EIF is considered a soft marker for Down syndrome, it has very low sensitivity, specificity, and LR [9]. *Up to 30% of Asian fetuses can have an EIF as a normal finding* [10].

6.6.1 Diagnosis and Management

- In isolated EIF, aneuploidy screening should be performed. Amniocentesis is not required in women who are screened negative for Down syndrome [5].
- Isolated EIF does not warrant referral for a fetal echocardiography. An extended basic cardiac examination is sufficient.

- When EIF is associated with other abnormal findings, detailed evaluation in a fetal medicine unit followed by genetic counseling is recommended. Decision for amniocentesis should be guided by the co-existing findings.

6.6.2 Outcome and Postnatal Follow Up

An isolated EIF has no effect on the baby. The patient should be reassured and advised routine obstetric follow-up. Repeat cardiac evaluation in the third trimester or after birth is unnecessary.

6.7 Mild Pyelectasis

Mild pyelectasis is defined as renal pelvis measurements between 4 and 7 mm (some consider 5 mm as the lower limit) [5]. Fetal renal pelvis diameter varies with the state of maternal hydration and the degree of distension of fetal bladder.

Isolated mild pyelectasis is seen in 1% of normal fetuses versus 2% of fetuses with Down syndrome, giving it a poor sensitivity and specificity. Therefore, in the absence of other risk factors, the possibility of Down syndrome remains small and does not justify invasive testing [11].

6.7.1 Diagnosis and Management

- Renal pelvis is imaged in the transverse view of the fetal abdomen with the spine anterior. The maximum anteroposterior measurement should be taken (see Fig. 6.8).
- Measurements below 4 mm are normal and should not be reported, even if the renal pelvis looks 'prominent'. Renal pelvis measuring >10 mm is not a soft marker for aneuploidy, but may be a sign of lower urinary tract obstruction.

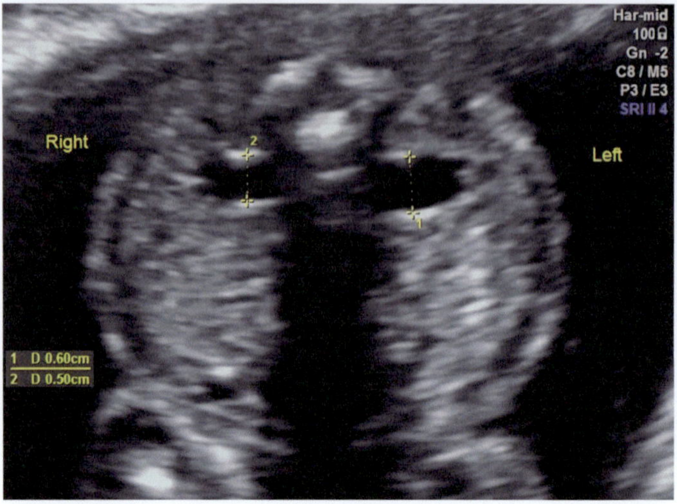

Fig. 6.8 Axial section showing bilateral mild pyelectasis

- Isolated mild fetal pyelectasis in women who are screened negative for Down syndrome does not warrant amniocentesis [5].
- All fetuses with renal pelvis ≥4 mm should be followed up at 32 weeks. If the renal pelvis measures ≥7 mm in the third trimester, postnatal ultrasound follow-up is required.
- Dilatation of renal calyces or ureters significantly increases the likelihood of an obstructive pathology. These fetuses require a post-natal ultrasound, irrespective of renal pelvis diameter.

6.7.2 Outcome and Postnatal Follow-Up

Mild pyelectasis usually corrects by the third trimester. If pyelectasis persists in the third trimester, neonatal renal ultrasound should be performed in the first week of birth. If this is normal, it should be repeated after 6 weeks. Postnatal problems are seen when renal pelvis diameter is >10 mm in the third trimester, the commonest being pelvi-ureteric junction obstruction and vesico-ureteric reflux. Though a few infants may require antibiotic prophylaxis or surgery, the overall prognosis remains good [12].

6.8 Mild Ventriculomegaly

The mean axial diameter of the atrium of the lateral cerebral ventricles ranges between 6.4 and 7.6 mm throughout gestation [13]. Fetal ventriculomegaly (VM) is defined as measurement of lateral ventricles (LV) more than 10 mm. Mild VM is used to indicate an atrial width of 10–15 mm, while borderline ventriculomegaly refers to a subgroup with an atrial width of 10–12 mm.

In addition to CNS malformations and fetal infection, ventriculomegaly may be associated with genetic abnormalities. About 5% of fetuses with isolated mild VM have an abnormal karyotype, most commonly Down syndrome. An additional 10–15% fetuses have abnormalities detected on chromosomal microarray [13, 14].

6.8.1 Diagnosis and Management

- The near-field LV is difficult to measure due to acoustic shadowing by the overlying skull bone. Hence, the far-field LV is usually measured.
- Image should be zoomed such that the fetal skull occupies the whole screen. LV should be measured in the transventricular axial plane.
- The calipers should be positioned on the internal margin of the medial and lateral walls of the atria, at an axis perpendicular to the long axis of the lateral ventricle. Measurement should be taken at the widest part of the lateral ventricle near the posterior portion (glomus) of the choroid plexus. Figure 6.9 demonstrates the correct placement of calipers.
- When mild VM is detected, a detailed fetal evaluation including neurosonography should be performed to rule out other malformations.
- Amniocentesis with chromosomal microarray is recommended in all cases of apparently isolated mild VM, even if maternal serum screening shows low risk of aneuploidy. Amniotic fluid PCR for CMV and toxoplasmosis should also be considered.
- Third-trimester ultrasound and long-term neonatal follow-up are important.

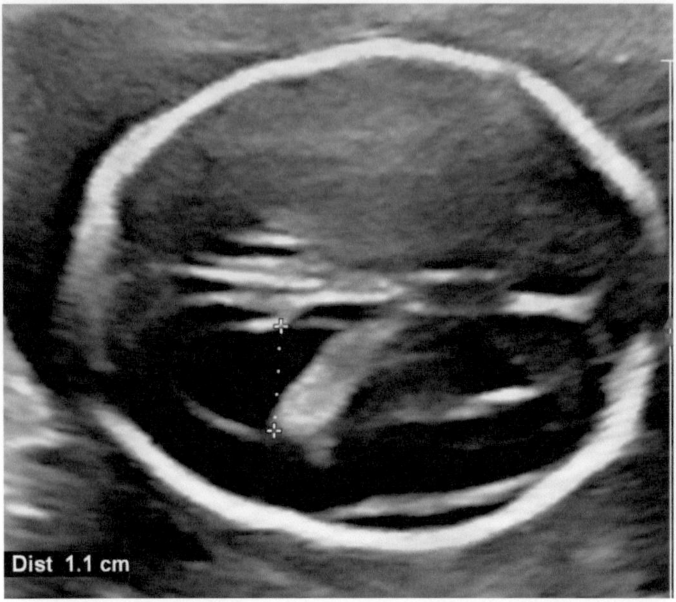

Fig. 6.9 Axial transventricular section showing measurement of LV. Mild ventriculomegaly is noted (11 mm)

6.8.2 Outcome and Postnatal Follow-Up

Progression of ventricular dilatation occurs in 16% of fetuses with isolated mild VM detected in the second trimester. Furthermore, 13% of fetuses will have additional CNS abnormalities which are not picked up at the anomaly scan. Isolated mild VM which does not worsen in the third trimester is associated with a delayed or abnormal neurodevelopment in 11% of children. There is very limited data on the incidence and severity of actual handicap among these children, which adds a degree of uncertainty to prenatal counseling [13, 14].

6.9 Single Umbilical Artery

Single umbilical artery (SUA) is defined as the absence of one of the two arteries in the umbilical cord. Single umbilical artery occurs in 0.5% of all fetuses, with atresia of the left artery being more common. Isolated SUA is not associated with an increased risk of chromosomal abnormalities. In non-isolated cases the incidence of aneuploidy (trisomy 18, 13, and triploidy) increases from 4% when one additional abnormality is present to 50% for fetuses with multiple coexisting abnormalities [15].

6.9.1 Diagnosis and Management

- Umbilical arteries can be imaged by positioning the color flow Doppler box on the fetal bladder (Figs. 6.10 and 6.11). One artery should be seen coursing on either side. They can also be demonstrated on color flow imaging of the umbilical cord.
- First-trimester diagnosis of SUA has a lower accuracy and presents difficulties in ruling out associated anomalies. Counting of umbilical arteries is therefore not considered an essential part of first-trimester obstetric scan.

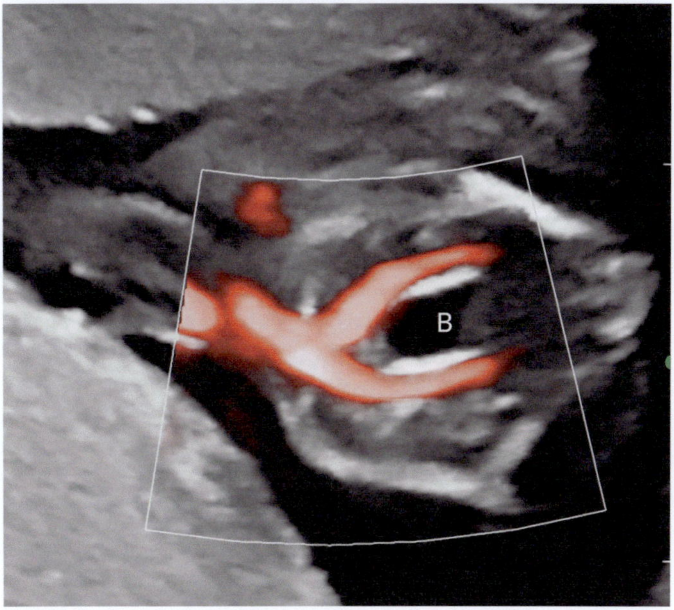

Fig. 6.10 Color Doppler interrogation of fetal bladder (*B*) showing two umbilical arteries (one on each side)

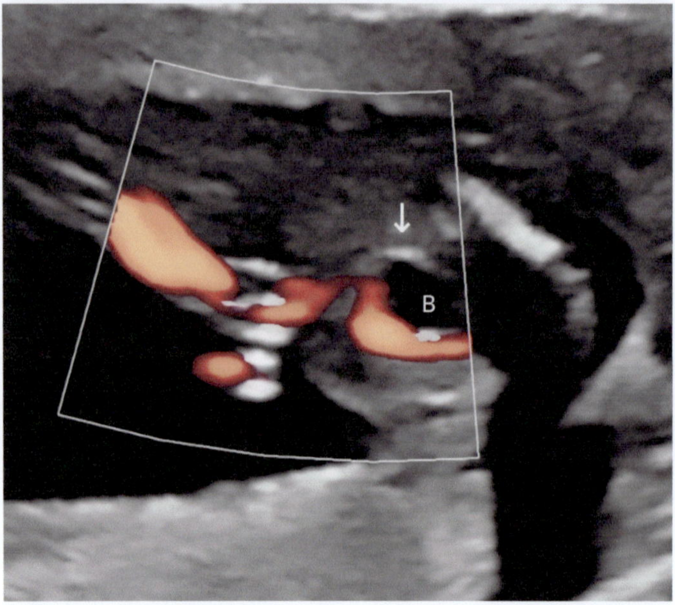

Fig. 6.11 Single umbilical artery. The second artery is missing (*arrow*). *B* bladder

- A diagnosis of SUA should prompt detailed evaluation of the fetus including kidneys, aorta, and heart (extended basic cardiac examination). Fetal echocardiography is not routinely warranted [5].
- Invasive testing is not indicated in isolated SUA [5].
- All fetuses with SUA should be evaluated in the third trimester for interval growth and any evolving anomalies. Weekly surveillance after 36 weeks is strongly recommended.

6.9.2 Outcome and Postnatal Follow-Up

There is controversy on whether isolated SUA is associated with IUGR, preterm labor, and adverse perinatal outcomes [16–18]. In the author's personal experience, isolated SUA has an excellent prognosis. If the third-trimester scan is normal, a postnatal clinical examination of the neonate is sufficient.

6.10 Short Femur and Short Humerus

Short femur length (FL) and short humeral length (HL) are both independent markers for Down syndrome, particularly short HL. For use in aneuploidy screening, a shortened femur or humerus is diagnosed when the ratio of observed to expected length is <0.9 [19]. Short FL and HL are *not* considered as soft markers when they occur as a part of growth restriction or skeletal dysplasia. Constitutional shortening also needs to be ruled out with respect to race, ethnicity, and parental short stature. Short humerus, particularly when isolated, is unlikely to be detected, as it is not part of screening ultrasound.

6.10.1 Diagnosis and Management

- Measurement of FL or HL should be performed with the bone perpendicular to the ultrasound beam. The epiphysial cartilage should be visible, but not included in the measurement.
- If short femur or humerus is noted, the fetus should be assessed for other features of skeletal dysplasia, including assessment of other long bones for length, fractures, bending, and abnormal mineralization. The skull, thorax, and spine should be evaluated. The height of both parents should be noted.
- Aneuploidy screening, preferably NIPT, should be offered [5].
- Decision for invasive testing will depend on other findings on ultrasound and the outcome of counseling.
- A third-trimester interval growth scan is recommended.

6.10.2 Outcome and Postnatal Follow-Up

Outcome depends on associated conditions like skeletal abnormalities, growth restriction, and aneuploidy. Isolated mild shortening has a good prognosis.

6.11 Thickened Nuchal Fold

Nuchal fold refers to the fetal skin on the posterior part of the fetal neck. The term used for its measurement in the second trimester is 'nuchal fold thickness' rather than 'nuchal translucency.'

Nuchal fold thickness is considered normal when it is <5 mm between 14 and 17 + 6 weeks and <6 mm between 18 and 24 weeks. Thickened nuchal fold (TNF) is a very significant second-trimester soft marker. The risk of chromosomal defects when a TNF is associated with structural malformations (35.5%) is much greater than that of an isolated TNF (3.7%). Besides Down syndrome, TNF is associated with other aneuploidies, pathogenic CNVs, single gene defects like Noonan syndrome, and structural malformations [20, 21].

6.11.1 Diagnosis and Management

- Nuchal fold thickness is measured in the trans-cerebellar plane. A transverse plane of the fetal head is obtained with the cavum septum pellucidum, thalami, and cerebellum. Calipers should be placed on the *outer* edge of the occipital bone and the *outer* edge of the skin in the midline (Fig. 6.12).
- Pregnant women with TNF should undergo a genetic sonogram along with measurement of long bones and fetal echocardiography.
- If TNF is an isolated finding, NIPT or amniocentesis should be offered [5].
- Amniocentesis with karyotyping should be offered in all cases of non-isolated TNF. Chromosomal microarray (CMA) should be considered if karyotype is normal.
- Close surveillance throughout the third trimester is recommended.

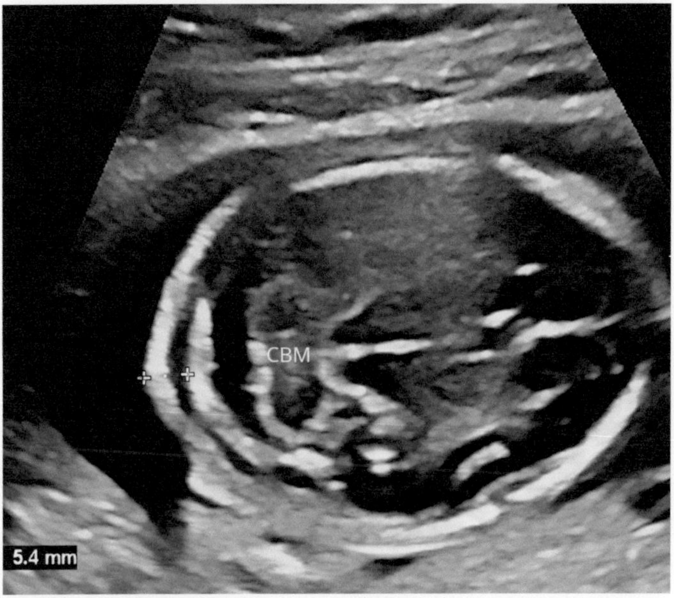

Fig. 6.12 Correct technique for measuring nuchal fold thickness (5.4 mm in this case). *CBM*—cerebellum

6.11.2 Outcome and Postnatal Follow-Up

Prognosis of a fetus with TNF depends on the associated genetic and structural abnormalities. Adverse pregnancy outcomes are increased when the TNF >10 mm. A good outcome is expected in fetuses with isolated TNF <10 mm. Isolated cases should be followed up for at least a year after birth [20].

6.12 Multiple Soft Markers

When one soft marker is detected, the fetus should be systematically evaluated to look for additional markers. Presence of multiple soft markers has a synergistic effect on the risk of aneuploidies and pathogenic CNVs [22]. This holds true even in the absence of major structural malformations. Konin and coworkers, in a study of 14,119 structurally normal fetuses, reported the risk of aneuploidy to be 0.58%, 1.84%, and 15% when the number of soft markers was 1, 2, and ≥ 3, respectively [23].

6.12.1 Diagnosis and Management

- Most of the soft markers discussed previously are associated with trisomy 21 except for CPC and SUA. These two markers, when non-isolated, are associated with trisomy 18 and other aneuploidies.
- When either a CPC or SUA is present along with a trisomy 21-related soft marker (e.g., mild pyelectasis), they should be reported as 2 isolated markers, rather than as multiple markers.
- In the presence of multiple markers, if at least one marker is strongly associated with aneuploidy (e.g., TNF or ARSA), amniocentesis should be offered.
- If none among the multiple markers are significantly associated with aneuploidy, NIPT versus invasive testing should be discussed. Women who already have a negative NIPT result require no further evaluation.
- Absence of markers should not be used to reduce the risk calculated from maternal serum screening.

6.12.2 Outcome and Postnatal Follow-Up

Once genetic abnormalities are ruled out, the outcome and follow-up depends on the specific markers present.

6.13 Key Message

1. No pregnancy should be terminated solely because of the presence of fetal soft markers.

References

1. Borenstein M, Minekawa R, Zidere V, Nicolaides KH, Allan LD. Aberrant right subclavian artery at 16 to 23 + 6 weeks of gestation: a marker for chromosomal abnormality. Ultrasound Obstet Gynecol. 2010;36(5):548–52.
2. Xue H, Zhang L, Yu A, Lin M, Guo Q, Xu L, Huang H. Prenatal genetic analysis of fetal aberrant right subclavian artery with or without additional ultrasound anomalies in a third level referral center. Sci Rep. 2023;13(1):3414.
3. Scala C, Leone Roberti Maggiore U, Candiani M, Venturini PL, Ferrero S, Greco T, Cavoretto P. Aberrant right subclavian artery in fetuses with Down syndrome: a systematic review and meta-analysis. Ultrasound Obstet Gynecol. 2015;46(3):266–76.
4. Cusick W, Shevell T, Duchan LS, Lupinacci CA, Terranova J, Crombleholme WR. Likelihood ratios for fetal trisomy 21 based on nasal bone length in the second trimester: how best to define hypoplasia? Ultrasound Obstet Gynecol. 2007;30(3):271–4.
5. Prabhu M, Kuller JA, Biggio JR. Society for Maternal-Fetal Medicine Consult Series #57: evaluation and management of isolated soft ultrasound markers for aneuploidy in the second trimester. Am J Obstet Gynecol. 2021;225(4):B2–B15.
6. Paladini D, Donarini G, Bottelli L, Rossi A, Coltri A, Fulcheri E. Isolated, persisting, large choroid plexus cysts should warrant neurosonographic follow-up. Ultrasound Obstet Gynecol. 2021;57(6):1006–8.
7. Slotnick RN, Abuhamad AZ. Prognostic implications of fetal echogenic bowel. Lancet. 1996;347(8994):85–7.
8. De Oronzo MA. Hyperechogenic fetal bowel: an ultrasonographic marker for adverse fetal and neonatal outcome? J Prenat Med. 2011;5(1):9–13.
9. Rodriguez R, Herrero B, Bartha JL. The continuing enigma of the fetal echogenic intracardiac focus in prenatal ultrasound. Curr Opin Obstet Gynecol. 2013;25(2):145–51.
10. Shipp TD, Bromley B, Lieberman E, Benacerraf BR. The frequency of the detection of fetal echogenic intracardiac foci with respect to maternal race. Ultrasound Obstet Gynecol. 2000;15(6):460–2.
11. Orzechowski KM, Berghella V. Isolated fetal pyelectasis and the risk of Down syndrome: a meta-analysis. Ultrasound Obstet Gynecol. 2013;42(6):615–21.
12. Ahmad G, Green P. Outcome of fetal pyelectasis diagnosed antenatally. J Obstet Gynaecol. 2005;25(2):119–22.
13. Melchiorre K, Bhide A, Gika AD, Pilu G, Papageorghiou AT. Counseling in isolated mild fetal ventriculomegaly. Ultrasound Obstet Gynecol. 2009;34(2):212–24.

14. Alluhaybi AA, Altuhaini K, Ahmad M. Fetal ventriculomegaly: a review of literature. Cureus. 2022;14(2):e22352.
15. Dagklis T, Defigueiredo D, Staboulidou I, Casagrandi D, Nicolaides KH. Isolated single umbilical artery and fetal karyotype. Ultrasound Obstet Gynecol. 2010;36(3):291–5.
16. Kim HJ, Kim JH, Chay DB, Park JH, Kim MA. Association of isolated single umbilical artery with perinatal outcomes: systemic review and meta-analysis. Obstet Gynecol Sci. 2017;60(3):266–73.
17. Mailath-Pokorny M, Worda K, Schmid M, Polterauer S, Bettelheim D. Isolated single umbilical artery: evaluating the risk of adverse pregnancy outcome. Eur J Obstet Gynecol Reprod Biol. 2015;184:80–3.
18. Caldas LM, Liao A, Carvalho MH, Francisco RP, Zugaib M. Should fetal growth be a matter of concern in isolated single umbilical artery? Rev Assoc Med Bras (1992). 2014;60(2):125–30.
19. Nyberg DA, Resta RG, Luthy DA, Hickok DE, Williams MA. Humerus and femur length shortening in the detection of Down's syndrome. Am J Obstet Gynecol. 1993;168(2):534–8.
20. Li L, Fu F, Li R, Liu Z, Liao C. Prenatal diagnosis and pregnancy outcome analysis of thickened nuchal fold in the second trimester. Medicine (Baltimore). 2018;97(46):e13334.
21. Malniece I, Grasmane A, Inashkina I, Stavusis J, Kreile M, Miklasevics E, Gailite L. The fetal phenotype of Noonan syndrome caused by severe, cancer-related PTPN11 variants. Am J Case Rep. 2020;21:e922468.
22. Hu T, Tian T, Zhang Z, Wang J, Hu R, Xiao L, Zhu H, Lai Y, Wang H, Liu S. Prenatal chromosomal microarray analysis in 2466 fetuses with ultrasonographic soft markers: a prospective cohort study. Am J Obstet Gynecol. 2021;224(5):516.e1–16.
23. Konin A, Poojary D, Hosmani A, Radhakrishnan P. VP30.03: prevalence of multiple fetal soft markers on ultrasound at 16 + 0–24 + 6 weeks and their association with fetal aneuploidies. Ultrasound Obstet Gynecol. 2021;58:221.

Invasive Testing for Aneuploidy

7

7.1 Introduction

Invasive testing through chorionic villus sampling (CVS) and amniocentesis forms an integral part of prenatal diagnosis. Maternal serum screening only provides an estimate of the probability that the fetus is affected by aneuploidy. Despite noninvasive prenatal testing (NIPT) being a highly sensitive screening test, false-positive results can occur. Hence, the decision to terminate a pregnancy should never be taken without direct fetal sampling. This chapter primarily focuses on invasive testing in singleton pregnancy. Specific concerns related to twin pregnancies are addressed in Chap. 8.

Amniocentesis for prenatal diagnosis of genetic disorders was first performed in the late 1960s when ultrasound was not routinely available. This procedure was performed after 17 weeks, as it was considered reasonably possible to aspirate amniotic fluid at this gestation. Because of the blind nature of this technique, failure to obtain amniotic fluid was not infrequent and the procedure-related miscarriage rate was approximately 2%. As ultrasound guidance became the norm, the procedure-related fetal loss fell by half [1, 2].

The promise of an earlier diagnosis led to the popularity of CVS. This enthusiasm was dampened by studies reporting increased limb defects when CVS was performed before 10 weeks

© The Author(s), under exclusive license to Springer Nature Singapore Pte Ltd. 2023

A. Kamat, *Down Syndrome Screening*,
https://doi.org/10.1007/978-981-99-7758-1_7

Table 7.1 Indications for invasive testing in the first and second trimester

Indications
Known parental balanced translocation.
Known parental carrier status for a genetic condition.
Previous child with a genetic abnormality.
Maternal serum screening shows a high-risk (screen-positive) result.
NIPT shows a screen-positive or a no-call result.
Raised nuchal translucency.
Structural abnormality in the fetus.
Presence of second-trimester soft markers.
Suspected fetal infection.

of gestation. With improvement in ultrasound resolution, use of finer needles, and increased knowledge of the feto-placental interface, complication rates following both amniocentesis and CVS have drastically reduced. Subsequent studies have also shown that limb defects are not increased when CVS and amniocentesis are performed after 10 weeks and 15 weeks, respectively [3].

There are several indications for performing invasive testing in the first and second trimester (see Table 7.1).

The second part of making a prenatal genetic diagnosis involves laboratory testing. In this chapter, we will discuss only those genetic tests that are used to detect common aneuploidies, viz. karyotyping, fluorescence in situ hybridization (FISH), and quantitative fluorescent polymerase chain reaction (QF-PCR). Finer technical details of genetic testing procedures have been intentionally omitted to avoid overwhelming the clinician for whom this book is written.

7.2 Amniocentesis

Amniocentesis refers to the aspiration of amniotic fluid under ultrasound guidance. Amniocentesis is performed for the diagnosis of genetic conditions, infections, metabolic defects, and for confirming lung maturity. It also has a therapeutic role to relieve maternal discomfort in polyhydramnios and to administer drugs to the fetus, e.g., thyroxine.

7.2.1 Preparation and Counseling

Prior to performing amniocentesis, a thorough counseling session with the pregnant woman and her partner is mandatory. The procedure should be explained in detail regarding the risks associated, the time taken for reporting and management of pregnancy following normal and abnormal reports. Wherever indicated, discussion about NIPT versus invasive testing should be conducted. It is also important to highlight that only specific disorders are being sought. The rare possibility of a failed culture (if karyotyping is being done) must also be mentioned. An informed written consent should then be obtained.

A screening ultrasound examination should be performed prior to the procedure to document fetal cardiac activity and gross malformations. In addition, liquor amount, placental position, cord insertion, and cervical length should be noted. A short cervix can predispose the patient to miscarriage; this is likely to be blamed on the invasive procedure if not picked up earlier.

7.2.2 Materials

- Amniocentesis needle: The needle should not be thicker than 20-gauge to minimize the risk of amniotic fluid leak. While a spinal needle can be used, it is sometimes difficult to reach the amniotic cavity in obese women, particularly between 15 and 16 weeks. It is preferable to use a 12–15 cm 22-gauge needle with an echogenic tip specially designed for amniocentesis.
- Syringes: 2 and 20 mL.
- Sterile test tubes for transport (no medium required).
- Sterile drapes, gauze, probe cover.
- Povidone iodine solution for skin disinfection.

7.2.3 Procedure

- The patient is painted and draped. Depending upon the position of the uterus desired for easier needle access, the bladder may need to be emptied.
- Chemoprophylaxis is not typically recommended, but this decision should be made on a case-by-case basis. Local anesthesia is not required when using a 22-gauge needle.
- Amniocentesis can be performed either by the freehand technique or through a needle guide attached to the ultrasound probe. The freehand technique allows slight corrections in the needle path prior to entering the uterus. Under constant ultrasound visualization, the needle is gently advanced toward a pool of amniotic fluid. The needle path should be away from maternal bowel and bladder, the placenta, and fetal parts, particularly, fetal eyes.
- The intended path of the needle must be planned carefully (Fig. 7.1), as multiple entries increase the risk of amniotic fluid

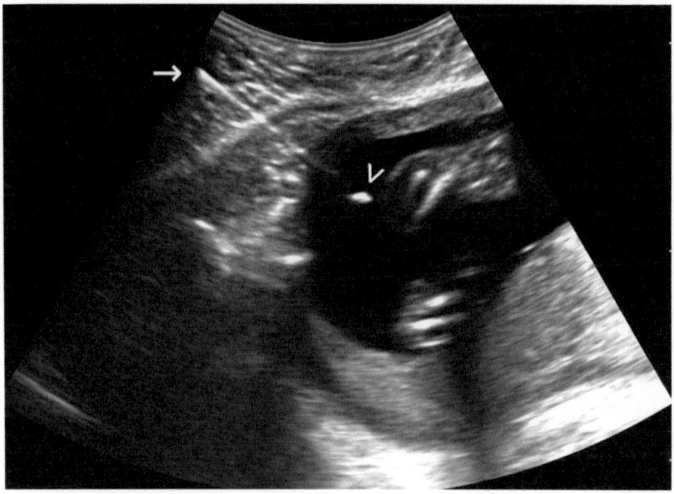

Fig. 7.1 Amniocentesis needle path under transabdominal USG guidance. The needle has been inserted 0.5 cm away from the TAS probe, and advanced in the imaging plane of the transducer at an angle of approximately 45°. Note the point in the image where the needle appears (*arrow*). Also note that the needle tip lies roughly in the center of the image (*arrowhead*)

leak and miscarriage. The final entry into the amniotic cavity is performed with a quick thrust to avoid tenting of the amnion. Once entry is confirmed, the needle tip should not be moved from side to side, as this can cause tearing of the amniotic membrane.

- In case of no other option, a transplacental entry may be performed in Rh-positive women. In such cases, the entry should be distant from the cord insertion to avoid serious injury to the cord vessels. A transplacental entry significantly increases the possibility of a bloody tap.
- The needle stylet is removed, the 2-cc syringe is attached and 2 mL of amniotic fluid is aspirated and discarded. A 20-cc syringe is then used to aspirate 15–20 cc of amniotic fluid, which is immediately transferred to labeled sterile tubes. The needle is gently withdrawn after disconnecting the syringe from it.
- In Rh-negative women, 300 μg anti-D immunoglobulin should be administered following the procedure.

7.2.4 Complications

Amniocentesis is a relatively safe procedure, and complications are rare in experienced hands. Evidence suggests that operators performing at least 50 procedures annually have lower complication rates.

Miscarriage Miscarriage rates range from 0.1 to 1%, with earlier studies reporting higher numbers. Better outcomes in recent years are likely due to better ultrasound resolution and training. It is to be noted that this miscarriage rate is over and above the background risk of pregnancy loss. Presently, the procedure-related risk of miscarriage in experienced hands appears to be 0.3% (95% CI, 0.11 to 0.49%). When corrected for pre-procedure aneuploidy risk, it is reduced to 0.12% (95% CI, −0.05 to 0.30%) [4].

Amniotic Fluid Leak This can occur in 1–2% of cases. In most patients, spontaneous sealing of membranes occurs and pregnancy continues uneventfully. This contrasts with the outcomes seen after spontaneous preterm rupture of membranes, wherein a preexisting utero-cervical pathology or intra-amniotic infection is the cause of the amniotic leak.

Fetal Injuries Various fetal injuries have been reported in the literature, including trauma to the fetal brain, eyes, and skin [5–7]. Overall, these are extremely rare, and can be prevented by continuous visualization of the needle tip throughout the procedure.

Maternal Injuries and Risk of Infection Again, these are only reported anecdotally in the literature. Rare cases of maternal death have been reported following septic shock after amniocentesis, which highlights the importance of sterility, despite it being a percutaneous procedure [8].

7.2.5 Early Amniocentesis

Amniocentesis between 10 and 14 weeks called 'early amniocentesis' emerged in the late 1990s as an option to CVS. This procedure has been abandoned because of a 15% risk of amniotic fluid leak with secondary complications like talipes equinovarus (caused by anhydramnios) and miscarriage [3].

7.3 Chorionic Villus Sampling

Chorionic villus sampling refers to the aspiration of chorionic villi for the purpose of prenatal diagnosis. It is best performed between 10 and 13 weeks of gestation. While late CVS (also called placental biopsy) is possible, obtaining an adequate sample is difficult and requires more skill as the placenta becomes more organized.

7.3.1 Pros and Cons of CVS Compared to Amniocentesis

CVS provides a definitive diagnosis at an earlier gestation. This gives the couple additional time for decision-making in case of abnormal results. Termination of an abnormal pregnancy is also safer and easier, especially in case of patients with previous cesarean section. Early diagnosis may help in timely fetal treatment, e.g., prevention of female pseudohermaphroditism in fetal 21-hydroxylase deficiency. CVS also provides a better sample when isolation and sequencing of DNA is needed.

CVS is a technically difficult procedure compared to amniocentesis, with a steeper learning curve. The fetal loss rate is operator-specific depending upon the number of procedures performed annually. While improved imaging and refinement of technique has brought the fetal loss rate very close to that of amniocentesis, it still remains slightly higher. Diagnostic error may also arise due to confined placental mosaicism, and cross-contamination can occur when sampling twin pregnancies.

7.3.2 Preparation and Counseling

A detailed first-trimester ultrasound and parental counseling are mandatory before the procedure. Placental position should be checked both with a full bladder and an empty bladder to plan the needle path. The aim is to align the placenta vertically to make sampling easier.

7.3.3 Materials

- CVS needle: A 15–20 cm long 18–20 G needle with an echogenic tip is used for transabdominal CVS. Transcervical CVS requires a special CVS catheter.
- Syringes: 20 mL syringe with lock.
- Sterile test tubes with transport medium.
- Sterile petri dish for washing the aspirated villi.

- Local anesthetic: Lignocaine 5 mL diluted to 1%.
- Sterile drapes, gauze, probe cover.
- Povidone iodine solution for skin disinfection.

7.3.4 Transabdominal CVS

- Chemoprophylaxis may be administered as per institutional policy (we administer a single dose of third-generation cephalosporin). Depending upon the position of the uterus desired for easier needle access, the bladder may need to be emptied.
- In Rh-negative women, 300 μg anti-D immunoglobulin should be administered.
- The patient is placed in a supine position, painted, and draped. Ultrasound scanning is done to confirm cardiac activity and the position of placenta.
- The needle entry point should be planned such that the needle can be inserted parallel to the long axis of the placenta. This allows for the needle movement over a larger distance through the substance of the placenta, thus ensuring an adequate sample (Fig. 7.2).
- An 18 or 20 G needle is inserted under constant ultrasound visualization into the placenta, and the stylet is withdrawn. A 20 mL syringe with a 3 cc of transport medium is attached to the needle and locked. A constant suction is applied and the needle is moved through the substance of the placenta for about ten times. Slight change in the direction of the needle allows the operator to widen the area sampled.
- The needle is completely withdrawn from the placenta, uterus, and the maternal abdominal wall, without letting go of the suction.
- Following the procedure, the villi are washed in the same medium in a Petri dish, and then transferred to labeled sterile tubes containing fresh medium for transport to the laboratory.

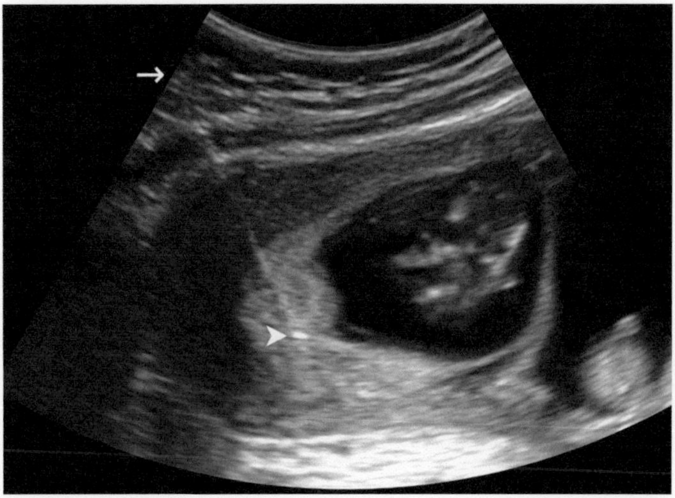

Fig. 7.2 Transabdominal CVS needle path for a posterior placenta. The needle has been inserted 0.5 cm away from the transducer, and advanced in the imaging plane at an angle of approximately 60°. Note the point in the image where the needle appears (*arrow*) and the echogenic needle tip in the placental substance (*solid arrowhead*)

7.3.5 Transcervical CVS

- The patient is placed in a lithotomy position, painted, and draped. Chemoprophylaxis and anti-D may be given if needed. The vagina is cleaned with povidone iodine solution and a speculum is inserted. Continuous transabdominal ultrasound scanning is performed by a second ultrasound operator.
- The CVS catheter with its stylet is bent slightly to make its shape conform to the intended path. The catheter is introduced through the cervical canal into the placenta, staying away from the amniotic cavity (Fig. 7.3).
- After withdrawing the stylet, a 20-cc syringe with a Luer lock containing the transport medium is connected, and the catheter is rapidly moved back and forth for about 10 times to aspirate the villi. The aspirated sample is then washed and transported, as described above.

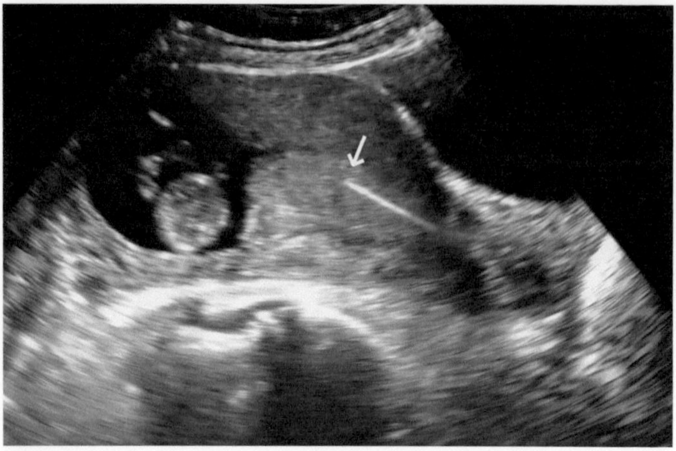

Fig. 7.3 Transcervical CVS. The placenta is in the lower segment. The catheter can be clearly visualized within the placental substance (*arrow*)

7.3.6 Transabdominal Versus Transcervical CVS

The route for performing CVS needs to be decided based on the placental position. A vertically situated placenta in the anterior or posterior uterine wall is ideal for a transabdominal approach. A placenta in the lower segment is easier to sample transcervically. Uterine fibroids, adenomyosis, maternal obesity, or vaginal infection influence the decision, as do operator preference and experience. Finally, in twins with distant placentas, each placenta may need a different approach.

Fetal loss rates remain comparable with both approaches. Transcervical sampling is associated with an increased chance of spotting per vaginum. Regarding procedure-related discomfort, obese women find transabdominal CVS to be more painful, while transcervical CVS is more painful in nulliparous women [9].

7.3.7 Complications

Miscarriage The miscarriage rate following CVS is slightly higher than amniocentesis, though the difference is not significant. In a recent systematic review and meta-analysis, the weighted procedure-related risk of miscarriage following CVS was only 0.20% (95% CI, −0.13 to 0.52%) [4]. Operator experience and the annual number of cases performed affect miscarriage risk. The inverse relationship between operator experience and fetal loss is more for CVS compared to amniocentesis, as CVS is a technically difficult procedure.

Limb Reduction Defects Limb reduction defects have been reported with early CVS (performed before 10 weeks of gestation). Procedures from the tenth week onwards do not show this trend [3].

Maternal Injuries and Risk of Infection These are extremely rare in experienced hands.

7.3.8 Diagnostic Errors in CVS

Chorionic villus sampling assumes that the placenta accurately reflects the fetal genetic constitution, an assumption that may rarely be incorrect. In about 0.1% of cases, the placental cell lines may show mosaicism not present in the fetus, called confined placental mosaicism (CPM). Therefore, unusual chromosomal aneuploidies and polyploidy reported on CVS should be confirmed by amniocentesis.

Chorionic villi consist of two types of cells. The cytotrophoblastic cells are the rapidly dividing cells which can be used for rapid analysis of common aneuploidy within 24–72 h. The mesenchymal core cells require to be cultured before analysis, but provide a better metaphase spread for more accurate results. Unfortunately, mesenchymal core cell culture can be contaminated by the growth of maternal decidual cells. On rare occasions, a discrepancy may be observed in the results obtained from rapid analysis and those obtained from culture. In such cases, amniocentesis should be performed rather than acting on the CVS results.

Despite these concerns, it is emphasized that CVS provides an accurate genetic analysis of the fetus in the first trimester, and CPM is exceedingly rare.

7.4 Karyotyping

A karyotype is a photographic representation of the complete set of chromosomes of an individual visible under a light microscope. Karyogram is a structured reporting of the karyotype, where the chromosomes are arranged in their numerical order (see Figs. 1.4 and 1.5 in Chap. 1). A normal human karyotype indicates that all 23 chromosome pairs are present, and each chromosome has the correct size, shape, banding pattern, and location of the centromere. In addition, there should be no extra chromosomes or satellites.

7.4.1 Methodology

1. *Cell Culture:* The sample is added to culture flasks containing nutrients and growth factors to stimulate cell division and growth. In CVS samples, the villi must be thoroughly washed before culture to remove all traces of blood. Typically, the cells are cultured for 8–12 days to allow them to multiply sufficiently for analysis.
2. *Halting cell division:* After the fetal cells have sufficiently multiplied, colchicine is added to halt cell division at metaphase or prometaphase when the DNA is most condensed and the chromosomes are most conspicuous.
3. *Isolation of cells:* This is accomplished by centrifuging the cultured sample to separate the cells from the fluid.
4. *Harvesting of chromosomes:* The isolated cells are treated with a hypotonic solution to cause the cells to swell. This facilitates the spreading of chromosomes.
5. *Chromosome staining:* Chromosomes are made visible and highlighted through staining. All chromosomal proteins must be digested and eliminated for the stain to bind properly, which is achieved by using an enzyme like trypsin.
6. Although a variety of dyes can be employed for staining, Giemsa stain is the most frequently used. Giemsa staining produces light and dark bands called 'G-bands.' The light bands

correspond to euchromatin, the loosely coiled, transcriptionally active portion of DNA rich in guanine-cytosine (GC) pairs. The dark bands represent heterochromatin, the densely packed, less active form of DNA rich in adenine-thymine (AT) pairs. Approximately 90% of all chromatin is euchromatin.

7. *Chromosome Analysis*: The chromosomes are examined under a microscope. The unique patterns produced by G-banding enable identification of specific chromosomes, which are then compared to a reference karyotype to look for any numerical or structural aberrations. Several automated systems are available for this purpose.

7.4.2 Pros

Karyotyping can identify aneuploidy with 100% sensitivity and specificity (except for the rare possibility of confined placental mosaicism in CVS samples). Translocation Down syndrome can be distinguished from free trisomy 21, which helps in counseling for the next pregnancy. Partial chromosomal gains or losses are detected, provided they are of sufficient size to be visible under a microscope.

7.4.3 Cons

Karyotyping is a labor-intensive technique which takes a reporting time of 2 weeks because of the time taken for culture. The accuracy of a karyotype report depends on the skill of the reporting geneticist. Other problems seen are slow growth, bacterial contamination, and culture failure, leading to a delay in result or no result.

Karyotyping cannot detect submicroscopic duplications or deletions. Therefore, if the fetus has an anomaly known to be associated with a microdeletion, a chromosomal microarray (CMA) is preferred.

Karyotyping may also detect benign findings like pericentric inversion of chromosome 9. This normal variant can cause considerable anxiety when detected in prenatal samples.

7.5 Fluorescence In Situ Hybridization (FISH)

Fluorescence in situ hybridization (FISH) is a technique used to detect specific DNA sequences within a cell by using DNA probes labeled with a fluorescent dye. Aneuploidy can be detected by using chromosome-specific DNA probes which light up under the fluorescence microscope, showing the number of copies of that chromosome. As FISH can be performed on interphase chromosomes, culture is not required, and results are available within 1–2 days. This technique can also detect structural chromosomal abnormalities and microdeletion syndromes.

7.5.1 Methodology

1. The amniotic fluid sample is centrifuged to get the cell pellet. In the case of a CVS sample, the chorionic villi are thoroughly washed to remove blood. The cells are fixed on a slide.
2. DNA probes labeled with fluorescent dyes are added to the slide and the slides are kept for overnight hybridization. For rapid aneuploidy detection, unique fluorescent colors are used for chromosomes 13, 18, 21, X, and Y.
3. After hybridization, the slide is washed to remove any unbound probes.
4. A fluorescence microscope is then used to examine the slide for the fluorescent signals. The number of signals of a particular color observed corresponds to the number of copies of that specific chromosome. For example, in trisomy 21, 3 fluorescent signals will be detected instead of 2, indicating that 3 copies of chromosome 21 are present in the cell (Fig. 7.4).
5. Several cells are examined to look for the possibility of mosaicism.

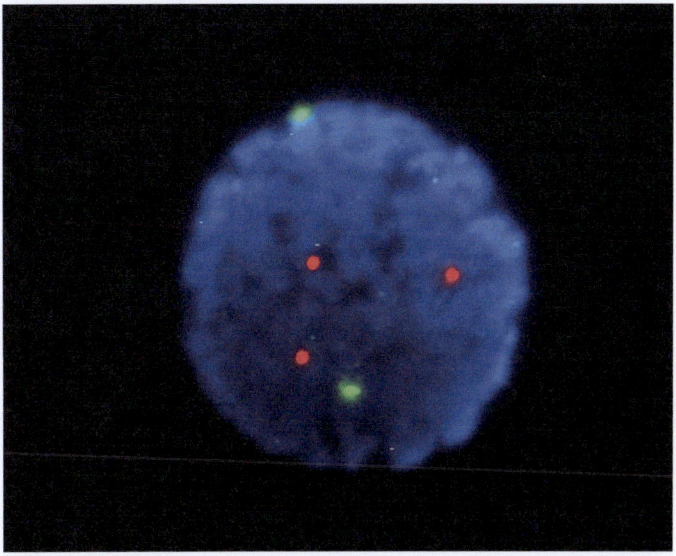

Fig. 7.4 Fluorescence in situ hybridization (FISH) of interphase nucleus from a fetus showing trisomy 21. Each green spot corresponds to a probe specific for chromosome 13, while the red spots correspond to probes specific for chromosome 21

7.5.2 Pros

Fluorescence in situ hybridization can be directly performed on the raw sample without the need for culture. Therefore, rapid results can be obtained in 24–48 h. This is especially useful in cases of amniocentesis after 20 weeks of gestation. FISH also provides insurance in cases of culture failure, where karyotyping is not possible. Maternal cell contamination and bacterial contamination rarely affect FISH results.

7.5.3 Cons

FISH technique provides information on the presence or absence of only those DNA sequences for which probes have been used. It does not provide information about other chromosomes, deletions, duplications, or point mutations. As the chromosomal structure cannot be evaluated, it does not distinguish free trisomy from a translocation.

The accuracy of FISH results can be influenced by the quality of the sample, the probes, and the hybridization conditions. Cross-hybridization, incomplete probe penetration, or probe degradation can rarely cause false-positive or false-negative results.

7.6 Quantitative Fluorescent Polymerase Chain Reaction (QF-PCR)

QF-PCR uses a polymerase chain reaction to amplify specific regions of DNA known as *small tandem repeats*. These are unique to each chromosome and can be counted by attaching fluorescent probes specific to each target sequence. The quantity of fluorescence-labeled DNA at each target is compared to that expected from a normal cell having a diploid chromosomal complement, and this ratio indicates whether a chromosome is extra or missing from the cell.

7.6.1 Methodology

1. The amniotic fluid sample is centrifuged to get the cell pellet. In the case of a CVS sample, the chorionic villi are thoroughly washed to remove blood.
2. As this is a DNA-based molecular test, maternal cell contamination must be ruled out before reporting results.
3. *DNA extraction:* Using techniques like column-based or bead-based purification, the fetal DNA is extracted.
4. *PCR amplification:* After checking the quality, the extracted DNA is amplified using PCR. The PCR reaction includes a fluorescent-labeled probe specific to the target region.
5. *Fluorescence detection:* Fluorescent signals from each target area are identified and quantified. These signals are plotted on a graph, wherein the strength of each signal produces a peak (Fig. 7.5).

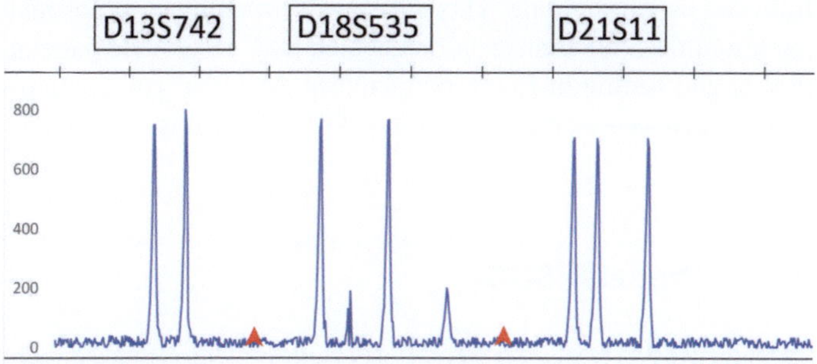

Fig. 7.5 QF-PCR electropherogram showing trisomy 21. Three spikes are detected by the probe set D21S11, which is specific for chromosome 21

6. The number of peaks produced by the fluorescent signals indicates the number of chromosome copies present in the cell.
7. A diploid cell having 2 copies of chromosome 21 will produce 2 equal-sized peaks for chromosome 21. In trisomy 21, there will either be three distinct peaks or one of the two peaks will be twice the expected size.
8. In monosomy X (Turner syndrome), there will be only one peak for the X chromosome, and no peak corresponding to the Y chromosome.

7.6.2 Pros

Like FISH, QF-PCR provides rapid results within 24–48 h. It is highly accurate for aneuploidy detection, with recent studies showing a 100% concordance to karyotyping [10]. It is less expensive compared to FISH or conventional karyotyping for aneuploidy detection.

7.6.3 Cons

QF-PCR can only detect numerical chromosomal aberrations. It cannot detect structural abnormalities, microdeletions, or single gene defects. A positive prenatal QF-PCR result should always be followed by karyotyping. This will detect structural chromosomal abnormalities, like translocations, which may necessitate parental testing and testing in future pregnancies. Maternal cell contamination can have a significant effect on QF-PCR as it is a molecular-based test.

7.7 Prenatal-BOBs

Prenatal-BoBs (BACs-on-Beads) is a multiplex array-based technique which uses microspheres that are coated with fluorescent chemicals. Each bead is coupled to bacterial artificial chromosomes (BACs), which are large pieces of bacterial DNA. DNA from prenatal samples is extracted, labeled, hybridized to the BOBs, and washed. The fluorescent signals emitted are then quantitatively analyzed [11].

Prenatal-BOBs assay scores over QF-PCR in detecting chromosomal structural abnormalities. It can also detect common microdeletions and microduplications, which are not possible with karyotyping. The shortcomings include its inability to detect polyploidy, maternal contamination, and low-level mosaicism. Prenatal-BOBs assay is not widely used in clinical practice [12].

7.8 Maternal Cell Contamination

Maternal cell contamination (MCC) is a serious problem which can negatively impact the accuracy of prenatal genetic diagnosis. MCC occurs at the time of sampling, but its effect depends on sample processing techniques used by labs.

The likelihood of MCC during CVS is more than amniocentesis, as it is difficult to separate the maternal decidua from the chorionic villi. For amniocentesis, MCC is associated with operator inexperience, difficult procedures, transplacental needle entry, number of needle entries, and a visibly bloody tap. Contamination can be reduced by aspirating the first 2–5 cc with a separate syringe and discarding it. MCC can be present even when the aspirated amniotic fluid appears clear [13].

Uncultured amniotic fluid has a higher chance of MCC, as the cell culture process increases amniocyte concentration, but not that of maternal blood cells. Culture of CVS samples can have an opposite effect, especially if the villi have not been washed well before transport. This is because maternal decidual cells get enriched in culture along with trophoblasts.

MCC can affect the results of karyotype and FISH, but the highest impact is on QF-PCR, as it can amplify contaminant cells with a concentration as low as 0.1%. Specific testing for MCC therefore becomes mandatory as a part of quantitative molecular testing [13].

7.9 Differences Between Karyotyping, FISH, and QF-PCR

Table 7.2 summarizes the important differences between karyotyping, FISH, and QF-PCR for prenatal detection of aneuploidy.

Table 7.2 Differences between karyotyping, FISH, and QF-PCR

	Karyotyping	FISH	QF-PCR
Technique	Light microscopy	Fluorescence microscopy	Molecular fluorescence test
Method	Qualitative	Qualitative	Quantitative
Culture required	Yes	No	No
Typical turnaround time (TAT)	14 days	2 days	2 days
Chromosomes detected	All	Few (typically 13, 18, 21, X, and Y)	Few (typically 13, 18, 21, X, and Y)
Chromosome structure	Detected	Not detected	Not detected
Sensitivity	100%	>99%	~100%
Maternal cell contamination	Less likely	Less likely	More likely
Relative cost	High	High	Low

7.10 Key Messages

1. Both CVS and amniocentesis are relatively safe procedures in experienced hands, when performed after 10 weeks and 15 weeks, respectively.
2. Amniotic fluid leak after amniocentesis is usually self-limiting.
3. CVS provides an earlier diagnosis and a better sample for DNA sequencing, but is technically more difficult.
4. Sampling route for CVS depends on the placental position, operator preference, and maternal factors like obesity, fibroids, and vaginal infection.
5. Amniocentesis is preferred over CVS in structurally normal fetuses with a high-risk NIPT result, because of the possibility of CPM.
6. Detailed counseling is mandatory prior to performing any invasive procedure.
7. Rapid aneuploidy tests like FISH and QF-PCR provide results within 2 days.
8. Karyotyping should be ordered along with FISH or QFPCR to detect chromosomal structural abnormalities like translocations. This helps to decide the need for parental testing and fetal testing in subsequent pregnancies.
9. QF-PCR results are most affected by MCC.
10. The probability of MCC increases with operator inexperience, difficult procedures, multiple needle entries, and transplacental entry in case of amniocentesis.

Acknowledgment The author thanks Ms. Shivanjali Kapse for sharing her insights on laboratory techniques.

References

1. Jacobson CB, Barter RH. Intrauterine diagnosis and management of genetic defects. Am J Obstet Gynecol. 1967;99(6):796–807.

2. Tabor A, Philip J, Madsen M, Bang J, Obel EB, Nørgaard-Pedersen B. Randomised controlled trial of genetic amniocentesis in 4606 low-risk women. Lancet. 1986;1(8493):1287–93.
3. Evans MI, Wapner RJ. Invasive prenatal diagnostic procedures 2005. Semin Perinatol. 2005;29(4):215–8.
4. Salomon LJ, Sotiriadis A, Wulff CB, Odibo A, Akolekar R. Risk of miscarriage following amniocentesis or chorionic villus sampling: systematic review of literature and updated meta-analysis. Ultrasound Obstet Gynecol. 2019;54(4):442–51.
5. Squier M, Chamberlain P, Zaiwalla Z, Anslow P, Oxbury J, Gould S, McShane MA. Five cases of brain injury following amniocentesis in midterm pregnancy. Dev Med Child Neurol. 2000;42(8):554–60.
6. Naylor G, Roper JP, Willshaw HE. Ophthalmic complications of amniocentesis. Eye (Lond). 1990;4(Pt 6):845–9.
7. Papi L, Farusi F, Teti G, Dini V, Romanelli M. Cutaneous foetal injuries related to amniocentesis. J Wound Care. 2013;22(10 Suppl):S23–6.
8. Elchalal U, Shachar IB, Peleg D, Schenker JG. Maternal mortality following diagnostic 2nd-trimester amniocentesis. Fetal Diagn Ther. 2004;19(2):195–8.
9. Wax JR, Davies NP, Watson WJ, Cartin A, Pinette MG, Chard R, Carpenter M. Pain associated with chorionic villus sampling: transabdominal vs transcervical approach. Am J Obstet Gynecol. 2009;201(4):400.e1–3.
10. Silva M, de Leeuw N, Mann K, Schuring-Blom H, Morgan S, Giardino D, Rack K, Hastings R. European guidelines for constitutional cytogenomic analysis. Eur J Hum Genet. 2019;27(1):1–16.
11. García-Herrero S, Campos-Galindo I, Martínez-Conejero JA, Serra V, Olmo I, Lara C, Simón C, Rubio C. BACs-on-Beads technology: a reliable test for rapid detection of aneuploidies and microdeletions in prenatal diagnosis. Biomed Res Int. 2014;2014:590298.
12. Choy KW, Kwok YK, Cheng YK, Wong KM, Wong HK, Leung KO, Suen KW, Adler K, Wang CC, Lau TK, Schermer MJ, Lao TT, Leung TY. Diagnostic accuracy of the BACs-on-Beads™ assay versus karyotyping for prenatal detection of chromosomal abnormalities: a retrospective consecutive case series. BJOG. 2014;121(10):1245–52.
13. Schrijver I, Cherny SC, Zehnder JL. Testing for maternal cell contamination in prenatal samples: a comprehensive survey of current diagnostic practices in 35 molecular diagnostic laboratories. J Mol Diagn. 2007;9(3):394–400.

Aneuploidy Screening in Twins

8

8.1 Introduction

Multiple pregnancies have increased sharply in the last three decades, in parallel with the increased use of assisted reproductive techniques (ART). An increase in median age at marriage has also contributed to this rise, as spontaneous twinning is more common in older women.

At present, the global twinning rate is 12 twin deliveries per 1000 deliveries, resulting in the birth of 1.6 million twin pairs each year. The spontaneous twinning rates are 1.5% for dizygotic twins and 0.4% for monozygotic twins, and ART significantly increases the incidence of both [1]. Transferring multiple embryos frequently results in dizygotic twins. Monozygotic twins, on the other hand, arise from the splitting of the zygote caused by disruption of the zona pellucida at the time of intra-cytoplasmic sperm injection (ICSI).

Screening for Down syndrome and other aneuploidies in twins has unique challenges and limitations. This chapter discusses the intricacies of serum screening, NIPT, and invasive testing in twin pregnancies. In this context, vanishing twin and selective fetal reduction are also discussed.

© The Author(s), under exclusive license to Springer Nature Singapore Pte Ltd. 2024

A. Kamat, *Down Syndrome Screening*,
https://doi.org/10.1007/978-981-99-7758-1_8

8.2 Zygosity and Chorionicity

The genetic profile of a twin fetus is determined by its zygosity. Dizygotic twins (fraternal twins) result from the fertilization of two ova by two sperms, and therefore have distinct genetic profiles. Their gender may be the same or different, purely by chance. Overall, two-thirds of all twins are dizygotic. On ultrasound, all dizygotic gestations are dichorionic-diamniotic (Fig. 8.1). While discordant fetal gender confirms dizygotic twinning, zygosity cannot be determined on ultrasound when both twins are of the same gender and the placentas are close to each other. In dizygotic twins, the risk of aneuploidy of each twin is independent of the other.

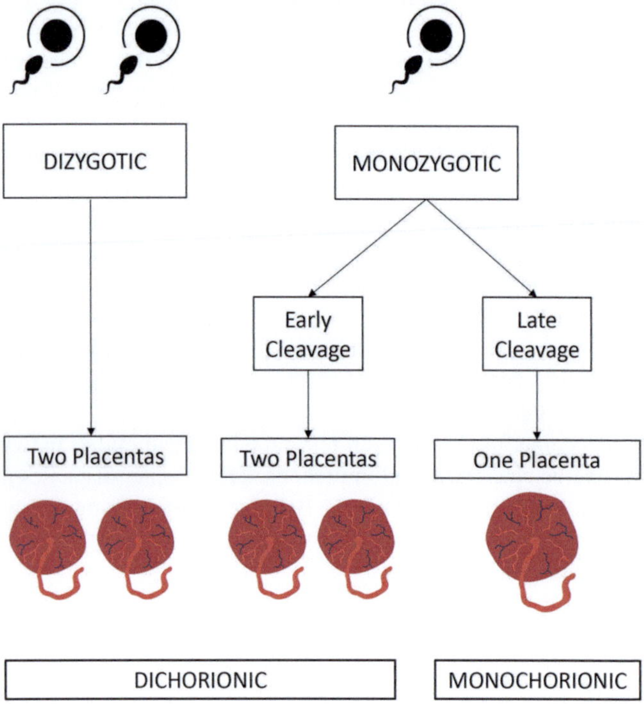

Fig. 8.1 Relationship between zygosity and chorionicity

Monozygotic twins arise from the splitting of a single fertilized ovum, with the day of cleavage determining the chorionicity and amnionicity. They can either be dichorionic-diamniotic (just like all dizygotic twins), monochorionic-diamniotic or, rarely, monochorionic-monoamniotic. Monozygotic twins have identical genes irrespective of the number of placentas and amniotic sacs. Hence, with a few rare exceptions, the fetuses are both euploid or both aneuploid.

Chorionicity refers to the number of placentas in a pregnancy. Dichorionic (DC) twins have two separate placentas which are often distant from each other. When the placentas are touching, there is a thick membrane between them and a wedge of chorionic tissue at their junction, forming the lambda ('λ') sign. Monochorionic (MC) twins arise from a single fertilized ovum and, hence, share a common placenta. Ultrasound features of MC twins include a thin inter-twin membrane and lack of a chorionic wedge at its junction with the placenta, giving rise to the 'T' sign.

Chorionicity is easily diagnosed before 14 weeks of gestation, with an accuracy close to 100%. Indeed, no first-trimester ultrasound is complete without clear documentation of chorionicity. In the second trimester, identification of the 'λ' and the 'T' sign becomes progressively difficult, and the accuracy drops to 86% [2].

Twins of uncertain chorionicity should be clinically managed like MC twins with close surveillance. However, for aneuploidy screening, they must be assessed individually, like DC twins. Risk calculation should be fetus-specific by using the NT value of each fetus. If invasive testing is required, both the fetuses must be sampled independently.

8.2.1 Post-Zygotic Non-disjunction in Monochorionic Twins

Non-disjunction is the failure of sister chromatids to separate during cell division. Non-disjunction can occur after the sperm has fused with the ovum (at the time of the first cell division of the zygote). In singletons, this produces a mosaic individual having a mixture of euploid and aneuploid cell lines. If the zygote splits into two after non-disjunction, it can produce genetically distinct monozygotic twins. One twin can have a normal genotype, while the other twin can be a mosaic or have an aneuploidy such as trisomy 21.

It must be emphasized that this occurrence is exceedingly rare, with only sporadic cases reported in the literature. Hence, for practical purposes, all MC twins should be considered as identical twins. However, this possibility should be mentioned when counseling for invasive procedures in MC twins to decide whether to sample only one fetus or both.

8.3 Maternal Age and Aneuploidy Risk

As with a singleton pregnancy, the risk of aneuploidy in a twin pregnancy increases with maternal age. The higher incidence of aneuploidy seen in twins is partly because multiple pregnancies are more common in older women. In a study published in 1990, Rodis et al. estimated that a 33-year-old woman with twins has the same risk of giving birth to a Down syndrome baby as that of a 35-year-old woman with a singleton pregnancy. The authors recommended chorionic villus sampling (CVS) or amniocentesis for all women above the age of 33 with twin pregnancies [3].

Maternal age alone cannot be used to screen for Down syndrome in twins for two reasons. First, using a maternal age-based cutoff of 33 years would result in an extraordinary number of invasive procedures, as a significant proportion of twins are born to older women. Second, maternal age alone has a sensitivity of only 30% for detection of Down syndrome in twins, making it quite unacceptable in practice [4].

8.4 Pregnancy-Specific Risk and Fetus-Specific Risk

In singleton pregnancies, the probability of birth of a child with Down syndrome is the same as the risk calculated for that fetus. In twins, the risk calculation is more complex as there are two fetuses to consider. A twin fetus has a lower chance of having Down syndrome compared to a singleton fetus. This is because of the high probability of a vanishing twin or a miscarriage when one twin is aneuploid. Despite this, the overall risk of Down syndrome is higher in twins compared to singletons for two reasons. First, older women are more likely to give birth to twins, both by spontaneous conception and ART. Second, having two fetuses instead of one statistically doubles the chance of the woman giving birth to an aneuploid baby.

We can consider two types of risks in twins:

- Fetus-specific risk: the risk of one particular fetus having Down syndrome.
- Pregnancy-specific risk: the risk of the pregnancy resulting in the birth of at least one child with Down syndrome.

8.4.1 Dichorionic Twins

As explained earlier, DC twins can either be dizygotic (fraternal) or monozygotic (identical) twins. Approximately 10% of DC twins are monozygotic and should have their risk calculated as MC twins. However, this is nearly impossible to ascertain on ultrasound. In all DC twins, we therefore calculate a fetus-specific risk for each baby, which more accurately reflects the probability of that fetus being aneuploid. Fetus-specific risk has the same false-positive rate as that for a singleton pregnancy, but with lower sensitivity.

The pregnancy-specific risk is the sum-total of the risks of the two fetuses. This is akin to the fact that the more the number of children a woman has throughout her life, the higher the chance that at least one of them will have Down syndrome. In DC twins, calculating a pregnancy-specific risk produces a high false-positive rate (FPR). For example, achieving a detection rate of 88% for Down syndrome using pregnancy-specific risk and a cut-off of 1:300 results in a screen-positive rate of 10% for DC twins [5]. The increased number of invasive procedures would increase the procedure-related pregnancy losses.

8.4.2 Monochorionic Twins

Monochorionic twins arise from a single fertilized ovum (monozygotic). Since both the fetuses are genetically identical, we do not calculate a separate risk for each fetus. Instead, a pregnancy-specific risk is calculated which applies to both fetuses.

8.5 Nuchal Translucency and Nasal Bone

Nuchal translucency (NT) is the most powerful tool for aneuploidy detection in twins. The distribution of NT according to gestational age is similar for singletons and twins. A combination of maternal age and NT can detect Down syndrome in twins with an overall sensitivity of 75% for a 5% FPR [6]. Unlike maternal serum markers which are not fetus-specific, NT provides an individual risk estimate for each fetus. Besides being highly reproducible, NT is unaffected by the number of fetuses and co-twin demise. In MC twins, however, the FPR is slightly higher since an increased NT can also be a sign of impending TTTS. Strict guidelines should be followed for assessment of NT (as described in Chap. 2) to avoid introducing observational errors.

8.5.1 Aneuploidy Risk Calculation Using NT

While using NT and maternal age to calculate risk of aneuploidy in twins, the following guidelines should be followed:

- In case of discordant sizes, the crown-rump length (CRL) of the larger twin is used to assign gestational age. It is assumed that the larger twin is appropriate for gestational age, as macrosomia is uncommon in the first trimester.
- MC twins are genetically identical, so two different risks cannot be calculated from discordant NT measurements. Instead, an average of the two measurements is used as the NT value for both fetuses to calculate a single common aneuploidy risk.

- Discordance in NT in MC twins is a sign of evolving twin-to-twin transfusion syndrome (TTTS) rather than discordant karyotype, and increased surveillance is recommended from 16 weeks onward.
- In DC twins, the risk for each fetus is separately calculated using its own NT value. Even if one fetus is screen positive and the other screen negative, both fetuses should be sampled at the time of invasive testing (see below).

8.5.2 Addition of Nasal Bone

The nasal bone provides additional fetus-specific data, which improves the efficacy of combined FTS in twins. Addition of NB to maternal age and NT increases the sensitivity to 89% for a 5% FPR [7]. Evaluating NB status is particularly helpful in triplets and higher order gestations where maternal serum markers cannot be used. It is emphasized that NB assessment is technically difficult compared to NT and must be performed only by trained and certified operators.

8.6 Maternal Serum Screening

Aneuploidy screening in twins using maternal serum markers raises several complex issues. Strict methodology is of utmost importance to avoid errors in screening. While the sensitivity of NT-based screening in twins is like singletons, biochemical screening is not as accurate because of several factors:

1. It is impossible to estimate the contribution of each individual placenta to the total level of a maternal serum marker.
2. As a normal placenta secretes more PAPP-A compared to an aneuploid one, it can bring the total PAPP-A level close to the median, thus masking the abnormality.
3. The placenta of a vanishing twin or reduced fetus also secretes serum markers at low but indeterminable levels.

4. Discordant placental size itself may cause disproportionate secretion of serum markers.
5. Zygosity affects the aneuploidy risk, but cannot be confirmed by ultrasound.
6. ART is another confounding factor as it independently alters levels of serum markers.
7. Aneuploidy risk calculation in twins is based on extrapolation of studies in singletons. There is a paucity of data specific to twins.

8.6.1 First-Trimester Combined Screening (FTS)

Levels of maternal serum markers are raised because of the presence of two placentas in DC twins, and a large placenta in MC twins. The median β-hCG value in a twin pregnancy is 2.0 MoM (multiples of median) compared to singleton pregnancy. The median PAPP-A value differs according to chorionicity. In MC twins, the MoM correction factor for PAPP-A is 1.8, while it is 2.2 in DC twins [8]. The aneuploidy risk calculation software usually makes this adjustment, provided correct information is fed into it.

Combined FTS is the screening method of choice for both MC and DC twins. Addition of serum markers to NT increases the sensitivity for Down syndrome screening from 75% to 80% while maintaining a 5% FPR. Using PAPP-A and β-hCG without NT (double marker test) is not recommended because of the poor detection rate (50% DR for a 5% FPR) [6]. As mentioned earlier, adding nasal bone status to combined screening further improves the sensitivity.

8.6.2 Second-Trimester Screening

As in the first trimester, second-trimester serum marker levels are higher in twin pregnancies. Compared to singleton pregnancies, the MoM values for alpha-fetoprotein, hCG, unconjugated estriol, and inhibin A are 1.6, 1.84, 1.99, and 2.13, respectively [7].

Second-trimester screening lacks fetus-specific variables for risk calculation, and therefore performs poorly compared to FTS. Muller and coworkers reported that the detection rate of Down syndrome using second-trimester serum screening was only 55% for an 8% screen-positive rate [9]. Despite outperforming screening by maternal age alone, triple and quadruple marker tests are not ideal for screening in twins. If offered to a patient with no previous screening and no NT scan, pre-test counseling about low DR and high FPR is recommended. If the first-trimester NT value is available (and combined FTS has not been done), risk estimation using maternal age and NT may be a better option.

8.6.3 Integrated Screening

There is a scarcity of data regarding integrated serum screening in multiple pregnancies. Combining integrated screening with NT could improve detection rates, but this has not been validated. As of now, integrated screening is not recommended in multiple pregnancies.

8.6.4 Second-Trimester Genetic Sonogram

As in singletons, use of soft markers to modify the risk of Down syndrome has not been validated in twins, and should not be performed. In case a soft marker is detected in one fetus at the time of the anomaly scan, the woman should be referred to a fetal medicine unit for detailed ultrasonography to look for additional findings. Further management should be based on recommendations for that specific marker (see Chap. 6). If amniocentesis is required, both fetuses should be sampled, irrespective of whether the soft marker is present in one or both.

8.6.5 Effect of Vanishing Twin

Vanishing twin occurs when there is an early fetal demise of one fetus in a twin pregnancy. In a vanishing twin, the placenta continues to function for a considerable time after fetal demise and produces serum markers. Since the markers secreted by the vanishing twin's placenta cannot be separately measured, serum screening becomes inaccurate.

With a vanishing twin, the median value for free β-hCG is like singleton pregnancy, as free β-hCG has a very short half-life. Median values of PAPP-A remain high, both in cases with an empty gestational sac (1.16 MoM), and those with a fetal pole (1.18 MoM). In the latter case, PAPP-A levels decline slowly, taking up to 8 weeks to reach singleton levels [10]. In the case of a vanishing twin, screening can be performed using maternal age with NT and β-hCG. If PAPP-A is included, screening efficacy can be maintained by correcting its levels based on the time interval between the embryonic demise and blood sampling [10]. Combined screening has a higher sensitivity in the absence of a second fetal pole. As most labs do not provide specific corrections for vanishing twin, it may be prudent to calculate aneuploidy risk using only maternal age and NT.

Among second-trimester serum markers, total hCG and unconjugated estriol do not change significantly. Maternal serum alpha-fetoprotein is raised and so is inhibin A [11]. If the twin has vanished early in the first trimester, and neither the fetus nor the placenta is seen on ultrasound, a quadruple marker test can be done.

8.7 Amniocentesis and CVS

As with screening, the presence of two fetuses complicates invasive testing in twin gestations. The most important concerns are:

- Fetal identification errors.
- Difficulty in assessing chorionicity.
- Increased risk of procedure-related loss.
- Subsequent management in case of discordant karyotypes.

8.7.1 Identification and Labeling

Definitive labeling of fetuses prior to invasive procedures cannot be overstated. If the two fetuses are discordant for aneuploidy, the abnormal fetus must be correctly identified in order to avoid accidental reduction of the normal one. If the affected fetus cannot be identified with certainty after the invasive test result, repeat sampling of both fetuses needs to be done prior to reduction.

Every center must have a strictly defined protocol for labeling fetuses. It is best to avoid using the terms 'twin 1' and 'twin 2', as this may be interpreted as the presenting and non-presenting twin. A common convention is to label the fetuses alphabetically (Fetus A, B, C, etc.) starting from the fetus close to the cervix and going clockwise. It is important to use as many details as possible for labeling each fetus such as (1) Position with respect to cervix, (2) Right or left side, (3) Placental position and cord insertion, (4) Presence of soft markers such as a single umbilical artery. If prenatal gender determination is legally allowed, it can be used whenever the fetuses are gender discordant.

Errors in identification and labeling are more likely to occur in certain situations:

1. Labeling is done prior to 10 weeks.
2. Incomplete information is used for labeling.
3. Re-labeling is done at subsequent scans as per operator's convenience.
4. Apparent shift in fetal positions caused by filling and emptying of maternal bladder.
5. Long interval between screening ultrasound and invasive testing or between invasive testing and fetal reduction.
6. Different operators performing the screening ultrasound, invasive testing, and fetal reduction.
7. After fetal reduction, if the amniotic sac of the reduced fetus collapses, the remaining fetuses can shift positions.

8.7.2 Amniocentesis

Just prior to amniocentesis, a detailed ultrasound should be performed to label the fetuses and reevaluate chorionicity, growth, and anatomy. The parents must be counseled in detail, regarding the technique, the risk of fetal loss, and the possibility of needing a subsequent fetal reduction.

Amniocentesis is performed after 15 weeks of gestation. The general rule of the thumb is to sample both sacs, even in twins discordant for anomaly. There are three techniques which can be used for sampling:

Sequential two-puncture technique: This technique involves two separate punctures away from each other into the two sacs. Two different needles are used to avoid cross-contamination. This technique is universally followed.

Simultaneous two-puncture technique: The two punctures are performed simultaneously by two operators, while the third operator monitors the path of both needles. This technique is too cumbersome, requires multiple operators, and is not widely used.

Single puncture technique: In this technique, one sac is sampled first. The needle is then advanced into the second sac and the first few milliliters of amniotic fluid are aspirated and discarded. A new syringe is used to aspirate the second sample through the same needle. Despite the advantage of a reduced number of entries into the uterus, there is a higher risk of cross-contamination and a theoretical risk of iatrogenic conversion to monoamniotic twins.

The use of dyes has been suggested in order to avoid sampling the same sac twice. After sampling one sac, the dye is injected before withdrawing the needle. Methylene blue is not recommended because of its association with increased risk of small bowel atresia and fetal loss. Indigo carmine is a safer alternative, though occasional cases of jejunal atresia have been reported following its use. Dyes, if at all used, should be restricted to higher order multiples, where there is a greater possibility of repeat sampling of the same sac [12, 13].

8.7.3 Chorionic Villus Sampling

Chorionic villus sampling (CVS) in twins is a difficult procedure, both technically and for follow-up decisions, and must be performed by the most experienced operator available. Errors in identification of the abnormal twin in the case of discordant karyotypes are far more likely following CVS. This is because considerable growth and change in relative position may have occurred by the time the CVS result is available.

While performing transabdominal CVS, it is advisable to sample the placenta close to each cord insertion and away from the membrane insertion. Separate needles should be used for each placenta and the intended paths planned beforehand. Despite these precautions, contamination or sampling errors occur in 3–4% of cases. Sampling errors are highest when the two placentas touch each other, or access to one placenta is technically difficult. The transcervical approach is also possible for twins. However, it carries a higher risk of contamination, and the subsequent need for amniocentesis. Sometimes, a combination of the two approaches may be required depending on the accessibility of the placentas.

8.7.4 Fetal Loss Following Invasive Procedures

Fetal loss following amniocentesis or CVS in twins is higher compared to singleton pregnancy. Overall risk of pregnancy loss caused by amniocentesis in twins is reported to be 1.6%, while that following CVS is reported to be 3.2% [14, 15]. These risks are over and above the background risk of spontaneous pregnancy loss in twins, which in itself, is higher than singleton pregnancies. Fetal loss rates are higher with inexperienced operators, multiple needle entries, transplacental amniocentesis, and following fetal reduction after the diagnostic procedure. However, a recent meta-analysis suggests that the procedure-related fetal loss rates in twins may be much lower than previously reported [16].

8.7.5 Amniocentesis Versus CVS

- Amniocentesis is technically easier in twins.
- Amniocentesis is associated with a lower risk of fetal loss and a lower risk of cross-contamination when the two placentas are close together.
- CVS provides a better sample whenever sequencing of DNA is required.
- CVS provides an earlier diagnosis for planning selective fetal reduction.
- Overall, both techniques are acceptable, and this choice should be made considering ultrasound findings in each case, operator experience, and the woman's choice.

8.7.6 Single Versus Double Sampling

Dichorionic twins can be dizygotic or monozygotic. If maternal serum screening shows a high risk of aneuploidy, it is not possible to determine which placenta is producing the abnormal markers. Therefore, sampling of both fetuses is performed even if they are discordant for anomaly or aneuploidy screening result.

In MC twins, the decision is more controversial as they are supposed to be genetically identical. There are two caveats to this rule. First, post-zygotic non-disjunction may produce genetically discordant MC twins. This is a very rare occurrence, with only sporadic cases reported. Second, chorionicity may be wrongly diagnosed at a later gestation, if it has not been accurately determined in the first trimester. For these reasons, most centers offer double sampling at the time of amniocentesis in MC twins. When chorionicity is confirmed in the first trimester, and the two fetuses are concordant for growth and anatomic survey, it is acceptable to sample a single sac [17].

When performing CVS in MC twins, it is acceptable to do either single or double sampling. Most centers prefer to take a single sample as post-zygotic non-disjunction is a very rare event. If a single sample is being taken, the woman must still be informed about the rare possibility of discordant karyotypes. Single sampling must be avoided if there is any doubt about chorionicity. For double sampling, the sampling sites should be as far away from each other as possible and close to the cord insertion of each fetus. One can also wait till 15 weeks and perform amniocentesis, thus reducing the chances of cross-contamination.

8.8 Noninvasive Prenatal Testing

Once NIPT became established as a highly sensitive screening test for singleton pregnancies, researchers looked for its application in multiple pregnancies. As women with twin pregnancies are older (especially those resulting from ART), they have an increased risk of giving birth to an aneuploid fetus. Maternal serum screening has lower accuracy in twins. In addition, invasive testing often involves sampling errors and has a higher risk of fetal loss. A noninvasive cfDNA test would therefore be an ideal way to test for aneuploidy in women with twin pregnancies. Despite several encouraging reports, NIPT in twins faces unique challenges and limitations.

8.8.1 Limitations of NGS-Based NIPT

Uncertain zygosity: Inability to confirm zygosity with ultrasound (in same-gender twins) makes it challenging to assign abnormal cfDNA levels to one or both fetuses.

Compensation by the co-twin placenta: The quantity of cfDNA released into maternal blood depends on the rate of apoptosis of synciotrophoblasts, and frequently, this is different for each placenta. Sometimes, one placenta may produce larger than normal amounts of cfDNA, while the other placenta accounts for less than the critical 4% fetal fraction required for diagnosis. As aneuploidy is associated with a low cfDNA production, the cfDNA from the normal twin can mask that produced by the aneuploid twin. Sensitivity for trisomy 13 and 18 is especially lower in twins as both these aneuploidies significantly reduce cfDNA production.

Vanishing twin: When there is the demise of one of the twin fetuses, its placenta continues to release cfDNA into maternal blood. This cfDNA cannot be quantified separately from that of the live twin. If fetal demise has occurred recently, the contribution of cfDNA from its placenta can be even greater than the normal placenta because of rapid cell death. Also, it is far more likely that the dead fetus is genetically abnormal compared to the surviving one. An unknown proportion of vanishing twins may also be diagnosed as singleton pregnancies. This is likely to affect NIPS results, as a correction for twin pregnancies will not be considered while mapping the cfDNA to each chromosome. Careful documentation of the gestational sac number in early pregnancy can prevent this error to some extent.

Nonidentical MC twins: In theory, NIPT should have a high sensitivity in MC twins because of one large placenta releasing large amounts of cfDNA. Post-zygotic nondisjunction can rarely lead to the formation of non-identical MC twins and introduce errors in NIPT results.

Performing single nucleotide polymorphism (SNP)-based NIPT in twins can theoretically identify individual sources of cfDNA and mitigate the above problems to a great extent. However, large-scale validation studies are still needed.

8.8.2 Test Performance of NIPT for Common Trisomies

The performance of NIPT to detect common trisomies in twins is slightly inferior to that in singletons. In a systematic review by Khalil and coworkers, the pooled detection rate (DR) of 12 studies (including their own) for trisomy 21 was 95% for an FPR of 0.09. The DR for trisomy 18 was 82% for an FPR of 0.08, while for trisomy 13, it was 80% for an FPR of 0.13. The main limitations of the included studies were the small sample size, retrospective design, and use of stored samples in some studies [18]. Similarly, the meta-analysis by the Nicolaides group reported that the pooled weighted DR and FPR were 99.0% and 0.02% for trisomy 21, 92.8% and 0.01% for trisomy 18, and 94.7% and 0.10% for trisomy 13, respectively [19].

Finally, the efficacy of NIPT in screening for sex chromosomal abnormalities, rare autosomal trisomies, and submicroscopic abnormalities in twins is unknown. Large-scale prospective studies are required before it can be recommended.

8.9 Aneuploidy Screening and Selective Fetal Reduction

Selective fetal reduction is performed for converting a higher order multiple pregnancy to either a twin pregnancy or a singleton pregnancy (depending on chorionicity, abnormalities in the fetus, and patient wishes). Fetal reduction is also employed in twins who are discordant for anomaly or karyotype.

8.9.1 Aneuploidy Testing Before Fetal Reduction

Aneuploidy risk assessment of all fetuses prior to selective reduction lowers the chance of retaining an aneuploid fetus. While serum screening is not reliable in higher order multiples, we can calculate a fetus-specific risk for each fetus using maternal age and NT. Addition of NB, tricuspid regurgitation, and ductus venosus Doppler improves the screening sensitivity. Documentation of chorionicity of all fetuses is of paramount importance.

Chorionic villus sampling of all fetuses prior to reduction does not significantly increase the risk of miscarriage following fetal reduction. As common aneuploidies are ruled out in the retained fetuses, the risk of spontaneous fetal demise is low, and this balances out the risk posed by the CVS procedure. As CVS must be performed shortly before fetal reduction, rapid testing for chromosomes 13, 18, 21, X, and Y by fluorescence in situ hybridization (FISH) is the preferred method. The disadvantages of this approach include the increased complexity of the procedure, the increased cost, and the need to have a genetic laboratory close to the center with facilities to perform overnight FISH [20].

Monochorionic twins, which are discordant for anomaly (or rarely karyotype), may also require fetal reduction. Injection of potassium chloride or lignocaine cannot be used to reduce one fetus of a MC pair because of shared placental circulation. Selective fetal reduction in MC twins can be achieved by interstitial laser, radiofrequency ablation, or bipolar cord coagulation. These procedures are expensive and have their own risk of fetal loss and preterm delivery. All these issues must be discussed prior to double sampling of MC twins.

8.9.2 Aneuploidy Testing After Fetal Reduction

Aneuploidy testing may occasionally be needed in the second trimester following selective reduction, when one of the retained fetuses is diagnosed with a structural malformation. In such cases, amniocentesis of all the retained fetuses needs to be performed, followed by reduction of the abnormal fetus if necessary. Second-trimester fetal reduction has a higher risk of miscarriage.

8.10 Key Messages

1. Zygosity, not chorionicity, determines whether the twins are genetically identical.
2. All MC twins are monozygotic, therefore assumed to be genetically identical, the rare exception being of post-zygotic non-disjunction.
3. Dichorionic twins can be monozygotic or dizygotic. All DC twins and twins with uncertain chorionicity are considered non-identical for aneuploidy screening.
4. A fetus-specific risk is calculated in DC twins, while a pregnancy-specific risk is calculated in MC twins.
5. Discordant NT in MC twins is a predictor for evolving TTTS.
6. Combined first-trimester screening is the screening method of choice in twins.

7. Maternal age + NT ± Nasal bone is also an acceptable alternative to combined screening. It is the only method which can be used in vanishing twins and higher order multiples.
8. Second-trimester serum screening has a lower sensitivity in twins.
9. Unambiguous labeling of fetuses is mandatory prior to any invasive procedure.
10. Double sampling is mandatory in DC twins. In MC twins, the decision of single versus double sampling should be taken on a case-to-case basis.
11. While NIPT appears to be efficacious for diagnosing common trisomies in twins, there is limited data on its performance.
12. NIPT in twins should be performed with caution, having understood its limitations.

References

1. Monden C, Pison G, Smits J. Twin peaks: more twinning in humans than ever before. Hum Reprod. 2021;36(6):1666–73.
2. Stenhouse E, Hardwick C, Maharaj S, Webb J, Kelly T, Mackenzie FM. Chorionicity determination in twin pregnancies: how accurate are we? Ultrasound Obstet Gynecol. 2002;19(4):350–2.
3. Rodis JF, Egan JF, Craffey A, Ciarleglio L, Greenstein RM, Scorza WE. Calculated risk of chromosomal abnormalities in twin gestations. Obstet Gynecol. 1990;76(6):1037–41.
4. Odibo AO, Lawrence-Cleary K, Macones GA. Screening for aneuploidy in twins and higher-order multiples: is first-trimester nuchal translucency the solution? Obstet Gynecol Surv. 2003;58(9):609–14.
5. Sebire NJ, Snijders RJ, Hughes K, Sepulveda W, Nicolaides KH. Screening for trisomy 21 in twin pregnancies by maternal age and fetal nuchal translucency thickness at 10-14 weeks of gestation. Br J Obstet Gynaecol. 1996;103(10):999–1003.
6. Spencer K. Screening for trisomy 21 in twin pregnancies in the first trimester using free beta-hCG and PAPP-A, combined with fetal nuchal translucency thickness. Prenat Diagn. 2000;20(2):91–5.
7. Bender W, Dugoff L. Screening for aneuploidy in multiple gestations: the challenges and options. Obstet Gynecol Clin N Am. 2018;45(1):41–53.

8. Spencer K, Kagan KO, Nicolaides KH. Screening for trisomy 21 in twin pregnancies in the first trimester: an update of the impact of chorionicity on maternal serum markers. Prenat Diagn. 2008;28(1):49–52.
9. Muller F, Dreux S, Dupoizat H, Uzan S, Dubin MF, Oury JF, Dingeon B, Dommergues M. Second-trimester down syndrome maternal serum screening in twin pregnancies: impact of chorionicity. Prenat Diagn. 2003;23(4):331–5.
10. Chaveeva P, Wright A, Syngelaki A, Konstantinidou L, Wright D, Nicolaides KH. First-trimester screening for trisomies in pregnancies with vanishing twin. Ultrasound Obstet Gynecol. 2020;55(3):326–31.
11. Huang T, Boucher K, Aul R, Rashid S, Meschino WS. First and second trimester maternal serum markers in pregnancies with a vanishing twin. Prenat Diagn. 2015;35(1):90–6.
12. McFadyen I. The dangers of intra-amniotic methylene blue. Br J Obstet Gynaecol. 1992;99(2):89–90.
13. Brandenburg H. The use of synthetic dyes for identification of the amniotic sacs in multiple pregnancies. Prenat Diagn. 1997;17(3):281–2.
14. Millaire M, Bujold E, Morency AM, Gauthier RJ. Mid-trimester genetic amniocentesis in twin pregnancy and the risk of fetal loss. J Obstet Gynaecol Can. 2006;28(6):512–8.
15. Appelman Z, Furman B. Invasive genetic diagnosis in multiple pregnancies. Obstet Gynecol Clin N Am. 2005;32(1):97–103. ix.
16. Di Mascio D, Khalil A, Rizzo G, Buca D, Liberati M, Martellucci CA, Flacco ME, Manzoli L, D'Antonio F. Risk of fetal loss following amniocentesis or chorionic villus sampling in twin pregnancy: systematic review and meta-analysis. Ultrasound Obstet Gynecol. 2020;56(5):647–55.
17. Audibert F, Gagnon A. No. 262-prenatal screening for and diagnosis of aneuploidy in twin pregnancies. J Obstet Gynaecol Can. 2017;39(9):e347–61.
18. Khalil A, Archer R, Hutchinson V, Mousa HA, Johnstone ED, Cameron MJ, Cohen KE, Ioannou C, Kelly B, Reed K, Hulme R, Papageorghiou AT. Noninvasive prenatal screening in twin pregnancies with cell-free DNA using the IONA test: a prospective multicenter study. Am J Obstet Gynecol. 2021;225(1):79.e1–79.e13.
19. Judah H, Gil MM, Syngelaki A, Galeva S, Jani J, Akolekar R, Nicolaides KH. Cell-free DNA testing of maternal blood in screening for trisomies in twin pregnancy: updated cohort study at 10-14 weeks and meta-analysis. Ultrasound Obstet Gynecol. 2021;58(2):178–89.
20. Evans MI, Andriole S, Britt DW. Fetal reduction: 25 years' experience. Fetal Diagn Ther. 2014;35(2):69–82.

9 Integrated, Contingent, and Sequential Stepwise Screening

9.1 Introduction

Maternal serum screening can be performed either in the first trimester (11–13 + 6 weeks) or in the second trimester (15–22 weeks). First-trimester screening (FTS) is performed using nuchal translucency (NT) with PAPP-A and free β-hCG, with or without nasal bone (NB). Second-trimester screening (STS) is performed with the quadruple screening test (Quad screen) which includes β-hCG, alpha-fetoprotein (AFP), unconjugated estriol, and inhibin A. The triple test is no longer recommended because of its poor sensitivity.

Despite being safe, economical, and easy to implement, these screening tests have a 5% false-positive rate (FPR) in order to achieve a detection rate (DR) of approximately 85% [1]. This means that out of all women undergoing these screening tests, a significant number still need invasive testing. Two-step screening is one method to improve the sensitivity and reduce the FPR. The first step usually involves screening with NT, PAPP-A, and free β-hCG. *The risk calculated from the first step is used as the baseline (*a-priori*) risk for the second step instead of maternal age-related risk.*

© The Author(s), under exclusive license to Springer Nature Singapore Pte Ltd. 2023

A. Kamat, *Down Syndrome Screening*,
https://doi.org/10.1007/978-981-99-7758-1_9

Table 9.1 Down syndrome screening models

Single-step screening	
First trimester • Dual marker test (without NT)[a] • Combined first-trimester screening	Second trimester • Triple test[a] • Quadruple test
Two-step screening	
Non-disclosure of first-trimester screening result • Integrated screening • Serum integrated screening	Disclosure of first-trimester screening result • Sequential stepwise screening • Contingent screening (intermediate risk approach) – With maternal serum markers – With NIPT – With first trimester ultrasound markers[a] – With second-trimester genetic sonogram[a] – Independent two-step screening[a]

[a] These screening approaches are no longer recommended in clinical practice

This chapter discusses the various options available for two-step screening for Down syndrome. Each screening model is described, followed by its advantages and disadvantages. A two-step strategy is not the minimal standard of care for Down syndrome screening. It requires healthcare providers to understand the correlation between first- and second-trimester variables. It is logistically difficult and requires detailed counseling at every step. Most centers should stick to simple single-step screening, which can be successfully implemented with minimal resources. Table 9.1 lists the various modalities for Down syndrome screening which involve maternal serum testing in the first trimester, second trimester, or both.

9.2 Definitions

Different screening models exist based on the two-step approach. A scrutiny of the published literature indicates that the use of terms is not consistent among various authors. It is essential to define each screening model from the outset.

Integrated screening (non-disclosure sequential screening): Blood sampling is performed in the first and the second trimester. An integrated risk is calculated using maternal age, NT, PAPP-A, β-hCG, unconjugated estriol, and inhibin A. Screening result is reported only after the second test.

Serum integrated screening: Same as integrated screening, but without NT.

Sequential stepwise screening: Result of FTS is informed to the pregnant woman. All *low-risk* women undergo repeat blood sampling in the second trimester and the final risk is calculated using the integrated test (see above).

Contingent screening (intermediate risk approach): Result of FTS is informed to the woman. The risk is reported as high, low, or intermediate. All *intermediate-risk* women undergo repeat blood sampling and Down syndrome screening either through an integrated test or NIPT. Ultrasound markers were earlier used for contingent screening, but this is no longer recommended.

Independent two-step screening: First-trimester and second-trimester screening is done independently using maternal age-related risk as the baseline risk each time. The pregnant woman receives separate screening reports in each trimester. Invasive testing is advised if either report shows a high-risk result. This approach is not recommended because of an unacceptably high FPR.

9.3 Integrated Screening

The integrated screening model includes nuchal translucency along with both first- and second-trimester markers in a single calculation to estimate the risk of aneuploidy. Though it is a cumbersome method, it is associated with the highest sensitivity for a given false positive rate.

9.3.1 Integrated Screening Methodology

- A blood sample is taken following the 11–13 + 6 weeks scan.
- Screening result is not calculated.
- Second blood sample is taken between 15 and 22 weeks.

- A statistical software calculates risk using maternal age, NT, PAPP-A, β-hCG, AFP, unconjugated estriol, and inhibin A. Nasal bone may also be included.
- Women who get a high-risk (screen-positive) result are offered invasive testing.
- Down syndrome DR = 90% for an FPR of 2.6% (risk cutoff, 1:245); DR = 85% for an FPR of 1.2% (risk cutoff, 1:120) [1, 2].

9.3.2 Serum-Integrated Screening Methodology

- Blood sample is taken between 11 and 13 + 6 weeks.
- NT and nasal bone are not required. This is useful when a trained sonologist is not available.
- Report is not released.
- Second blood sample is taken between 15 and 22 weeks.
- A statistical software calculates risk using maternal age, PAPP-A, β-hCG, AFP, unconjugated estriol, and inhibin A. Test result is issued.
- Women who get a high-risk (screen-positive) result are offered invasive testing.
- Down syndrome DR = 90% for a 5.3% FPR [1].

9.3.3 Pros and Cons

The integrated screening test offers a very high sensitivity and a low FPR, reducing the number of invasive procedures. By including both first- and second-trimester markers, their independent association with Down syndrome is utilized. An additional advantage is that every patient undergoing screening gets a risk assessment for open neural tube defects. The serum integrated test is useful in centers where certified NT operators are not available, or maternal habitus makes it difficult to get a correct NT measurement.

There are certain disadvantages as well. First, the screening result is not released until after the second-trimester blood sample, which increases the anxiety of the pregnant woman. If significantly abnormal marker levels are detected in the first trimester itself, it creates an ethical dilemma for the reporting lab. In such cases, definitive testing is delayed until the second-trimester test result is available. If first-trimester free β-hCG as well as second-trimester β-hCG are used, the relative dependence of the test on this marker increases disproportionately. As two blood samples must be tested, the cost of the test is significantly higher than single-step screening. Integrated screening is not recommended for multiple pregnancies. Finally, if the pregnant woman does not report for the second sample, no report can be generated.

9.4 Sequential Stepwise Screening

Sequential stepwise screening involves separate risk calculation in the first and second trimesters. *Patients who get a low-risk FTS report are subjected to STS*, with the risk calculated as in integrated screening.

9.4.1 Methodology

- First-trimester screening performed with maternal age + NT + PAPP-A + free β-hCG.
- Nasal bone may also be included.
- Result of FTS is informed to the woman.
- If FTS result is screen-positive, CVS or amniocentesis is offered.
- If FTS result is screen-negative, repeat blood sampling is performed at 16 weeks. The final risk is calculated by integrating first-trimester and second-trimester markers with maternal age and NT.
- The final risk is used to decide further management.
- Down syndrome DR = 95% for a 5% FPR [3, 4].

9.4.2 Pros and Cons

The sequential stepwise screening model maintains a high sensitivity for detection of Down syndrome, while also providing a screening result in the first trimester. This allows a greater flexibility for decision-making.

The disadvantage of this complicated approach is that despite getting a low-risk result in the FTS, the patient is still not reassured, and instead made to undergo another screening test for the same conditions. Thus, compliance becomes an important issue, besides the increased cost of screening.

9.5 Contingent Serum Screening (Intermediate Risk Approach)

Contingent serum screening is a stepwise screening which aims to find a middle ground between single-step and two-step screening by defining an intermediate risk group in which further testing is carried out [5].

9.5.1 Methodology

- First-trimester screening performed as usual with maternal age + NT + PAPP-A + free β-hCG.
- Result of FTS is informed to the woman.
- If the result is high risk, CVS or amniocentesis is offered.
- If the result is low risk, no further evaluation is done.
- If the result is intermediate risk, repeat blood sampling is performed at 16 weeks. The final risk is calculated by integrating first-trimester and second-trimester serum markers with maternal age and NT.
- The final risk is used to decide further management.
- Down syndrome DR = 88%–94% for a 5% FPR [3].

9.5.2 Pros and Cons

Using this approach, only 25% of women need to undergo a second-trimester screening [5]. This reduces the cost of the test and provides a definitive result to three-fourths of women in the first trimester itself. While it can be argued that these women would miss serum screening for ONTDs with MSAFP, the resolution offered by present-day ultrasound machines makes this screening redundant. In places where trained sonographers are not available, MSAFP screening would still make sense.

Certain issues need to be resolved before widely applying the contingent screening model, namely, (1) Defining the intermediate risk, which at present, is rather arbitrarily decided by the testing laboratories, (2) Selecting an acceptable number of cases missed by contingent screening which would have been picked up if integrated screening had been done in all patients, and, (3) Whether β-hCG should be measured in one or both trimesters. Aneuploidy screening, even with a single-step model, involves considerable counseling. Contingent screening with intermediate risk is a complex screening model which many pregnant women may find difficult to fully comprehend. About a quarter of women need to be recalled for a second test, which poses an additional logistic load for the testing laboratory.

9.6 Contingent Screening with First-Trimester USG Markers

Several first-trimester ultrasound markers are associated with an increased risk of Down syndrome. Absent nasal bone (NB), tricuspid regurgitation (TR), and reversed ductus venosus (DV) flow are observed in 36%, 67%, and 24% of trisomy 21 fetuses, respectively, though the figures vary widely among published reports [6–8]. It is possible to establish a contingent screening model in which these ultrasound markers are used in the intermediate risk group to refine the risk further.

9.6.1 Methodology

- First-trimester screening performed as usual with maternal age + NT + PAPP-A + free β-hCG.
- Result of FTS is informed to the woman.
- If the result is high risk, CVS, or amniocentesis is offered.
- If the result is low risk, no further evaluation is done.
- If the result is intermediate risk, either NB, TR, or DV, or all three are used to recalculate the FTS result as high risk or low risk using appropriate software.
- Risk calculated is used to decide further management.
- Down syndrome DR = 93–96% for an FPR of 4.3–5.6%; DR = 97% for an FPR of 4% when all 3 markers are used [9].

9.6.2 Pros and Cons

Despite a modest improvement in screening performance, there are several problems associated with this approach. Evaluation of NB, TR, and DV is technically difficult and highly prone to errors (see Chap. 2). Only sonographers who are formally trained and certified for these markers should report them. There is little evidence on which marker works best in a contingent approach. Finally, using ultrasound markers and NIPT can create a contingent-contingent approach, which further complicates the screening process.

At present, use of contingent screening using NB, TR, and DV flow should only be restricted to centers with trained and certified sonographers, strict protocols, and a continuous audit process.

9.7 Contingent Screening with Noninvasive Prenatal Testing (NIPT)

When used as a first-line screening tool for Down syndrome, NIPT has a sensitivity of 99.1% for a 0.1% FPR [10]. However, NIPT is not cost-effective at present and has several disadvantages when applied across the entire population (see Chap. 5). Using NIPT in contingent screening restricts its need to only 20–25% of women who get an intermediate risk result with combined FTS.

9.7.1 Methodology

- FTS is performed with maternal age + NT + PAPP-A + free β-hCG.
- Result of FTS is informed to the woman.
- If the result is high risk, CVS or amniocentesis is offered.
- If the result is low risk no further evaluation is done.
- If the result is intermediate risk, NIPT is performed. In contingent screening with NIPT, a patient who agrees to undergo FTS in principle agrees to undergo NIPT if FTS shows an intermediate risk result.
- Result of NIPT is used to decide further management.
- In case NIPT gives a no-call result, invasive testing is offered.
- Down syndrome DR = 98% for a 0.5% invasive testing rate (FPR depends on the percentage of no-call results of NIPT) [11].

9.7.2 Pros and Cons

This approach increases the DR and reduces the FPR and the number of women needing invasive testing. The benefits of NT scan are retained, including early detection of anomalies and screening for preeclampsia.

The main disadvantage of this approach is that the average screening cost per patient is high, because NIPT is a mandatory second step in women with screen-positive results.

9.8 Contingent Screening with Genetic Sonogram

Soft markers are unusual ultrasound findings which do not represent major structural abnormalities, but increase the risk of aneuploidy. A genetic sonogram is a structured examination of the fetus in the second trimester to detect soft markers.

9.8.1 Risk Modification Using Likelihood Ratios

Second-trimester soft markers can be used to modify the risk of Down syndrome which has been previously assigned from maternal age or combined FTS. This statistical calculation involves multiplying the previously calculated risk by a factor called as 'likelihood ratio' (LR) of each soft marker.

The LR for a soft marker indicates the number of times the risk would increase if that soft marker is present. Each soft marker has its own positive LR (when the marker is present) and negative LR (when the marker is absent). Positive LRs are >1, indicating an increase in risk when the marker is present. Negative LRs are <1, indicating a risk reduction when the marker is absent. When only one marker is present, the final risk is calculated by multiplying the existing risk with positive LR of that marker and negative LR of other markers.

To avoid the complicated calculations involving positive LRs and negative LRs, isolated marker LRs have been separately calculated. Whenever a soft marker is isolated, the baseline risk is simply multiplied by the isolated marker LR for that soft marker to obtain the final risk. Table 9.2 shows the positive LR, negative LR, and the isolated marker LR for each soft marker.

Let us consider an example below:

A 29-year-old woman undergoes combined FTS, and the FTS result shows a trisomy 21 risk of 1 in 500. At the 19 weeks ultrasound, an absent nasal bone is detected.

Table 9.2 Likelihood ratios of second-trimester ultrasound soft markers for Down syndrome [12, 13]

Marker	Positive LR	Negative LR	Isolated marker LR
Increased nuchal fold	23.3–49.0	0.8–0.82	3.79
Ventriculomegaly	25.0–27.5	0.94–0.95	3.81
Echogenic bowel	11.4–28.0	0.86–0.90	1.65
Absent/hypoplastic nasal bone	23.3–29.1	0.39–0.46	6.58
Aberrant right subclavian artery	19.0–21.5	0.71–0.73	3.94
Short humerus	4.8–5.0	0.74–0.90	0.78
Short femur	3.7–4.6	0.73–0.80	0.61
Mild pyelectasis	5.5–7.6	0.92–0.94	1.08
Intracardiac echogenic focus	5.8–6.3	0.75–0.80	0.95
No marker present	–	–	0.13

- Patient age: 29 years (age-related risk 1:1000).
- Combined first-trimester risk (NT + PAPP-A + free β-hCG) = 1:500 (This is now used as the baseline or a priori risk).
- Findings on second-trimester genetic sonogram: Absent nasal bone (isolated).
- Isolated marker LR for absent nasal bone = 6.58.
- Final risk = (a priori risk) × (isolated marker LR) = 1:500 × 6.58 = 1:76.
- The patient is now considered high risk for Down syndrome and offered amniocentesis.

9.8.2 Pros and Cons

Contingent screening by genetic sonogram appears tempting, as it can be performed at the time of the anomaly scan. It also avoids the risks and cost of invasive procedures or NIPT. However, there are several valid reasons why soft markers should not be used to refine the aneuploidy risk calculated by combined FTS.

1. Soft marker assessment can be subjective, e.g., echogenic bowel.
2. Some markers are transient findings and disappear at a later gestation, e.g., mild pyelectasis.
3. Performing a genetic sonogram requires highly trained specialists.
4. Markers like echogenic intracardiac focus and mild pyelectasis are commonly noted in normal fetuses.
5. There is a lack of universal agreement on defining values for certain markers, e.g., whether 5 mm or 6 mm should be used as a cutoff for thickened nuchal fold.
6. Genetic sonography assumes that all soft markers are independent of each other. There is paucity of data regarding their correlation. For example, short humerus and short femur are independent soft markers. But when both occur together, it may reflect either a skeletal dysplasia or constitutional shortening.
7. Isolated marker LRs are calculated by multiplying positive LR of the detected marker with negative LRs of all the other markers. This value changes depending on the number of soft markers being examined. The positive LRs also vary widely from study to study.
8. NB may be seen in the first trimester and appear hypoplastic in the second trimester.
9. When isolated, some markers have an LR below 1, leading to a statistical reduction in the baseline risk when they are present.
10. It is controversial whether fetal echocardiography should be included in a genetic sonogram.
11. Using a test with a lower sensitivity (genetic sonogram) to change the risk calculated by combined FTS may not be appropriate.
12. Gestational age at scan and maternal obesity affects the detection rate of soft markers.
13. Soft markers for Down syndrome have no significance in women with a low-risk result on NIPT.

9.8.3 Recommendations for Use of Soft Markers

A systematic search for soft markers in all pregnant women is unwarranted. If a soft marker is detected during an anomaly scan, guidelines for that specific marker should be followed, as detailed in Chap. 6. If multiple soft markers are present, amniocentesis is strongly recommended.

Soft markers should not be routinely used to recalculate the risk of Down syndrome. In women who are FTS screen positive, but are reluctant for amniocentesis, NIPT is the recommended test. Women getting low fetal fraction or no-call results on NIPT are at a higher risk of aneuploidy, and should be offered amniocentesis.

Nevertheless, a genetic sonogram still has some role to play in specific situations [14]:

- In countries where genetic testing is not easily available or where it is an out-of-pocket expense.
- In women with twins, especially those conceived by donor IVF. In these women, NIPT is expected to have a suboptimal performance. These women may also be reluctant to undergo invasive testing.
- Screening after co-twin demise or selective fetal reduction.

9.9 Independent Two-Step Screening

In the independent two-step screening method, each patient is offered both the first trimester combined screening test and the quadruple marker test. Each screening test is completely independent of the other, and maternal age is used as the baseline risk for each test. *This screening approach is not recommended.*

9.9.1 Methodology

- First-trimester screening performed as usual with maternal age + NT + PAPP-A + free β-hCG.
- Result of FTS is informed to the patient.
- If the result is screen-positive, CVS, or amniocentesis is offered.
- If the result is screen-negative, a quadruple test is done at 15–22 weeks *with maternal age-related risk considered as the baseline risk*. The results of first-trimester screening are completely disregarded.
- If the quadruple test shows a screen-positive result, CVS, or amniocentesis is offered.
- If the quadruple test is screen-negative, no further testing is done.

9.9.2 Pros and Cons

Repeating the screening test twice slightly improves the DR for Down syndrome. However, the FPR increases significantly, resulting in an unacceptably high number of invasive procedures.

9.10 Concluding Remarks

When Down syndrome screening was introduced, it was fairly straightforward. Women above the age of 35 were offered amniocentesis and those with a normal karyotype were reassured. Multi-step screening models have led to more complex logistics, counseling issues, and legal difficulties. Whichever method a center uses, the protocol must be the same for all patients and documented in writing to avoid medico-legal issues later. Both the physician and the patient must know, that despite using complex protocols, no screening test can be diagnostic. Occasional cases of Down syndrome will still be missed despite diligent screening.

Finally, the protocol followed at our center is as follows:

- Detailed ultrasound at 11–13 + 6 weeks is performed. If any obvious anomaly is detected or NT is >3 mm, invasive testing is offered.
- If the 11–13 + 6 weeks scan is normal, the woman is counseled about Down syndrome screening. If she refuses, no further evaluation is done until the anomaly scan.
- If the woman consents, first-trimester screening is performed with maternal age + NT + nasal bone + PAPP-A + free β-hCG.
- Result of FTS is informed to the woman.
- If the result is screen-positive (risk >1:250), NIPT or CVS or amniocentesis is offered.
- If the result is screen-negative (risk <1:1000), no further evaluation is done.
- If the result is intermediate risk (risk 1:250–1:1000), the woman is counseled and offered a choice between NIPT and contingent serum screening.
- If a high-risk result is obtained in the above step, amniocentesis is performed.
- If a low-risk result is obtained in the above step, no further testing is offered.

As aneuploidy screening is an out-of-pocket expense in India, women in the intermediate risk group are offered a choice between NIPT and contingent serum screening. Overall, very few women require invasive testing. We have found this screening model to work extremely well in our clinical practice.

Importantly, we are able to successfully implement a multi-step protocol, with counseling at each step, because ours is a dedicated fetal medicine unit. Most obstetric units would be better served by performing a single-step screening test, i.e., *either the combined FTS or the quadruple marker test depending on the gestational age at first visit.*

9.11 Key Messages

1. Women who have already undergone combined FTS should not be offered an independent quadruple marker test.
2. Multi-step screening protocols are only suitable for specialized clinics with experienced sonologists and counselors.
3. Contingent screening with NIPT offers a cost-effective option for including cfDNA screening in clinical practice.
4. Using second-trimester soft marker LRs to modify the risk obtained in the combined FTS is no longer recommended.

References

1. Wald NJ, Hackshaw AK, Walters J, Mackinson AM, Rodeck C, Chitty L. First and second trimester antenatal screening for Down's syndrome: the results of the serum, urine and ultrasound screening study (SURUSS). J Med Screen. 2003;10(2):56–104.
2. Wald NJ, Watt HC, Hackshaw AK. Integrated screening for Down's syndrome based on tests performed during the first and second trimesters. N Engl J Med. 1999;341(7):461–7.
3. American College of Obstetricians and Gynecologists' Committee on Practice Bulletins—Obstetrics; Committee on Genetics; Society for Maternal-Fetal Medicine. Screening for fetal chromosomal abnormalities: ACOG practice bulletin, number 226. Obstet Gynecol. 2020;136(4):e48–69.
4. Benn PA, Campbell WA, Zelop CM, Ingardia C, Egan JF. Stepwise sequential screening for fetal aneuploidy. Am J Obstet Gynecol. 2007;197(3):312.e1–5.
5. Wright D, Bradbury I, Benn P, Cuckle H, Ritchie K. Contingent screening for down syndrome is an efficient alternative to non-disclosure sequential screening. Prenat Diagn. 2004;24(10):762–6.
6. Moon MH, Cho JY, Lee YM, Jung SI, Yang JH, Kim MY, Ryu HM, Chung JH, Park SH. First-trimester screening for down syndrome; the role of nasal bone assessment in the Korean population. Prenat Diagn. 2007;27(9):830–4.
7. Falcon O, Faiola S, Huggon I, Allan L, Nicolaides KH. Fetal tricuspid regurgitation at the 11 + 0 to 13 + 6-week scan: association with chromosomal defects and reproducibility of the method. Ultrasound Obstet Gynecol. 2006;27(6):609–12.

8. Geipel A, Willruth A, Vieten J, Gembruch U, Berg C. Nuchal fold thickness, nasal bone absence or hypoplasia, ductus venosus reversed flow and tricuspid valve regurgitation in screening for trisomies 21, 18 and 13 in the early second trimester. Ultrasound Obstet Gynecol. 2010;35(5):535–9.
9. Illa M, Mula R, Arigita M, Grande M, Gonce A, Borobio V, Borrell A. Likelihood ratios to apply for nasal bone, ductus venosus and tricuspid flow at the 11-13 weeks' scan in down syndrome screening. Fetal Diagn Ther. 2013;34(2):116–20.
10. Gil MM, Quezada MS, Revello R, Akolekar R, Nicolaides KH. Analysis of cell-free DNA in maternal blood in screening for fetal aneuploidies: updated meta-analysis. Ultrasound Obstet Gynecol. 2015;45(3):249–66.
11. Nicolaides KH, Syngelaki A, Poon LC, Gil MM, Wright D. First-trimester contingent screening for trisomies 21, 18 and 13 by biomarkers and maternal blood cell-free DNA testing. Fetal Diagn Ther. 2014;35(3):185–92.
12. Aagaard-Tillery KM, Malone FD, Nyberg DA, Porter TF, Cuckle HS, Fuchs K, Sullivan L, Comstock CH, Saade GR, Eddleman K, Gross S, Dugoff L, Craigo SD, Timor-Tritsch IE, Carr SR, Wolfe HM, Bianchi DW, D'Alton ME. First and second trimester evaluation of risk (FASTER) research consortium. Role of second-trimester genetic sonography after down syndrome screening. Obstet Gynecol. 2009;114(6):1189–96.
13. Agathokleous M, Chaveeva P, Poon LC, Kosinski P, Nicolaides KH. Meta-analysis of second-trimester markers for trisomy 21. Ultrasound Obstet Gynecol. 2013;41(3):247–61.
14. Odibo AO, Ghidini A. Role of the second-trimester 'genetic sonogram' for down syndrome screen in the era of first-trimester screening and noninvasive prenatal testing. Prenat Diagn. 2014;34(6):511–7.

Putting It All Together: A Stepwise Approach

10

10.1 Introduction

This chapter provides a stepwise approach to Down syndrome screening in both singleton and multiple pregnancies. It is important to note that the recommendations presented here are based on widely accepted guidelines and are applicable in most settings. However, it is crucial to exercise discretion, as these recommendations may not be entirely suitable for every pregnant woman.

While this chapter may be used as a starting point for the study of this fascinating subject, the reader is urged to read the previous chapters to get a clear understanding of each step. By doing so, they will be better equipped to navigate through the complexities of aneuploidy screening.

10.2 Singleton Pregnancy

Down syndrome screening in singleton pregnancy is a relatively straightforward process, provided proper guidelines are followed. As the screening result is directly influenced by measurements like crown rump length (CRL) and nuchal translucency (NT), even a small error in measurement might put the patient at a risk

© The Author(s), under exclusive license to Springer Nature Singapore Pte Ltd. 2023

A. Kamat, *Down Syndrome Screening*,
https://doi.org/10.1007/978-981-99-7758-1_10

of fetal loss following an unnecessary referral for invasive testing. Nuchal translucency (NT) and nasal bone (NB) require the operator to be trained, certified, and periodically audited. Figure 10.1 illustrates the stepwise screening process in a singleton pregnancy.

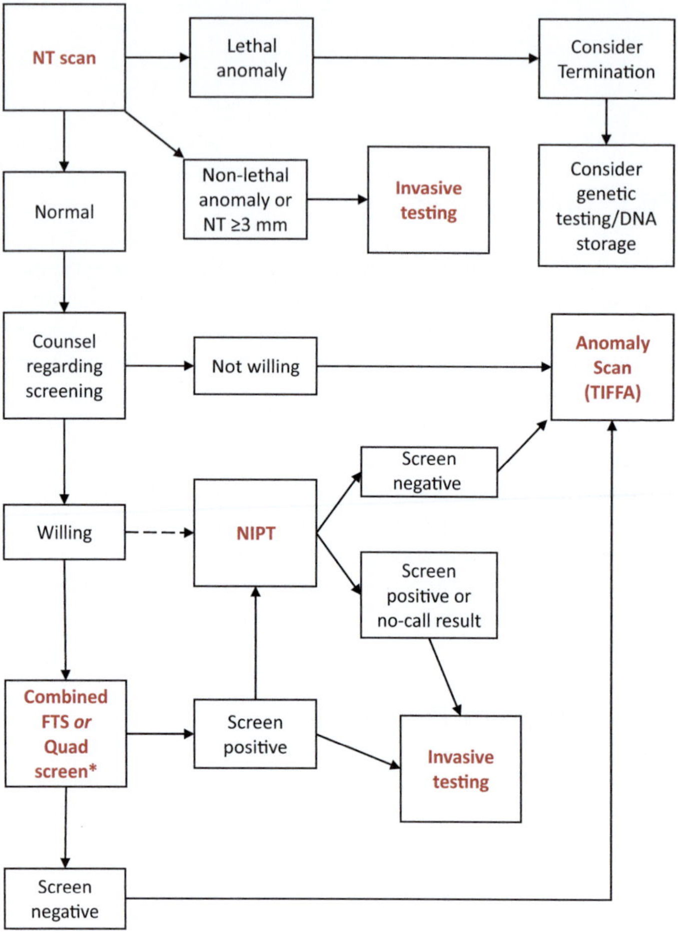

Fig. 10.1 Stepwise screening for aneuploidy in singleton pregnancy. * Note that the Quad screen should not be repeated in women who have already had a combined FTS result

10.2.1 Step 1: The 11–13 + 6 Weeks Scan

- All women should have an ultrasound scan between 11 and 13 + 6 weeks of gestation before aneuploidy screening.
- The ultrasound scan serves to establish or confirm the gestational age.
- Nuchal translucency (NT) measurement is an essential component of a first-trimester combined screening and should be performed strictly in accordance with established guidelines (see Chap. 2).
- If the NT value is above 3 mm, invasive testing should be offered.
- Nasal bone should only be assessed for its presence or absence. NB length should not be measured. NB should be interpreted only as a part of combined screening.
- If significant structural abnormalities are noted at the 11–13+6 weeks scan, invasive testing should be offered.
- The patient may directly opt for termination of pregnancy in case of a severe malformation. Testing of products of conception (POC) by FISH and/or microarray analysis should be offered. Maternal cell contamination is a major concern if karyotyping is performed.
- If invasive testing or testing of POC is being done, DNA storage should be offered. This is inexpensive and retains the fetal sample for future testing. DNA storage offers an additional advantage in situations where immediate genetic counseling may not be practical because of the emotional state of the couple.

10.2.2 Step 2: Before the Screening Test

- No woman should undergo aneuploidy screening without prior counseling (see Chap. 4).
- Counseling should include the following points:
  - The specific conditions being tested for (not 'mental retardation').
  - Age-related risk for the woman.

  - Difference between a screening test and a diagnostic test.
  - Limitations of the test.
  - Procedure following a high-risk result, including invasive tests and noninvasive prenatal test (NIPT).
  - That prenatal screening is optional.

- Details about counseling, along with the woman's choice should be documented in her records.
- If the woman does not wish to undergo aneuploidy screening, she should be offered a targeted anomaly scan at 20 weeks (Step 7).

10.2.3 Step 3: Maternal Serum Screening

- Combined first-trimester screening can be done between 11 and 13 + 6 weeks.
- Quadruple test can be done from 15 to 22 weeks, but is most accurate between 16 and 18 weeks. Quadruple test should not be offered to women who have already undergone combined first-trimester screening, as this significantly increases the false positive rate.
- Blood sample should be collected and shipped expeditiously as per the laboratory requirements (see Chap. 4).
- If the patient is receiving hCG injections, serum screening should be done 2 weeks after the last injection.

10.2.4 Step 4: After the Screening Test

- If screen negative, the woman should be offered a targeted anomaly scan at 20 weeks (Step 7).
- If screen positive, the woman should be offered either NIPT (Step 5) or invasive testing (Step 6), after explaining the pros and cons of both.

- In case intermediate risk is being reported, further testing depends on the institutional policy. If the contingent or integrated serum screening model is being followed, maternal serum is tested again in the second trimester. Otherwise, NIPT is offered (see Chap. 9). The woman may also request to have invasive testing done.

10.2.5 Step 5: Noninvasive Prenatal Testing (NIPT)

- Possibilities of low fetal fraction and no-call result should be explained before testing.
- NIPT is not a diagnostic test. Abnormal or screen-positive results need confirmation by amniocentesis.
- In the absence of structural abnormalities, low-risk NIPT results do not require further evaluation.

10.2.6 Step 6: Invasive Testing (CVS or Amniocentesis)

- Choice between CVS and amniocentesis should be taken individually for each patient depending upon the gestational age, position of the placenta, and the type of genetic test that needs to be performed.
- Both are relatively safe procedures in experienced hands.
- With CVS, the rare possibility of confined placental mosaicism should be explained.
- If invasive testing shows a normal karyotype, the woman should be offered a targeted anomaly scan at 20 weeks (Step 7).

10.2.7 Step 7: Targeted Imaging for Fetal Anomalies (TIFFA)

- A detailed scan should be performed at approximately 20 weeks to evaluate fetal growth and to look for structural malformations.

- A painstaking search for soft markers in low-risk patients is not recommended.
- Routine modification of aneuploidy screening risk with soft markers is not recommended.
- In women who have had a low-risk NIPT report or a normal karyotype, soft markers should not be considered from the point of view of aneuploidy risk. However, soft markers such as echogenic bowel, pyelectasis, ventriculomegaly, and shortening of long bones require follow-up in the third trimester to look for progression or evolution (see Chap. 6).
- Any structural abnormality known to be associated with aneuploidy (e.g., duodenal atresia) requires amniocentesis. Amniocentesis should be offered even if maternal serum screening or NIPT has shown low risk.

10.3 Twin Pregnancies

Screening in twin pregnancies is more complex, less sensitive, and highly dependent on chorionicity. Invasive testing in twins has a slightly higher risk of fetal loss. Thorough knowledge of the intricacies and limitations of screening in twins is necessary prior to embarking on this perilous task (see Chap. 8).

Most recommendations for stepwise screening in singleton pregnancy also apply to twin pregnancies. In this section, the differences between the two are highlighted. Figure 10.2 illustrates the stepwise screening process in twins.

10.3.1 Step 1: The 11–13 + 6 Weeks Scan

- Chorionicity should be definitively established at the 11–13 + 6 weeks scan. If reported earlier, it should be reconfirmed.
- In case of a difference between gestational age estimated from the last menstrual period and USG, gestational age should be assigned according to the CRL of the larger fetus. Dates should not be changed for pregnancies following ART.

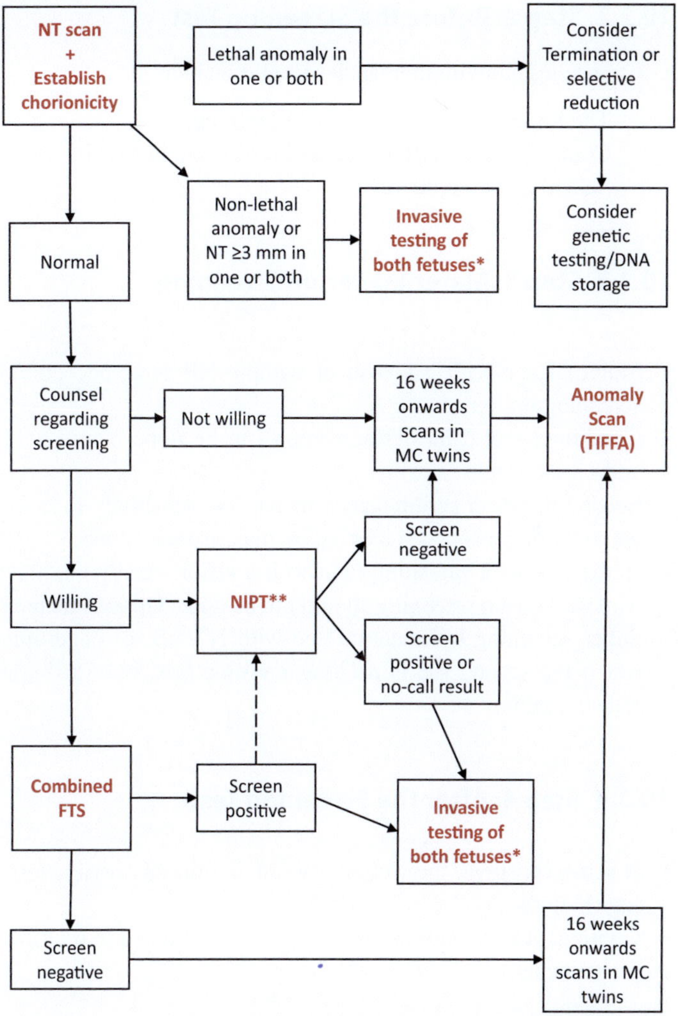

Fig. 10.2 Stepwise screening for aneuploidy in twin pregnancies. * In selected cases of monochorionic (MC) twins concordant for growth and anatomy, single sampling could be considered (see Chap. 8). ** NIPT in twins should be performed with caution, after having carefully considered the limitations

10.3.2 Step 2: Before the Screening Test

- Counseling in twin pregnancies should include:
  - The lower sensitivity of serum screening.
  - Complexities of NIPT and invasive testing in twins.
  - Selective fetal reduction.

10.3.3 Step 3: Maternal Serum Screening

- Maternal age with NT with or without NB is an acceptable screening option.
- Combined first-trimester screening can be done between 11 and 13 + 6 weeks.
- Second-trimester serum screening has low sensitivity in twins and only outperforms screening by maternal age alone.
- In the case of a vanishing twin with a visible fetal pole, first-trimester serum screening should not be done. Options include either screening by maternal age with NT/NB, or quadruple test if the second sac is no longer visible (i.e., only a single fetus remains).

10.3.4 Step 4: After the Screening Test

- If screen positive, the woman should be offered invasive testing (Step 6).
- Contingent or sequential screening is not validated in multiple pregnancies.

10.3.5 Step 5: Noninvasive Prenatal Testing (NIPT)

- Cell-free DNA screening should be performed with caution in twins after explaining its limitations.
- NIPT should not be performed for sex chromosome aneuploidies, rare autosomal trisomies, or submicroscopic abnormalities.

- NGS-based NIPT should not be offered in the presence of a vanishing fetus or in multiple pregnancies following a donor egg IVF cycle.
- A screen-positive NIPT result requires amniocentesis with the sampling of both sacs.

10.3.6 Step 6: Invasive Testing

- Decision-making in twins is complex. Issues like CVS versus amniocentesis and single versus double sampling need to be discussed.
- Labeling of twins prior to invasive testing should be unambiguous.
- Monochorionic (MC) twins may rarely have discordant genetic profiles.
- Fetal loss rate is expected to be slightly higher compared to singleton pregnancies.
- Double sampling should be offered in dichorionic (DC) twins.
- In MC twins, single versus double sampling should be discussed.

10.3.7 Step 7: Targeted Imaging for Fetal Anomalies (TIFFA)

- In DC twins, a detailed scan should be performed between 18 and 20 weeks to evaluate fetal growth and to look for structural malformations.
- MC twins should be evaluated and followed up as per current guidelines.
- Modification of aneuploidy risk by ultrasound soft markers is not recommended.

10.4 Higher Order Multiples

- First-trimester screening should be done using maternal age with NT.
- Assessment of NB, ductus venosus, and tricuspid valve improve the sensitivity of screening. A high degree of error is expected when these markers are evaluated without formal training, certification, and audit.
- Maternal serum screening and NIPT should not be performed in higher order multiples.
- Serum screening and NIPT should not be performed after selective fetal reduction to twins or singleton.

Special Situations in Aneuploidy Screening

11

11.1 Introduction

Prenatal screening is a valuable tool for the detection of Down syndrome and other aneuploidies. There are certain situations which require the screening protocols to be modified in order to be effective. This chapter focuses on the special situations in aneuploidy testing, including a previous affected child with Down syndrome, intrauterine growth restriction (IUGR), and presence of an anomaly. Other topics discussed are screening in pregnancies following assisted reproduction, preimplantation genetic testing, and testing of products of conception.

11.2 Previous Baby with Down Syndrome

A woman with a previous Down syndrome baby is often hesitant to attempt another pregnancy out of fear of giving birth to another affected child. With the currently available prenatal tests, it is possible to rule out aneuploidy in the subsequent pregnancies with a reasonable degree of accuracy.

© The Author(s), under exclusive license to Springer Nature Singapore Pte Ltd. 2023
A. Kamat, *Down Syndrome Screening*,
https://doi.org/10.1007/978-981-99-7758-1_11

11.2.1 Work Up for a Subsequent Pregnancy

- The index child should be examined by a clinical geneticist. At times, this may lead to the discovery of another reason for the child's subnormal intelligence rather than Down syndrome.
- Obtaining the karyotype of the index child is mandatory, even if the child has typical features of Down syndrome. The genetic basis of Down syndrome determines the need for parental testing, the recurrence risk, and the testing in subsequent pregnancies.
- If the index child's karyotype shows a translocation, both parents should be subjected to karyotyping.

This workup should ideally be performed in the pre-conceptional period as it gives adequate time for genetic counseling, decision-making, and parental testing. However, many women present directly in the first trimester, leading to time constraints for each step.

11.2.2 Nondisjunction Down Syndrome (Free Trisomy 21)

Nondisjunction Down syndrome in the index child is diagnosed when the karyotype shows 3 copies of chromosome 21. Recurrence risk for free trisomy 21 (as also for trisomy 13 and 18) is 1%.

In the subsequent pregnancy, all screening options should be discussed, viz., maternal serum screening, noninvasive prenatal testing (NIPT), and amniocentesis. *For maternal serum screening, the baseline (*a priori*) risk for screening is assumed to be recurrence risk (1%) or maternal age risk, whichever is higher.* As the detection rate of serum screening is significantly lower, most couples opt for either NIPT or amniocentesis. A familial tendency for nondisjunction of chromosome 21 has also been reported [1].

11.2.3 Translocation Down Syndrome

Translocation Down syndrome usually results from one parent having a balanced translocation (see Chap. 1). When one parent is a Robertsonian translocation carrier, the recurrence risk is determined by the carrier parent's sex and the specific chromosome involved. The risk of recurrence is 10–15% if the mother is a rob(14q;21q) carrier, and 5% if the father is a rob(14q;21q) carrier. When the parental translocation is (21q;21q), the recurrence risk is 100%, as all their gametes are unbalanced. In most cases, however, the Robertsonian translocation occurs de novo, with both parents having a normal karyotype. The recurrence risk in this setting is approximately 2–3% [2].

When a parent has a translocation, invasive testing should be offered in all subsequent pregnancies. This is because of the high risk of recurrence and the limited sensitivity of prenatal screening. As mentioned in Chap. 1, translocation may rarely be limited to the gonads in one parent, and peripheral blood cells may show a normal karyotype [3]. Hence, the option of definitive invasive testing must never be denied to parents of an affected child, even if their own blood karyotype is normal.

11.2.4 Mosaic Down Syndrome

Mosaic Down syndrome is thought to occur purely by chance. The risk of recurrence is the same or lower than free trisomy 21, and the guidelines for testing in subsequent pregnancies are also the same.

11.3 Fetal Growth Restriction and Aneuploidy

Fetal growth restriction (FGR) is one of the commonest problems that an obstetrician deals with. Out of all cases of FGR, only 8% have an underlying genetic etiology, half of them being trisomy 18,13, 21, and triploidy. Besides aneuploidy, FGR can be caused by deletions or duplications, single-gene disorders, and epigenetic expression changes. Most genetically abnormal fetuses also have structural abnormalities which provide a clue as to the etiology of FGR. Furthermore, these fetuses typically show growth restriction beginning in the first half of pregnancy [4, 5].

Genetic abnormalities in structurally normal fetuses with FGR can be difficult to suspect prenatally. A classic example is Down syndrome. Down syndrome fetuses often develop a growth lag in the second half of pregnancy. Other signs, like placental calcification, reduced liquor, and abnormal Doppler do not differ from other causes of FGR.

Even in cases of isolated FGR with a normal karyotype, submicroscopic deletions or duplications can be present in 4% of cases [4]. These can only be detected if chromosomal microarray analysis (CMA) is performed on the amniotic fluid sample. The disadvantage of performing CMA in FGR is the possibility of detecting variants of unknown significance (VOUS). These are unusual copy number variants that have not been specifically mapped to any known human disorder. When VOUS are detected in the setting of an otherwise isolated FGR, counseling becomes very difficult.

11.3.1 Indications for Genetic Testing

Fetal growth restriction is a common problem, while genetic abnormalities are extremely rare. Therefore, performing invasive testing in every case of FGR is hardly justifiable. The International Federation of Gynecology and Obstetrics (FIGO) recommends that karyotype or CMA may be offered when one or more of the following conditions are met [6]:

- Early-onset severe FGR (estimated fetal weight < third percentile).
- Presence of ultrasound findings associated with a genetic abnormality.
- When obvious signs of placental dysfunction are absent.
- When a genetic diagnosis will change the management.

Even in cases which do not meet the above criteria, the possibility of a genetic etiology cannot be eliminated. But, the yield of pathogenic findings and benefits of testing are likely to be low. Finally, in structurally normal fetuses with late-onset FGR (after 32 weeks), a genetic etiology is extremely unlikely [7].

11.4 Fetus with a Structural Malformation

Structural malformations may be detected either at the 11–14 weeks scan or, more likely, at the time of the anomaly scan. Genetic testing of the fetus should be offered if the malformation is known to be associated with a genetic abnormality. Table 11.1 gives a system-wise list of commonly detected anomalies and their probability of being associated with a chromosomal abnormality, when present as an isolated finding.

Genetic testing of an anomalous fetus has several benefits. In non-lethal malformations, it helps the couple to decide regarding termination or continuation of pregnancy. Even in lethal anomalies, genetic testing helps in counseling about recurrence risk and the need for parental testing.

The commonest genetic defects seen in malformed fetuses are trisomy 13, 18, and 21. Sex chromosomal abnormalities, triploidy, microdeletions, and microduplications can also have congenital abnormalities as part of the phenotype. Some malformations have a polygenic or multifactorial origin, and in more than half the cases, no specific cause can be detected. Multiple anomalies increase the risk of associated chromosomal abnormalities.

Combined first-trimester screening, quadruple marker test, and NIPT screen for common trisomies, but they are not diagnostic tests. Also, their scope is limited to the common trisomies. Invasive testing is mandatory if the couple opts for genetic testing in the presence of an anomaly [8]. CMA is better than karyotyping in anomalous fetuses; it detects 6% additional pathogenic findings [9]. FISH can quickly diagnose common aneuploidies and is useful when gestational age is advanced.

Table 11.1 Structural malformations and their risk of association with chromosomal abnormalities

System	High risk of chromosomal abnormalities	Low risk of chromosomal abnormalities (when isolated)
1. Brain and spine	Blake's pouch cyst Cephalocele Cerebellar abnormalities Corpus callosum agenesis Holoprosencephaly Macrocephaly Microcephaly Open spina bifida Ventriculomegaly	Absent septum pellucidum Acrania Arachnoid cyst Choroid plexus cysts Closed spinal dysraphism Hemimegaloencephaly Hydranencephaly Lissencephaly Porencephalic cyst Sacrococcygeal teratoma Schizencephaly Septo-optic dysplasia Vein of Galen aneurysm Mega cisterna magna
2. Face and neck	Anophthalmia/ Microphthalmia Cystic hygroma Ear abnormalities (difficult to detect) Facial clefts Hypotelorism Micrognathia Nasal abnormalities Nuchal edema	Cataract Congenital high airway obstruction syndrome* Dacryocystocele Epignathus Goiter Hypertelorism* Isolated unilateral cleft lip
3. Thorax	Diaphragmatic hernia Pleural effusion	Bronchogenic cyst Congenital pulmonary airway malformation Pulmonary agenesis Pulmonary sequestration

Table 11.1 (continued)

System	High risk of chromosomal abnormalities	Low risk of chromosomal abnormalities (when isolated)
4. Heart	Absent pulmonary valve syndrome Aberrant right subclavian artery Aortic arch abnormalities Aortic coarctation Atrioventricular septal defect Common arterial trunk Double-outlet right ventricle Hypoplastic left heart syndrome Pulmonary atresia with ventricular septal defect Tetralogy of Fallot Ventricular septal defect	Anomalous pulmonary venous connection Aortic stenosis Cardiac tumors Ebstein's anomaly Pulmonary stenosis Pulmonary atresia with intact ventricular septum Situs abnormalities Transposition of the great arteries Tricuspid dysplasia/atresia
5. Limbs	Arthrogryposis Clinodactyly Clubhands Ectrodactyly Polydactyly Syndactyly	Limb reduction defects* Skeletal dysplasia* Talipes
6. Abdominal wall	Omphalocele	Bladder or cloacal exstrophy Body stalk anomaly Gastroschisis
7. Gastrointestinal tract	Anorectal atresia Duodenal atresia Esophageal atresia	Abdominal cyst Small bowel atresia

(continued)

Table 11.1 (continued)

System	High risk of chromosomal abnormalities	Low risk of chromosomal abnormalities (when isolated)
8. Urogenital system	Ambiguous genitalia Urethral obstruction and megacystis	Horseshoe kidney Hydronephrosis Multicystic kidneys* Pelvic kidney Pelviureteral junction obstruction Polycystic kidneys* Renal agenesis Ureterovesical junction obstruction Urogenital sinus
9. Systemic	Hydrops	

Anomalies marked with an asterisk (*) may still be associated with non-chromosomal syndromes or single gene mutations.

In case of lethal anomalies, the couple may opt to terminate the pregnancy immediately. In such cases, CMA can be performed by sending a one-inch square full-thickness biopsy of the fetal skin along with placental biopsy (Sect. 11.7.2). CMA is preferred over karyotype because of the risk of maternal contamination during culture. Often, the emotional state of the couple may not permit immediate genetic counseling. Here, DNA storage is an excellent and an inexpensive option which should be offered. The opportunity to test the affected fetus is forever lost if DNA has not been stored.

11.5 Assisted Reproductive Technology (ART) and Aneuploidy

ART encompasses all fertility treatments in which either eggs or embryos are handled. In this section, we discuss the link between ART and aneuploidy, and the subtleties of screening such pregnancies.

11.5.1 Effect of ART Procedures on Incidence of Aneuploidy

ART is associated with a higher incidence of structural malformations and chromosomal abnormalities [10–12]. Advanced maternal age and twinning rate partly account for this observation. Couples with male subfertility or a history of recurrent pregnancy loss are also more likely to carry genetic mutations. Finally, a low oocyte yield or a poor fertilization rate may necessitate the transfer of a lower grade embryo, increasing the chance of an aneuploid pregnancy. (It is important to note, however, that the morphological grade of an embryo does not always correlate with its genetic constitution.) ART procedures like intracytoplasmic sperm injection (ICSI) or assisted hatching do not damage the embryo or increase the risk of aneuploidy [12, 13].

11.5.2 Considerations in Screening Pregnancies Conceived through ART

Maternal serum markers: Maternal serum markers are altered in pregnancies conceived by ART, with an increase in hCG and inhibin A levels, and a reduction in PAPP-A and estriol levels [14]. The software for risk calculation can apply correction factors based on the type of conception. It is the responsibility of the clinician to note this correctly on the requisition form.

Self-IVF and screening: Women undergoing IVF are older, and therefore more likely to give birth to a child with Down syndrome. Given the difficulty with which they have conceived, most women are reluctant to undergo invasive testing. These issues must be discussed and documented prior to offering a screening test. Irrespective of her age, it is perfectly acceptable if a woman declines aneuploidy screening. In women undergoing frozen transfer, the *maternal age on the day of the ovum pickup* (OPU) should be considered for screening, regardless of when the ET occurs. It is important to remember that cryopreserved oocytes and embryos do not age. *Gestational age should always be calcu-*

lated from the ET date. Maternal serum screening and noninvasive prenatal screening (NIPS) can be performed as in other women.

Donor eggs and sperm: Errors frequently occur when serum screening is performed in women who have undergone IVF using donor egg. *In such cases, the age of the donor on the day of donor OPU should be considered as 'maternal age' for screening purpose, and not that of the pregnant woman.* Gestational age should be calculated from ET, as in the case of self-IVF.

NIPT measures the total cell-free DNA in maternal blood, 90% of which is maternal in origin. Out of the fetal fraction, half the DNA is expected to resemble that of the mother. Hence, the performance of NIPT is significantly lower in pregnancies arising from donor egg IVF, and especially so in twin pregnancies (see Chap. 5). The source of the sperm does not affect aneuploidy screening. In pregnancies where donor sperm is used, serum screening and NIPT can be performed as usual.

Screening in women receiving hCG injections: Women in ART programs may receive hCG injections as a part of luteal phase support. Such treatment may be continued into the first trimester, and can interfere with combined screening, which uses β-hCG. Since hCG takes 10 days to get cleared from maternal blood, screening should not be performed within 2 weeks of receiving the last injection.

Multiple pregnancy: Multiple pregnancies frequently occur after ART, making aneuploidy screening a complex procedure. Intricacies of screening in multiple pregnancies are elaborated in Chap. 8.

11.6 Preimplantation Genetic Testing (PGT)

Preimplantation genetic testing (PGT) refers to the evaluation of the genetic makeup of each embryo before transfer. The origins of PGT trace back to the 1990s when it was used as an experimental procedure for sex selection and for identifying monogenic diseases. PGT involves close coordination between several units, including the embryology unit, embryo biopsy unit, cryopreservation unit, and genetic laboratory. The genetic laboratory should be close to the IVF unit, especially if rapid fluorescence in situ hybridization (FISH) is to be performed. Since PGT encompasses far more than testing for Down syndrome, it is discussed in a slightly broader context.

11.6.1 Indications for PGT

Routine PGT in all women undergoing IVF has not been shown to improve outcomes [15]. It may be considered in the following situations:

- One or both partners are carriers for a genetic abnormality.
- Family history of inheritable chromosomal abnormalities or hereditary cancer syndromes.

PGT has also been tried in cases of repeated implantation failures and recurrent pregnancy losses, but there is a lack of evidence as to whether this improves outcomes.

11.6.2 Embryo Biopsy for PGT

- The embryos are cultured with individual culture drop technique and not group embryo culture technique.
- Cumulus is meticulously removed.
- An opening is created in the zona pellucida either by mechanical drilling, chemical drilling (acid Tyrode's solution), or laser.
- Cells to be tested are removed by aspiration, extrusion, flow displacement, or single-needle biopsy technique.
- Cells are fixed on slides for aneuploidy testing using FISH. For testing monogenetic disorders, the cells are directly transferred to PCR tubes.

PGT can be performed by either polar body biopsy, day-3 cleavage stage biopsy, or blastocyst stage biopsy [16].

Polar body biopsy: Polar bodies are byproducts of oogenesis (see Chap. 1). Polar body biopsy can be performed either simultaneously or sequentially. Simultaneous biopsy involves removing both polar bodies concurrently. In a sequential biopsy, the second polar body is removed after assessing fertilization.

Polar body biopsy is relatively less invasive and permits an ET in the same cycle. Disadvantages include the time-consuming nature of the process, the inability to sample the paternal genetic contribution, and the higher likelihood of errors. Also, it is crucial to time the biopsy correctly. An early biopsy can damage spindle remnants, while degeneration of the polar body is likely if it is performed too late.

Cleavage stage biopsy: This is performed on day 3 embryos with at least six blastomeres. Thawed frozen embryos can also be biopsied, similar to fresh embryos. Meiotic errors in both gametes can be detected. Embryo transfer is possible in the same cycle, either on day 4 or at the blastocyst stage.

The disadvantage of this technique is the risk of embryo damage, reducing the number of viable blastocysts available for transfer. Mosaicism is also a concern, since a single embryo can have genetically distinct cell lines. Mosaicism is relatively more common in day-3 embryos, even in those that subsequently result in a normal baby. Presumably, the abnormal cell lines get filtered out in the later stages of development. Despite this, cleavage-stage biopsy remains a popular technique today.

Blastocyst stage biopsy: Blastocyst biopsy can be performed on day 5 or day 6 embryos. It involves the sampling of cells of the trophectoderm with or without the cells of the inner cell mass. This technique allows for morphological screening of blastocyst grade before selecting blastocysts for biopsy. Furthermore, a larger number of cells are available for testing.

One drawback is the potential occurrence of mosaicism between the cells found in the trophectoderm and those present in the inner cell mass. Also, fresh transfer is usually not possible because of the time taken for genetic testing. Survival of embryos after freeze-thaw cycle is lower after blastocyst biopsy compared to unbiopsied embryos. Still, this technique remains the most accurate of the three and is gradually replacing the other two [16].

11.6.3 Genetic Testing of Embryos

Once the embryo has been biopsied, there are three types of genetic tests that can be performed, depending on the indication for testing.

Preimplantation genetic testing for monogenic disorders (PGT-M): PGT-M was earlier known as *preimplantation genetic diagnosis (PGD).* This form of testing is used when the couple is known to carry a genetic defect, which needs to be ruled out in the embryo. The test is only for a specific mutation (e.g., spinal muscular atrophy, cystic fibrosis, or some hereditary cancer syndromes).

Preimplantation genetic testing for structural rearrangements (PGT-S): This is used to detect structural rearrangements within the chromosomes. It cannot detect balanced translocations.

Preimplantation genetic testing for aneuploidy (PGT-A): PGT-A was earlier known as *preimplantation genetic screening (PGS).* By using PGT-A, embryos can be screened for whole chromosome abnormalities, such as monosomy or trisomy. Since few cells are available for testing, DNA amplification is needed. Array comparative genomic hybridization and next-generation sequencing are used for this purpose. FISH can be also used if only a few chromosomes (e.g., chromosomes 13,18, and 21) are to be tested.

11.6.4 Noninvasive Preimplantation Genetic Testing (niPGT)

Noninvasive preimplantation genetic testing for aneuploidy (niPGT-A) represents the latest advance in screening embryos for aneuploidy before transfer. Two techniques are used to obtain DNA without removing any cells from the blastocyst.

Blastocentesis involves the aspiration of fluid from the blastocoel cavity with an ICSI needle to get fragments of DNA for testing. This technique is less invasive than an embryo biopsy.

Spent culture medium PGT (niPGT-SCM) involves testing of the medium in which the embryo has been cultured. Nucleic acids can cross the zona pellucida, but the exact mechanism by which the embryo ejects DNA into the culture medium is currently unknown. Some researchers claim that niPGT-A using spent culture medium is more reliable than blastocyst trophoectoderm biopsy [17]. However, these claims are yet to be verified in larger prospective trials.

Some limitations of niPGT are:

1. A large proportion of the DNA obtained comes from apoptotic cells and is therefore partially degraded and of poor quality.
2. Embryonic cells undergo a process called 'euploidization,' by which a mosaic cell ejects the abnormal DNA to become euploid. Both the blastocoel fluid and SCM contain higher proportion of these abnormal DNA bits compared to the embryo itself.
3. Current DNA amplification, sequencing, and bioinformatics systems are designed for prenatal samples (where a larger amount of genetic material is available). The number of false positives and false negatives is higher when the same are extrapolated to niPGT.

11.6.5 Prenatal Aneuploidy Screening Following Euploid ET

When PGT-M has been performed, confirmation by CVS or amniocentesis is strongly recommended. If PGT-A or niPGT-A were employed for universal screening of embryos prior to transfer, prenatal aneuploidy screening should be offered, but with cautious interpretation. The following broad guidelines can be followed [18]:

- PGT is still an evolving field, and a detailed counseling of the couple prior to screening is important.
- 11–13 + 6 weeks scan is recommended.

- There are two reasons why maternal serum screening should not be offered in pregnancies following PGT and euploid embryo transfer. First, the screening algorithms are based on maternal age-related risk, and not that following a euploid embryo transfer. Second, PGT is highly sensitive compared to serum screening.
- NIPT may be considered after proper counseling.
- If the 11–13 + 6 weeks scan shows a structural abnormality or raised NT, invasive testing should be offered.

11.6.6 Prenatal Aneuploidy Screening Following Mosaic ET

Diagnostic methods like NGS have led to more frequent detection of embryonic mosaicism with PGT. Some couples may opt for mosaic ET when euploid embryos are not available. Over 100 healthy children have been born following such transfers. Normal outcomes have been attributed to the segregation of the euploid and aneuploid cell lines; the euploid cells form the embryo, and the aneuploid cells either form the placenta or undergo apoptosis. Nevertheless, a normal outcome is not guaranteed, and thorough counseling and documentation are mandatory before mosaic ET [19].

The following points should be noted regarding prenatal aneuploidy testing in pregnancies achieved with mosaic ET [18]:

- 11–13 + 6 weeks scan is recommended.
- Neither maternal serum screening nor NIPT should be offered.
- CVS should not be offered because of the possibility of placental mosaicism.
- Amniocentesis with karyotyping is recommended in all cases.

11.7 Testing Products of Conception

Genetic testing of products of conception (POC) is a valuable diagnostic tool in pregnancies that have ended in a miscarriage or stillbirth, or have been terminated because of structural malformations. POC testing involves analyzing samples from embryonic tissue, placenta, umbilical cord, or the fetus. The purpose is to identify a genetic cause and predict the likelihood of its recurrence in future pregnancies.

11.7.1 Recurrent Pregnancy Loss

While a comprehensive discussion on recurrent pregnancy loss (RPL) is beyond the scope of this book, it is briefly explained below in the context of genetic testing:

- Sterile and gentle collection of the sample is essential.
- The POC should be washed in saline to remove clots and maternal contamination.
- If villi are identifiable, they should be sent for testing. If not, the entire POC can be sent after thorough rinsing.
- The sample should ideally be sent to the lab in a transport medium. If not available, it can be transported in saline or lactated Ringer's solution supplemented with a few drops of an antibiotic.
- Alcohol or formalin should not be used.
- The sample should not be frozen. It can be stored at 4–8 degrees Celsius until transportation. Immediate transport to the laboratory is desirable.
- If DNA-based test like QFPCR or microarray is ordered, maternal blood (4 ml in an EDTA bulb) should be sent for maternal cell contamination (MCC) testing.
- Correct labeling and sending a detailed clinical history are mandatory.

Testing of POC is often performed in couples with RPL when other causes have been ruled out. Though its role in improving outcomes in these women is debatable, it helps to explain the cause of miscarriage in half of the cases. It also helps to identify the subgroup of couples with unexplained RPL who may benefit from expectant management versus PGT [20].

The sample sent for testing in RPL is usually the POC from a failed early pregnancy. A large proportion of the cells are already in the dying phase, and failed culture results are common. As the decidual cells are more viable, they get enriched during culture, resulting in MCC. When a culture-based test like karyotype is performed, it may represent the cells of the mother rather than the POC, especially when the result shows two X chromosomes. Therefore, when testing POC in cases of RPL, the ideal test is CMA + FISH + MCC testing.

11.7.2 Abortus with Structural Malformations

Genetic testing should be offered when the fetus has a malformation with a possible genetic etiology. When there are severe malformations, the woman may choose to have the pregnancy terminated immediately without prenatal genetic testing. In such cases, testing of the abortus can still be offered. The following points should be noted:

- In a fetus with a complex malformation or skeletal dysplasia, an x-ray fetogram and autopsy are as important as genetic testing. High-throughput sequencing techniques (e.g., exome sequencing) generate a vast amount of genetic data. It is difficult to interpret this data without knowing the complete phenotype of the abortus. Variants of unknown significance (VOUS) are genetic mutations which may or may not produce a clinical effect in the individual. Without a clearly defined phenotype, it is impossible to label VOUS as pathological variants.
- Like POC, contamination should be avoided while sending the sample for testing.
- Biopsy should be taken from the fetal arm or thigh. The biopsy site should be cleaned with saline. Depending on the gestational age, a 0.5–1 square inch of full-thickness skin biopsy (including subcutaneous fat) is optimum. The sample should be rinsed in saline before being sent to the laboratory.
- A full-thickness placental biopsy of a similar size can be sent along *in a separate container.*

- The sample should be sent to the lab in a transport medium, or in saline or lactated Ringer's solution supplemented with an antibiotic.
- Alcohol or formalin should not be used.
- The sample should not be frozen. It can be stored at 4–8 degrees Celsius until transportation.
- If DNA-based test like QFPCR or microarray are ordered, maternal blood (4 ml in a purple-top EDTA bulb) should be sent for MCC testing.
- Correct labeling is mandatory. Clinical history and reports should accompany the sample. Details of previous affected pregnancies, all antenatal ultrasounds and x-ray fetogram (if available) should be sent.
- The findings of fetal autopsy should be informed to the genetic laboratory as soon as available. If the autopsy results are available after the genetic report has already been released, it should still be intimated to the laboratory. The autopsy findings can help in the reinterpretation of genotype, including reclassification of a variant from a VOUS to a pathogenic variant.

Structural malformations can be associated with mutations which are too small to be detected by karyotype or microarray. DNA should be stored as a precautionary measure, especially when initial testing identifies no abnormalities. This allows for the possibility of conducting advanced tests, like exome sequencing.

11.8 Key Messages

1. A detailed genetic workup of the index child including karyotyping is mandatory.
2. If the index child shows a translocation Down syndrome, parental testing followed by invasive testing in subsequent pregnancies should be offered.

3. For women with a previous child having free trisomy 21, the baseline (a priori) risk for screening is assumed to be recurrence risk (1%) or maternal age risk, whichever is higher.
4. Genetic testing of a growth-restricted fetus is likely to have a greater yield in the presence of structural malformations and absence of other signs of placental dysfunction.
5. Fetuses with structural malformations known to be associated with aneuploidy should undergo invasive testing. NIPT or maternal serum screening should not be offered.
6. In IVF with frozen ET, the maternal age on the day of the OPU should be considered for screening. Gestational age should be calculated from the ET date.
7. In donor-egg IVF, the age of the donor on the day of OPU should be considered as 'maternal age' for screening purposes.
8. Maternal serum screening should not be performed in structurally normal fetuses following a euploid ET. If anomalies are present, invasive testing should be offered.
9. Amniocentesis with karyotyping should be done for all pregnancies following a mosaic embryo transfer.
10. When testing products of conception, the ideal test is CMA + FISH + MCC testing.
11. DNA storage should be offered in abortuses with structural malformations.

Acknowledgment The author thanks Dr. Chandan Salunke for sharing his insights on PGT.

References

1. Gair JL, Arbour L, Rupps R, Jiang R, Bruyère H, Robinson WP. Recurrent trisomy 21: four cases in three generations. Clin Genet. 2005;68(5):430–5.
2. Kolgeci S, Kolgeci J, Azemi M, Shala-Beqiraj R, Gashi Z, Sopjani M. Cytogenetic study in children with down syndrome among kosova Albanian population between 2000 and 2010. Mater Sociomed. 2013;25(2):131–5.

3. Kovaleva NV. Germ-line transmission of trisomy 21: data from 80 families suggest an implication of grandmaternal age and a high frequency of female-specific trisomy rescue. Mol Cytogenet. 2010;3:7.
4. Wu X, He S, Li Y, Guo D, Chen X, Liang B, Wang M, Huang H, Xu L. Fetal genetic findings by chromosomal microarray analysis and karyotyping for fetal growth restriction without structural malformations at a territory referral center: 10-year experience. BMC Pregnancy Childbirth. 2023;23(1):73.
5. Meler E, Sisterna S, Borrell A. Genetic syndromes associated with isolated fetal growth restriction. Prenat Diagn. 2020;40(4):432–46.
6. Melamed N, Baschat A, Yinon Y, Athanasiadis A, Mecacci F, Figueras F, Berghella V, Nazareth A, Tahlak M, McIntyre HD, Da Silva CF, Kihara AB, Hadar E, McAuliffe F, Hanson M, Ma RC, Gooden R, Sheiner E, Kapur A, Divakar H, Ayres-de-Campos D, Hiersch L, Poon LC, Kingdom J, Romero R, Hod M. FIGO (international Federation of Gynecology and obstetrics) initiative on fetal growth: best practice advice for screening, diagnosis, and management of fetal growth restriction. Int J Gynaecol Obstet. 2021;152(Suppl 1):3–57.
7. Peng R, Yang J, Xie HN, Lin MF, Zheng J. Chromosomal and subchromosomal anomalies associated to small for gestational age fetuses with no additional structural anomalies. Prenat Diagn. 2017;37(12):1219–24.
8. Benachi A, Letourneau A, Kleinfinger P, Senat MV, Gautier E, Favre R, Bidat L, Houfflin-Debarge V, Bouyer J, Costa JM, Collaborative SEquençage a Haut Debit et Aneuploidies (SEHDA) Study Group. Cell-free DNA analysis in maternal plasma in cases of fetal abnormalities detected on ultrasound examination. Obstet Gynecol. 2015;125(6):1330–7.
9. Wapner RJ, Martin CL, Levy B, Ballif BC, Eng CM, Zachary JM, Savage M, Platt LD, Saltzman D, Grobman WA, Klugman S, Scholl T, Simpson JL, McCall K, Aggarwal VS, Bunke B, Nahum O, Patel A, Lamb AN, Thom EA, Beaudet AL, Ledbetter DH, Shaffer LG, Jackson L. Chromosomal microarray versus karyotyping for prenatal diagnosis. N Engl J Med. 2012;367(23):2175–84.
10. Boulet SL, Kirby RS, Reefhuis J, Zhang Y, Sunderam S, Cohen B, Bernson D, Copeland G, Bailey MA, Jamieson DJ, Kissin DM, States Monitoring Assisted Reproductive Technology (SMART) Collaborative. Assisted Reproductive Technology and Birth Defects Among Liveborn Infants in Florida, Massachusetts, and Michigan, 2000–2010. JAMA Pediatr. 2016;170(6):e154934.
11. Lv H, Diao F, Du J, Chen T, Meng Q, Ling X, Li H, Song C, Xi Q, Jiang Y, Xu Y, Tao S, Huang L, Wen M, Peng M, Liu C, Lu Q, He Y, Yin Y, Liu X, Xu B, Han X, Zhou K, Jiang T, Zhao Y, Ma H, Jin G, Xia Y, Liu J, Lin Y, Hu Z, Shen H. Assisted reproductive technology and birth defects in a Chinese birth cohort study. Lancet Reg Health West Pac. 2021;7:100090.

12. Hansen M, Kurinczuk JJ, Milne E, de Klerk N, Bower C. Assisted reproductive technology and birth defects: a systematic review and meta-analysis. Hum Reprod Update. 2013;19(4):330–53.
13. Jwa J, Jwa SC, Kuwahara A, Yoshida A, Saito H. Risk of major congenital anomalies after assisted hatching: analysis of three-year data from the national assisted reproduction registry in Japan. Fertil Steril. 2015;104(1):71–8.
14. Lambert-Messerlian G, Dugoff L, Vidaver J, Canick JA, Malone FD, Ball RH, et al. First- and second-trimester down syndrome screening markers in pregnancies achieved through assisted reproductive technologies (ART): a FASTER trial study. Prenat Diagn. 2006;26(8):672–8.
15. Harper JC, Aittomäki K, Borry P, Cornel MC, de Wert G, Dondorp W, Geraedts J, Gianaroli L, Ketterson K, Liebaers I, Lundin K, Mertes H, Morris M, Pennings G, Sermon K, Spits C, Soini S, Van APA M, Veiga A, Vermeesch JR, Viville S, Macek M Jr, on behalf of the European Society of Human Reproduction and Embryology and European Society of Human Genetics. Recent developments in genetics and medically assisted reproduction: from research to clinical applications. Eur J Hum Genet. 2018;26(1):12–33.
16. ESHRE PGT Consortium and SIG-Embryology Biopsy Working Group, Kokkali G, Coticchio G, Bronet F, Celebi C, Cimadomo D, Goossens V, Liss J, Nunes S, Sfontouris I, Vermeulen N, Zakharova E, De Rycke M. ESHRE PGT consortium and SIG embryology good practice recommendations for polar body and embryo biopsy for PGT. Hum Reprod Open. 2020;2020(3):hoaa020.
17. Huang L, Bogale B, Tang Y, Lu S, Xie XS, Racowsky C. Noninvasive preimplantation genetic testing for aneuploidy in spent medium may be more reliable than trophectoderm biopsy. Proc Natl Acad Sci U S A. 2019;116(28):14105–12.
18. Zwingerman R, Langlois S, Committee Opinion No. 406. Prenatal testing after IVF with preimplantation genetic testing for aneuploidy. J Obstet Gynaecol Can. 2020;42(11):1437–1443.e1.
19. Abhari S, Kawwass JF. Pregnancy and neonatal outcomes after transfer of mosaic embryos: a review. J Clin Med. 2021;10(7):1369.
20. Dahdouh EM, Kutteh WH. Genetic testing of products of conception in recurrent pregnancy loss evaluation. Reprod Biomed Online. 2021;43(1):120–6.

Case Studies: Decision-Making in Practice 12

12.1 Introduction

This chapter deals with the interpretation of complex screening results and difficult situations encountered in day-to-day practice. It highlights some common errors in risk calculation and reporting that can cause tremendous anxiety to pregnant women. It also underscores the importance of considering individual circumstances in the decision-making process.

The author has selected cases of interest from his own clinical practice. These cases show how screening tests work, their limitations, and the issues that can occur if screening is done without due diligence. Each case presents unique challenges and gives the reader the opportunity to navigate through the nuances involved. Prior to proceeding further, it is highly recommended that readers acquaint themselves with the material covered in the previous chapters.

12.2 Case 1: Screen-Positive Woman Refusing Further Testing

A 34-year-old primigravida, weighing 60 kg, has conceived spontaneously. She is a non-diabetic and a non-smoker. Her 11–13 + 6 weeks scan is within normal limits. She has undergone combined first-trimester screening (FTS) with a screen-positive result. The woman claims that she did not know exactly what the

© The Author(s), under exclusive license to Springer Nature Singapore Pte Ltd. 2023

A. Kamat, *Down Syndrome Screening*,
https://doi.org/10.1007/978-981-99-7758-1_12

blood test was for. She also does not wish to terminate a Down syndrome baby if it is structurally normal. She refuses to do any further testing because of cost and risk (of amniocentesis).

12.2.1 Combined FTS Report

Maternal characteristics Parity: Nulliparous Age in years: 34 Weight in kg: 60 Conception method: Spontaneous Diabetes: No	**Measurements at 11–13 + 6 weeks** Singleton pregnancy Fetal crown-rump length: 66 mm (12 + 6 weeks) Nuchal translucency: 2.3 mm Fetal heart rate: 166 bpm
Serum markers Serum PAPP-A: 2.34 IU/L (MoM = 0.74) Serum free β-hCG: 88.0 IU/L (MoM = 2.52)	
Risk from age + history Trisomy 21: 1 in 370 Trisomy 18: 1 in 833 Trisomy 13: 1 in 2500	**Combined FTS risk at term** Trisomy 21: **1 in 127** Trisomy 18: 1 in 10,000 Trisomy 13: 1 in 10,000
Result Summary The sample is SCREEN-POSITIVE for trisomy 21 (risk cutoff of 1:250).	

12.2.2 Comments

- It appears that pre-test counseling has not been effective in this case.
- Possible need for further testing should always be discussed prior to performing combined FTS.

12.2.3 Further Testing

- The woman and her partner should be counseled in detail about the pros and cons of NIPT and invasive testing.
- If NIPT or invasive testing returns a low-risk or normal result, it would help in alleviating the woman's anxiety for the rest of her pregnancy.

- She should also be explained that it is not possible to detect all structural malformations on prenatal ultrasound.
- Finally, her decision should be respected (and documented).

12.2.4 Follow-Up and Outcome

An extensive counseling session was conducted with the woman and her partner. They refused further testing for aneuploidy. Her ultrasound scans throughout pregnancy were normal. She delivered a normal baby at term.

12.3 Case 2: Intermediate Risk (Biochemical)

A 20-year-old primigravida, weighing 56 kg, has conceived spontaneously. She is a non-diabetic and a non-smoker. Her 11–13 + 6 scan is within normal limits. She has undergone a combined FTS which is reported as follows:

12.3.1 Combined FTS Report

Maternal characteristics Parity: Nulliparous Age in years: 20 Weight in kg: 56 Conception method: Spontaneous Diabetes: No	**Measurements at 11–13 + 6 weeks** Singleton pregnancy Fetal crown-rump length: 60 mm (12 + 3 weeks) Nuchal translucency: 1.0 mm Fetal heart rate: 160 bpm
Serum markers Serum PAPP-A: 1.02 IU/L (MoM = 0.37) Serum free β-hCG: 56.2 IU/L (MoM = 1.41)	
Risk from age + history Trisomy 21: 1 in 1400 Trisomy 18: 1 in 2500 Trisomy 13: 1 in 10,000	**Combined FTS risk at term** Trisomy 21 (combined): 1 in 1510 Trisomy 21 (biochemical): **1 in 750** Trisomy 18: 1 in 10,000 Trisomy 13: 1 in 10,000
Result Summary The sample is SCREEN-NEGATIVE for trisomy 13, 18, and 21 (risk cutoff of 1:250). Biochemical risk for trisomy 21 is in the INTERMEDIATE RISK zone.	

12.3.2 Comments

- Laboratories should be strongly discouraged from mentioning biochemical risk separately on the report. The combined risk has the biochemical component (serum marker levels) already factored in. Reporting a separate risk based on biochemistry alone unnecessarily increases patient anxiety.
- Low PAPP-A levels are noted (defined as <0.4 MoM). This is associated with an increased risk of preeclampsia and fetal growth restriction.

12.3.3 Further Testing

- No further testing for aneuploidy is necessary.
- Monitor the pregnancy for preeclampsia and growth restriction.

12.3.4 Follow Up and Outcome

Pregnancy was uneventful and resulted in the birth of a normal-weight baby.

12.4 Case 3: IVF Pregnancy with Raised NT and Megacystis

A 37-year-old primigravida, weighing 76 kg, has conceived through a self-cycle IVF. She is a diabetic. Her 11–13 + 6 weeks scan is showing an NT measurement of 4.5 mm, and fetal bladder size to be 8 × 10 mm. She is not keen on undergoing an invasive procedure as this is a precious pregnancy, and wishes to know if NIPT is an option for her. She is willing to accept a 99% certainty that her baby will be normal.

12.4.1 The 11–13 + 6 Weeks Scan Report

Singleton live fetus in intrauterine cavity. Fetal crown-rump length: 54 mm (12 + 0 weeks). Nuchal translucency: 4.5 mm. Fetal heart rate: 176 bpm. Fetal bladder persistently measures 8 × 10 mm, suggestive of fetal megacystis. Rest of fetal anatomy appears within normal limits.
Impression Raised NT > 99th percentile with fetal megacystis.

12.4.2 Comments

- The NT is significantly raised. Both the raised NT and megacystis are strongly associated with risk of chromosomal abnormalities, including sex chromosomal abnormalities, triploidy, and rare autosomal trisomies.
- NIPT is not a diagnostic test. It is a screening test with a high sensitivity for trisomy 13, 18, and 21. The 99% sensitivity of NIPT is only for trisomy 21.

12.4.3 Further Testing

- Invasive testing should be offered. The sample should be tested using FISH, followed by either karyotyping or a chromosomal microarray.
- DNA storage should be offered.

12.4.4 Follow-Up and Outcome

Amniocentesis was performed at 15 weeks with FISH and karyotyping, which confirmed trisomy 18 in the fetus. The couple opted to terminate the pregnancy.

12.5 Case 4: Screen-Positive Report Following Donor-Egg IVF

A 44-year-old primigravida, weighing 82 kg, has conceived through a donor-egg IVF cycle. She is a non-diabetic and a non-smoker. Her 11–13 + 6 scan is within normal limits. She has undergone a combined FTS which is reported as follows:

12.5.1 Combined FTS Report

<table>
<tr><td>Maternal characteristics
Parity: Nulliparous
Age in years: 44
Weight in kg: 82
Diabetes: No</td><td>Measurements at 11–13 + 6 weeks
Singleton pregnancy
Fetal crown-rump length: 70 mm (13 + 1 weeks)
Nuchal translucency: 1.1 mm
Fetal heart rate: 171 bpm</td></tr>
<tr><td>Serum markers
Serum PAPP-A: 1.60 IU/L (MoM = 0.45)
Serum free β-hCG: 38.1 IU/L (MoM = 1.58)</td><td></td></tr>
<tr><td>Risk from age + history
Trisomy 21: 1 in 36
Trisomy 18: 1 in 67
Trisomy 13: 1 in 208</td><td>Combined FTS risk at term
Trisomy 21: 1 in 46
Trisomy 18: 1 in 1429
Trisomy 13: 1 in 667</td></tr>
<tr><td colspan="2">Result Summary
The sample is SCREEN-POSITIVE for trisomy 21 (risk cutoff of 1:250).</td></tr>
</table>

12.5.2 Comments

- The conception method is not specified in the report.
- The results show that the risk of trisomy 21 from age + history is calculated to be 1:37. This is the maternal age-related risk at 44 years. Her own age has been erroneously used to calculate her aneuploidy risk, despite having conceived through donor-egg IVF.
- Donor's age should be used in the aneuploidy risk calculation. As egg donors are typically young women, it is likely that the corrected result will be screen-negative.

12.5.3 Further Testing

- If the corrected result is still screen-positive, then invasive testing should be offered.

12.5.4 Follow-Up and Outcome

The egg donor's age was 25 years. The corrected aneuploidy risks were 1 in 1667 for trisomy 21, and 1 in 10,000 for trisomy 13, and 18. No further testing was done; the baby was normal at birth.

12.6 Case 5: Contradictory Results on FTS and Quad Screen

A 31-year-old primigravida, weighing 47 kg, has conceived spontaneously. She is a non-diabetic and a non-smoker. The 11–13 + 6 weeks scan was within normal limits. Her combined FTS result was screen-negative. Her obstetrician offered her a quadruple marker test to be doubly sure. Quadruple marker is screen-positive for trisomy 21.

12.6.1 Combined FTS Report

Maternal characteristics	**Measurements at 11–13 + 6 weeks**
Parity: Nulliparous Age in years: 31 Weight in kg: 47 Conception method: Spontaneous Diabetes: No	Singleton pregnancy Fetal crown-rump length: 66 mm (12 + 6 weeks) Nuchal translucency: 2.2 mm Fetal heart rate: 158 bpm Fetal anatomy appears normal
Serum markers Serum PAPP-A: 2.92 IU/L (MoM = 0.72) Serum free β-hCG: 50.3 IU/L (MoM = 1.23)	

Risk from age + history	Combined FTS risk at term
Trisomy 21: 1 in 769 Trisomy 18: 1 in 2000 Trisomy 13: 1 in 5000	Trisomy 21: 1 in 1950 Trisomy 18: 1 in 10,000 Trisomy 13: 1 in 10,000
Result Summary The sample is SCREEN-NEGATIVE for trisomy 13, 18, and 21 (risk cutoff of 1:250).	

12.6.2 Quadruple Marker Test Report

Pregnancy details		Specimen details	
Parity: Nulliparous Age in years: 31 Weight in kg: 49 Conception method: Spontaneous Diabetes: No		Gestation at collection date: 19+ 3 weeks (BPD = 44 mm, HC = 164 mm).	
Test Name	**Value**	**Unit**	**Corrected MoM**
AFP	65.20	U/mL	1.18
β-hCG	53.90	Ng/mL	5.66
Inhibin A	312.53	Pg/mL	1.31
uE3	5.22	Nmol/L	0.81
Risk from age + history Trisomy 21: 1 in 800 Trisomy 18: 1 in 2000		**Quadruple screening risk at term** Trisomy 21: **1 in 171** Trisomy 18: 1 in 100,000 Neural tube defect: Low risk	
Result Summary The sample is SCREEN-POSITIVE for trisomy 21 (risk cutoff of 1:250).			

12.6.3 Comments

- Independent serum screening should never be repeated in the second trimester when it has already been done in the first trimester. If screening is to be done in both trimesters, an integrated or contingent screening model should be followed.
- The woman now has two screening reports showing contrary results.
- This scenario could have been avoided altogether by not doing a quadruple marker test (since the combined FTS result was screen-negative).

12.6.4 Further Testing

- Options include either recalculating the second-trimester risk using an integrated model or doing NIPT. Invasive testing should be done if the woman insists.

12.6.5 Follow-Up and Outcome

The couple insisted on an amniocentesis for confirmation. The fetal karyotype was normal. Unfortunately, she had an amniotic fluid leak 3 days following amniocentesis, and miscarried a week later.

12.7 Case 6: Advanced Maternal Age with NIPT Screen-Positive Result

A 42-year-old para 2, weighing 78 kg, has conceived spontaneously. She is a non-diabetic and a non-smoker. After a normal NT scan at 11 weeks, she opted for NIPT as a screening test. NIPT test results are screen-positive for trisomy 18. The woman desires to terminate the pregnancy as she already has two normal children, and she has read on a website that there is >99% chance that this baby will be severely abnormal.

12.7.1 NIPT Test Report

<table>
<tr><td colspan="2">Pregnancy details
Parity: 2
Age in years: 42
Weight in kg: 78
Conception method: Spontaneous
Gestational age: 11 + 1 weeks</td><td colspan="2">Fetal fraction
3.4%</td></tr>
<tr><td>Chromosome</td><td>Aneuploidy</td><td>LLR score</td><td>LLR score cutoff</td></tr>
<tr><td>Chromosome 21</td><td>Low risk</td><td>−0.81</td><td>≥2.5</td></tr>
<tr><td>Chromosome 18</td><td>High risk</td><td>3.9</td><td>≥3.0</td></tr>
</table>

Chromosome 13	Low risk	−2.1	≥3.0
Sex chromosomal abnormalities	Low risk		
Result Summary			
The sample is SCREEN-POSITIVE for trisomy 18.			

12.7.2 Comments

- NIPT is a screening test, not a diagnostic test.
- The fetal fraction is low (<4%). Low fetal fraction reduces performance of NIPT.
- The fetus is structurally normal, which is very unlikely if trisomy 18 is present.
- This can be a false-positive result. Placental mosaicism must be considered as a possibility.
- CVS is to be avoided as it cannot rule out confined placental mosaicism.

12.7.3 Further Testing

- Amniocentesis should be offered for confirmation of fetal karyotype before offering termination.

12.7.4 Follow-Up and Outcome

The fetal karyotype was normal on amniocentesis. The pregnancy was continued. Fetal growth restriction set in by 28 weeks. The woman required a cesarean delivery at 33 weeks because of an absent end-diastolic flow in the umbilical artery. The neonate weighed 1.3 kg and ultimately did well.

12.8 Case 7: Intermediate Risk and a No-Call NIPT Result

A 28-year-old primigravida, weighing 79 kg, has conceived spontaneously. She is a non-diabetic and a non-smoker. Her 11–13 + 6 weeks scan is within normal limits. Her combined FTS showed intermediate risk for trisomy 21. NIPT was done subsequently, and the laboratory released a no-call report. The repeat blood sample sent for NIPT is also showing the same.

12.8.1 Combined FTS Report

Maternal characteristics Parity: Nulliparous Age in years: 28 Weight in kg: 79 Conception method: Spontaneous Diabetes: No	**Measurements at 11–13 + 6 weeks** Singleton pregnancy Fetal crown-rump length: 65 mm (12 + 6 weeks) Nuchal translucency: 2.2 mm Fetal heart rate: 178 bpm Fetal anatomy appears normal
Serum markers Serum PAPP-A: 1.90 IU/L (MoM = 0.81) Serum free β-hCG: 52.1 IU/L (MoM = 1.73)	
Risk from age + history Trisomy 21: 1 in 966 Trisomy 18: 1 in 2000 Trisomy 13: 1 in 5000	**Combined FTS risk** Trisomy 21: **1 in 656** Trisomy 18: 1 in 10,000 Trisomy 13: 1 in 5000
Result Summary The sample is screened INTERMEDIATE RISK for trisomy 21 (risk cutoff of 1:250).	

12.8.2 NIPT Test Report (Repeat Sample)

Pregnancy details Parity: Nulliparous Age in years: 28 Weight in kg: 79 Conception method: Spontaneous Gestational age: 16 + 2 weeks		**Fetal fraction** 2.5%	
Chromosome	**Aneuploidy**	**LLR score**	**LLR score cutoff**
Chromosome 21	NA	NA	≥2.5
Chromosome 18	NA	NA	≥3.0
Chromosome 13	NA	NA	≥3.0
Sex chromosomal abnormalities	NA	NA	
Result Summary No result could be generated due to a low fetal fraction.			

12.8.3 Comments

- The contingent screening model with intermediate risk increases the test sensitivity, but also the screen-positive rate.
- A no-call NIPT result requires invasive testing, as aneuploidy itself can be a reason for the low fetal fraction.

12.8.4 Further Testing

- Amniocentesis should be offered for confirmation of fetal karyotype.

12.8.5 Follow-Up and Outcome

The fetal karyotype revealed a mosaicism for Turner syndrome. The woman opted to terminate the pregnancy.

12.9 Case 8: Hypoplastic Nasal Bone

A 40-year-old para 1, weighing 70 kg, has conceived through intrauterine insemination. She is a diabetic, but a non-smoker. Her 11–13 + 6 scan was within normal limits. In view of advanced age, she has opted for NIPT as a screening test, which has shown a screen-negative result. However, at her 19 weeks targeted anomaly scan, nasal bone (NB) length is 3 mm, and reported as hypoplastic. There are no other structural abnormalities or markers.

12.9.1 NIPT Test Report

<table>
<tr><td colspan="2">Pregnancy details
Parity: 1
Age in years: 40
Weight in kg: 70
Conception method: IUI
Gestational age: 13+ 2 weeks</td><td colspan="2">Fetal fraction
8.4%</td></tr>
<tr><td>Chromosome</td><td>Aneuploidy</td><td>LLR score</td><td>LLR score cutoff</td></tr>
<tr><td>Chromosome 21</td><td>Low risk</td><td>1.1</td><td>≥2.5</td></tr>
<tr><td>Chromosome 18</td><td>Low risk</td><td>−0.9</td><td>≥3.0</td></tr>
<tr><td>Chromosome 13</td><td>Low risk</td><td>−1.4</td><td>≥3.0</td></tr>
<tr><td>Sex chromosomal abnormalities</td><td>Low risk</td><td></td><td></td></tr>
<tr><td colspan="4">Result Summary
The sample is SCREEN-NEGATIVE for trisomies 13, 18, 21 and sex chromosomal abnormalities.</td></tr>
</table>

12.9.2 Targeted Anomaly Scan Summary

<table>
<tr><td>Single live fetus of 19 + 2 weeks.
FHR = 145/minute
Fetal growth and liquor: Normal
Nasal bone measures 3 mm (0.6 MoM, <5th percentile)
No structural abnormalities.
No other soft markers for aneuploidy.</td></tr>
<tr><td>Impression
Hypoplastic nasal bone</td></tr>
</table>

12.9.3 Comments

- Hypoplastic NB is a soft marker for common trisomies, mostly trisomy 21.
- In the absence of other malformations, it is acceptable to do no further testing if NIPT shows a screen-negative result. If the woman insists, invasive testing may be done.
- Hypoplastic NB does not cause any cosmetic defects in euploid fetuses.

12.9.4 Further Testing

- Further testing is not mandatory.

12.9.5 Follow-Up and Outcome

The couple opted not to do invasive testing. Pregnancy was uneventful and resulted in the birth of a normal baby.

12.10 Case 9: DCDA Twins Discordant for NT

A 30-year-old primigravida, weighing 74 kg, has conceived on ovulation induction. She is a non-diabetic and a non-smoker. Her 11–13 + 6 weeks scan shows dichorionic (DC) twins with NT values 1.2, and 2.7, respectively. Rest of the findings on ultrasound are within normal limits. She has undergone a combined FTS which is reported as follows.

12.10.1 Combined FTS Report

Maternal characteristics Parity: Nulliparous Age in years: 30 Weight in kg: 74 Conception method: Ovulation drugs Diabetes: No	**Measurements at 11–13 + 6 weeks** Dichorionic twin pregnancy *Fetus A (Right sided, Placenta anterior and right lateral)* Crown-rump length: 67 mm (13 + 0 weeks) Nuchal translucency: 1.2 mm Fetal heart rate: 166 bpm Fetal anatomy appears normal *Fetus B (Left sided, Placenta anterior and left lateral)* Crown-rump length: 64 mm (12 + 5 weeks) Nuchal translucency: 2.7 mm Fetal heart rate: 172 bpm Fetal anatomy appears normal
Serum markers Serum PAPP-A: 3.62 IU/L (MoM = 0.67) Serum free β-hCG: 66.4 IU/L (MoM = 1.13)	**Risk from age + history** Trisomy 21: 1 in 909 Trisomy 18: 1 in 2000 Trisomy 13: 1 in 10,000
Combined FTS risk at term (fetus A) Trisomy 21: 1 in 5000 Trisomy 18: 1 in 10,000 Trisomy 13: 1 in 10,000	**Combined FTS risk at term (fetus B)** Trisomy 21: **1 in 182** Trisomy 18: 1 in 10,000 Trisomy 13: 1 in 1686
Result Summary Fetus A: The sample is SCREEN-NEGATIVE for trisomy 21, 18, and 13 (risk cutoff of 1:250). Fetus B: The sample is SCREEN-POSITIVE for trisomy 21 (risk cutoff of 1:250).	

12.10.2 Comments

- Dichorionic twins can be monozygotic if the embryo splits early. Hence, testing of both fetuses is recommended, even though only one fetus appears to be at high risk for aneuploidy.
- NIPT is not recommended in DC twins with discordant findings, as the karyotypes can be discordant. The cfDNA from the normal placenta can mask the cfDNA from the aneuploid placenta, as aneuploidy is associated with a reduced fetal fraction.

12.10.3 Further Testing

- Invasive testing of both fetuses should be offered.

12.10.4 Follow-Up and Outcome

CVS was done with double sampling; QFPCR and karyotyping were ordered. Fetus A was euploid, while fetus B was found to have trisomy 21. The women opted for selective fetal reduction. The pregnancy continued uneventfully, and a normal baby was born at term.

12.11 Case 10: Unexpected Outcome Following a Screen-Negative Result

A 34-year-old primigravida, weighing 67 kg, has conceived spontaneously. She is a non-diabetic and a non-smoker. Her 11–13 + 6 weeks scan is within normal limits. She has undergone a detailed counseling regarding aneuploidy screening and testing. Besides combined FTS, NIPT was also mentioned as a screening option. She opted for combined FTS.

12.11.1 Combined FTS Report

Maternal characteristics	**Measurements at 11–13 + 6 weeks**
Parity: Nulliparous Age in years: 34 Weight in kg: 67 Conception method: Spontaneous Diabetes: No	Singleton pregnancy Fetal crown-rump length: 56 mm (12 + 1 weeks) Nuchal translucency: 1.2 mm Nasal bone is present Fetal heart rate: 160 bpm Fetal anatomy appears normal
Serum markers Serum PAPP-A: 1.53 IU/L (MoM = 0.76) Serum free β-hCG: 48.0 IU/L (MoM = 1.28)	

Risk from age + history	**Combined FTS risk at term**
Trisomy 21: 1 in 370	Trisomy 21: 1 in 5000
Trisomy 18: 1 in 833	Trisomy 18: 1 in 10,000
Trisomy 13: 1 in 2500	Trisomy 13: 1 in 10,000
Result Summary The sample is SCREEN-NEGATIVE for trisomy 13, 18 and 21 (risk cutoff of 1:250).	

12.11.2 Comments

- Combined first-trimester screening (FTS) shows a low risk of trisomy 13, 18, and 21.

12.11.3 Further Testing

- No further testing for aneuploidy is necessary.

12.11.4 Follow-Up and Outcome

All ultrasound scans throughout the pregnancy were normal. The woman delivered at 39 weeks. The baby had features of Down syndrome. Karyotyping of the baby confirmed free trisomy 21.

The couple had been counseled in detail prior to undergoing the combined FTS. The difference between a screening test and invasive testing was also discussed. They accepted the fact that screening tests can miss some cases of Down syndrome.

12.11.5 Present-Day Status

At the time of writing this book, the girl is 3 years old, and doing well. The mother has undergone special educator training. She has also started a social media group to support mothers of Down syndrome children and women who choose to continue a Down syndrome pregnancy. She has remained in touch with the author, and continues to provide regular updates about her daughter's achievements.

This case highlights two important points. First, a low-risk screening result and normal ultrasounds do not rule out Down syndrome with certainty. Second, the importance of a detailed pre-test counseling cannot be overstated.

13 Trisomy 18, Trisomy 13, and Other Aneuploidies

13.1 Introduction

Rapid development of technology for prenatal diagnosis has been fueled by the need to detect Down syndrome. There are several other genetic abnormalities which can be detected concurrently. This chapter covers the genetics, natural history, and prenatal diagnosis of trisomy 18, trisomy 13, monosomy X, and triploidy. Several rarer genetic disorders also share clinical findings with these aneuploidies. It is therefore very difficult to predict the genotype of an anomalous fetus solely based on ultrasound findings. Rare genetic disorders are beyond the scope of this book.

13.2 Trisomy 18: Edwards Syndrome

Edwards syndrome is the second most common autosomal trisomy after Down syndrome, with a prevalence of 1 in 6000 at birth, and a male:female ratio of 0.6. Nearly all affected fetuses have multiple congenital abnormalities, leading to diagnosis and termination of pregnancy in most cases. Spontaneous fetal loss is also common in trisomy 18. The actual prevalence of this syndrome in the fetus may, therefore, be significantly higher than reported [1].

© The Author(s), under exclusive license to Springer Nature Singapore Pte Ltd. 2023

A. Kamat, *Down Syndrome Screening*,
https://doi.org/10.1007/978-981-99-7758-1_13

13.2.1 Genetic Basis

In over 95% of fetuses with Edwards syndrome, there is an extra copy of an entire chromosome 18. This extra chromosome is of maternal origin in 90% of cases; the causative mechanism is non-disjunction during meiosis II or, less frequently, during meiosis I. Like trisomy 21, the risk of trisomy 18 is higher in older women. In the remaining 10% of cases, the extra chromosome is of paternal origin; this error almost always results from postzygotic non-disjunction.

Trisomy 18 mosaicism accounts for a small proportion of cases of Edwards syndrome. Such fetuses display a varying degree of phenotypic features, ranging from near normal anatomy to lethal malformations. The percentage of aneuploid cells does not correlate well with the expressed phenotype. Trisomy 18 can rarely result from the triplication of the long arm of chromosome 18, particularly the portion from 18q11.2 to the terminus. The phenotype, again, is variable [1].

13.2.2 First-Trimester Ultrasound

In over 90% of cases, diagnosis is suspected at the 11–13 + 6 weeks scan because of the presence of severe malformations (though pinpointing the exact aneuploidy may be difficult). Nuchal translucency (NT) is increased with a mean value of 5.4 mm, and this finding should prompt a detailed fetal assessment. A systematic evaluation of fetal anatomy in the first trimester is more effective at detecting trisomy 18 than maternal serum screening [2]. Anomalies typically detected in the first trimester include:

- *Head:* posterior fossa cysts, abnormal intracranial translucency.
- *Face:* absent nasal bone, retrognathia.
- *Neck:* enlarged nuchal translucency, cystic hygroma.
- *Heart:* tricuspid regurgitation, structural abnormalities.
- *Abdomen:* omphalocele (Fig 13.1a), abnormal ductus venosus course.

- *Spine:* open neural tube defect.
- *Limbs:* club hands or clenched hands, radial ray anomaly (Fig 13.1b).
- *Urogenital:* megacystis.
- Hydrops.
- Early growth restriction.

13.2.3 Second-Trimester Ultrasound

Abnormalities which are possible to diagnose in the first trimester become clearer in the second trimester. *Additional anomalies* which can be diagnosed after 18 weeks include:

- *Head:* Dandy-Walker variants, agenesis of the corpus callosum (Fig. 13.1c), strawberry-shaped skull, choroid plexus cysts.
- *Face:* micrognathia.
- *Heart:* septal defects (Fig. 13.1d), polyvalvular defects.
- *Abdomen:* diaphragmatic hernia.
- *Limbs:* Clenched hands with overlapping digits, rocker-bottom feet.
- *Urogenital:* horseshoe kidney, cystic renal dysplasia.
- *Umbilical cord:* single umbilical artery.

A combination of early growth restriction and multiple malformations (especially limb anomalies) is the classical profile of a fetus with Edwards syndrome. A fetus with isolated choroid plexus cysts or an isolated single umbilical artery is unlikely to be a trisomy 18 fetus.

13.2.4 Maternal Screening

Both PAPP-A and β-hCG are significantly lower in trisomy 18 (see Table 3.1). Combined first-trimester screening (FTS) has a sensitivity of 67% for a false-positive rate (FPR) of 5.8%. Trisomy 18 can also be screened for by the quadruple marker test (detection rate 84%) as values of alpha-fetoprotein and unconjugated

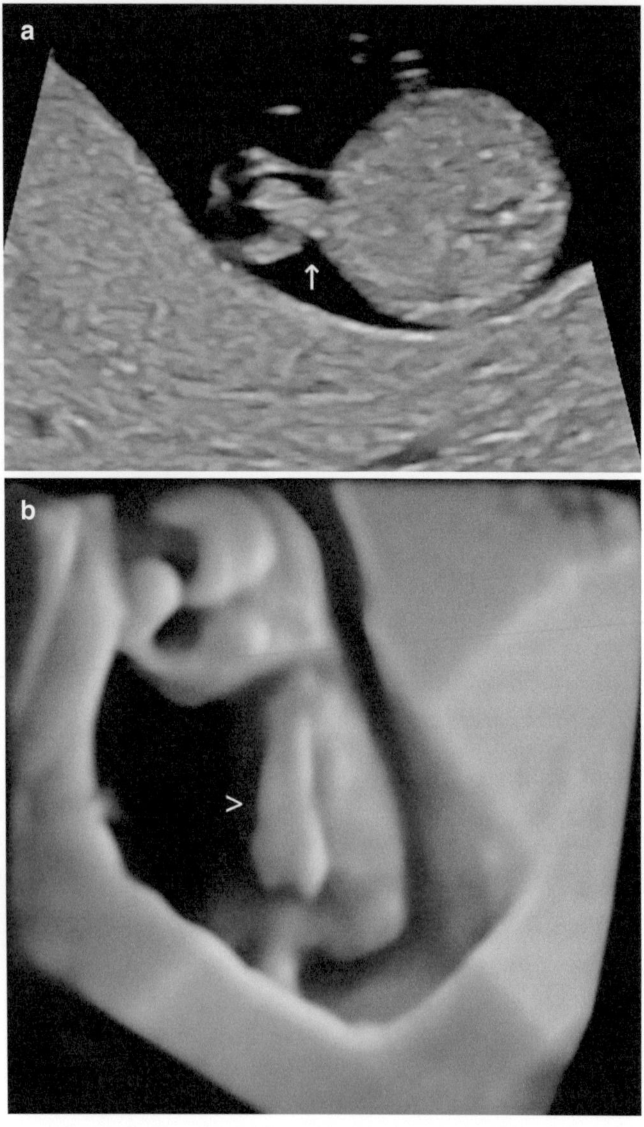

Fig. 13.1 Trisomy 18. (**a**) Omphalocele in a 13-week fetus. Note the herniation of small bowel into the base of the umbilical cord (*arrow*). (**b**) Radial ray anomaly (3D surface rendering). Note that the forearm is almost absent (*arrowhead*). (**c**) Complete agenesis of corpus callosum with abnormal course of the pericallosal artery (**d**) Ventricular septal defect (*solid arrowhead*)

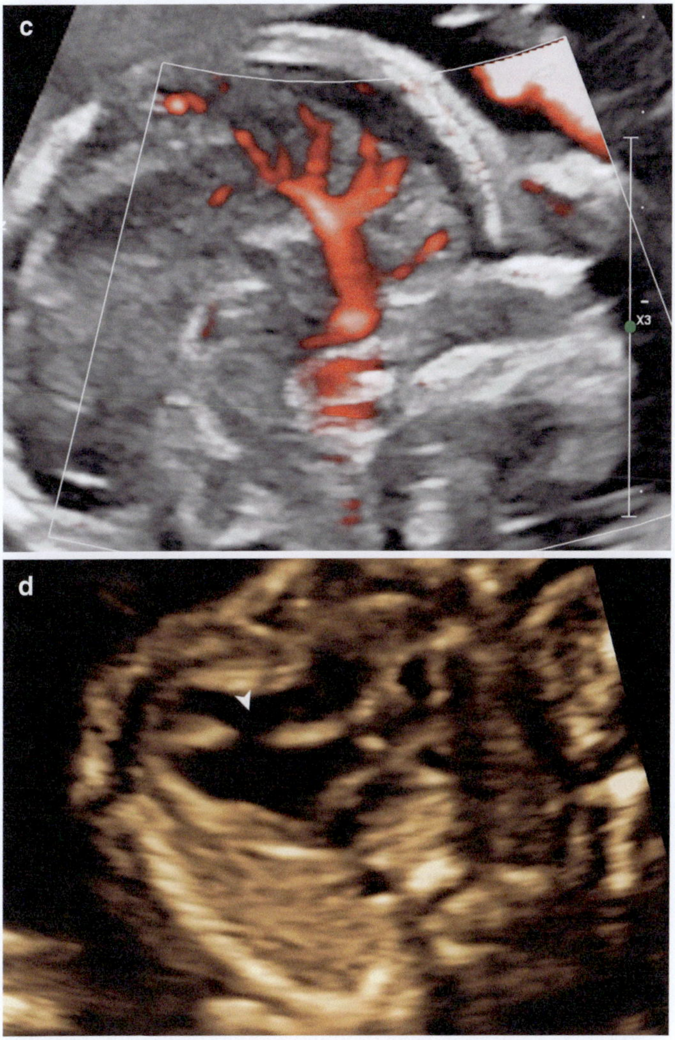

Fig. 13.1 (continued)

estriol are low (in addition to β-hCG). Noninvasive prenatal testing (NIPT) is highly accurate with sensitivity of 98% and a specificity of >99% [3–5]. Despite this, most cases are diagnosed following invasive testing done for structurally malformed fetuses.

13.2.5 Can Structurally Normal Fetuses Have Trisomy 18?

Unlike trisomy 21 fetuses, trisomy 18 fetuses have multiple and severe malformations which can be picked up on ultrasound. So, should invasive testing be offered to trisomy 18 screen-positive women without obvious fetal anomalies? It is worthwhile discussing some of the published research on this.

- Bundy et al. (1986) described ultrasound findings in 12 fetuses with trisomy 18 and reported detection rates of 50% and 100% in the second and third trimester, respectively. Five fetuses had their first ultrasound scan in the third trimester, with IUGR and oligohydramnios in 3 of them. The relatively poor sensitivity is likely due to the poor imaging resolution at that time and the retrospective nature of the study [6].
- Yeo et al. (2003) published a study with 38 fetuses with trisomy 18 and reported 4 or more sonographically demonstrable anomalies in each fetus. Choroid plexus cysts were present in 50% of affected fetuses, but in no case was this an isolated finding. A systematic, targeted anomaly scan was performed on all fetuses. Despite a retrospective review of prenatal sonograms, they reported a 100% sensitivity [7].
- Bronsteen et al. (2004) published a case series of 49 fetuses with trisomy 18. The percentage of fetuses with ultrasound abnormalities was 88% at 17 weeks, 93% at 18 weeks, and 100% at 19 weeks. The commonest abnormalities were of the brain, heart, and limbs [8].
- Yang et al. (2005) reported 30 cases of trisomy 18, all of which were identified by a systematic, targeted scan, with 83% of fetuses presenting with cardiac defects [9].

- Watson et al. (2008), in a retrospective review of 98 genetically confirmed cases, reported finding ultrasound abnormalities in only 94% of fetuses. Addition of fetal biometry below fifth percentile increased the sensitivity to 97%. Choroid plexus cysts were present in 39 fetuses, but in all cases, they were associated with another anomaly or significant IUGR [10].
- Lai et al. (2010) reported 69 cases of trisomy 18 confirmed by karyotype over a 10-year period at a single center. Detection rate by ultrasound scan was 92.7% in the first trimester and 100% in the second trimester [11].
- However, Becker et al. (2019) in a large study at a tertiary care institution, reported a sensitivity of only 95% for trisomy 18 detection by ultrasound. Only 76% fetuses were detected prior to 20 weeks gestation. All sonographic exams met the recommended standards. Two fetuses had bilateral choroid plexus cysts as the only finding [12].
- Finally, Chen et al. (2022) reported a case of a structurally normal fetus with mosaic trisomy 18 at amniocentesis. The baby was phenotypically normal at 7 months after birth, and the abnormal trisomy 18 cell line was seen to decrease progressively after birth [13].

So, should women with a positive trisomy 18 serum screen and a structurally normally fetus be offered further testing? This debate is unlikely to have a definite verdict soon. Nevertheless, some inferences can be derived from the various studies. It is possible to achieve a detection rate close to 100% by ultrasound alone, provided:

1. Ultrasound is done after 19 weeks of gestation.
2. Scanning is done with a specific aim of detecting trisomy 18.
3. A systematic genetic sonogram is performed by an experienced sonographer.
4. Ultrasound scan includes fetal echocardiography and evaluation of small parts.
5. Abnormal fetal biometry is included as a marker for trisomy 18.

As of now, whenever combined FTS or quadruple marker test shows high risk for trisomy 18, the woman should be counseled about genetic sonogram. The possibility of an occasional missed case and a lower sensitivity for mosaic and partial trisomy 18 fetuses should be discussed. Screen-positive fetuses with any anomaly, IUGR, or soft marker should directly undergo invasive testing. NIPT is an excellent option for trisomy 18 screen-positive women when the fetus shows normal growth and anatomy. If NIPT is screen positive for trisomy 18 in a structurally normal fetus, amniocentesis rather than CVS should be offered in order to bypass the possibility of placental mosaicism.

13.2.6 Natural History and Obstetric Management

Intrauterine fetal demise occurs in over 60% of fetuses with Edwards syndrome from the time of diagnosis until term. Those diagnosed in the first trimester and those with severe anomalies have the highest mortality rate [14].

Among those that are born alive, only 5–10% survive till their first birthday. With full resuscitation (short of cardiac surgery), the 1-year survival increases to 25% [15]. All children with a complete trisomy 18 have severe physical and neurological handicap. Long-term outcome is worse when this syndrome is diagnosed prenatally.

In 2020, the Support Organization For Trisomy group reported that their oldest living member with full trisomy 18 had turned 40 years old. Long-term survival after intensive neonatal care in trisomy 18 has several implications. Edwards syndrome can no longer be strictly considered as a lethal disorder and this information needs to be provided to couples who face this prenatal diagnosis. Couples who are pro-life may choose to continue pregnancy and opt for full neonatal resuscitation. In other couples, prenatal diagnosis to allow safe termination of pregnancy assumes paramount importance, as there is no certainty of a quick neonatal death.

13.2.7 Risk of Recurrence

Risk of recurrence in the next pregnancy is expected to be 1%.

13.3 Trisomy 13: Patau Syndrome

The trisomy 13 syndrome or the Patau syndrome is the third most common autosomal trisomy, with a prevalence of 1 in 12,000 at birth [16]. Trisomy 13 usually presents as multiple congenital abnormalities in the fetus. Compared to the other trisomies, there is a higher predisposition for midline and craniofacial anomalies.

13.3.1 Genetic Basis

Most cases of Patau syndrome occur because of an extra copy of part or whole of chromosome 13. In 75% of cases of Patau syndrome, a complete extra chromosome is present. This extra copy is usually of maternal origin and arises from non-disjunction during meiosis II. The remaining 25% of cases result from a Robertsonian translocation, most commonly rob(13q;14q). Occasionally, a mosaicism for trisomy 13 is noted with a varying expression of phenotypic features.

13.3.2 First-Trimester Ultrasound

Like trisomy 18, ultrasound is more sensitive than maternal serum screening for the diagnosis of trisomy 13. NT is increased with a mean value of 4 mm. Other typical features which can be identified in the first trimester are:

- *Head:* holoprosencephaly (Fig. 13.2a), posterior fossa cysts.
- *Face:* midline clefts, proboscis, cyclopia, retrognathia, absent nasal bone.
- *Neck:* enlarged nuchal translucency, cystic hygroma.
- *Heart:* tricuspid regurgitation, structural abnormalities, tachycardia.

- *Abdomen:* abnormal ductus venosus course.
- *Limbs:* clenched hands.
- *Urogenital:* megacystis, echogenic kidneys.
- Hydrops.
- *Growth:* early growth restriction.

13.3.3 Second-Trimester Ultrasound

Additional abnormalities which are more likely to be detected in the second trimester are:

- *Head:* agenesis of corpus callosum, cerebellar abnormalities.
- *Face:* bilateral cleft lip and palate (Fig. 13.2b), microphthalmia (Fig. 13.2c) and anophthalmia.
- *Heart:* septal defects, anomalous pulmonary venous connections, hypoplastic left heart.
- *Abdomen:* diaphragmatic hernia.
- *Limbs:* polydactyly (Fig. 13.2d).
- *Urogenital:* cystic renal dysplasia.
- *Umbilical cord:* single umbilical artery.
- *Growth:* fetal growth restriction.
- *Liquor:* polyhydramnios.

Although Patau syndrome shares many common findings with Edwards syndrome, its classic profile is a fetus with severe midline craniofacial defects and polydactyly.

13.3.4 Maternal Screening

Nuchal translucency should always be included in the first-trimester screening as the NT is significantly higher in trisomy 13 fetuses. Both PAPP-A and β-hCG values are significantly lower. Combined screening has a sensitivity of 91% for a cutoff of 1:100 and a false-positive rate of 5%. Addition of fetal heart rate further improves the sensitivity to 93% [17]. The quadruple test has a poor sensitivity for trisomy 13 as the second-trimester serum markers are not significantly altered.

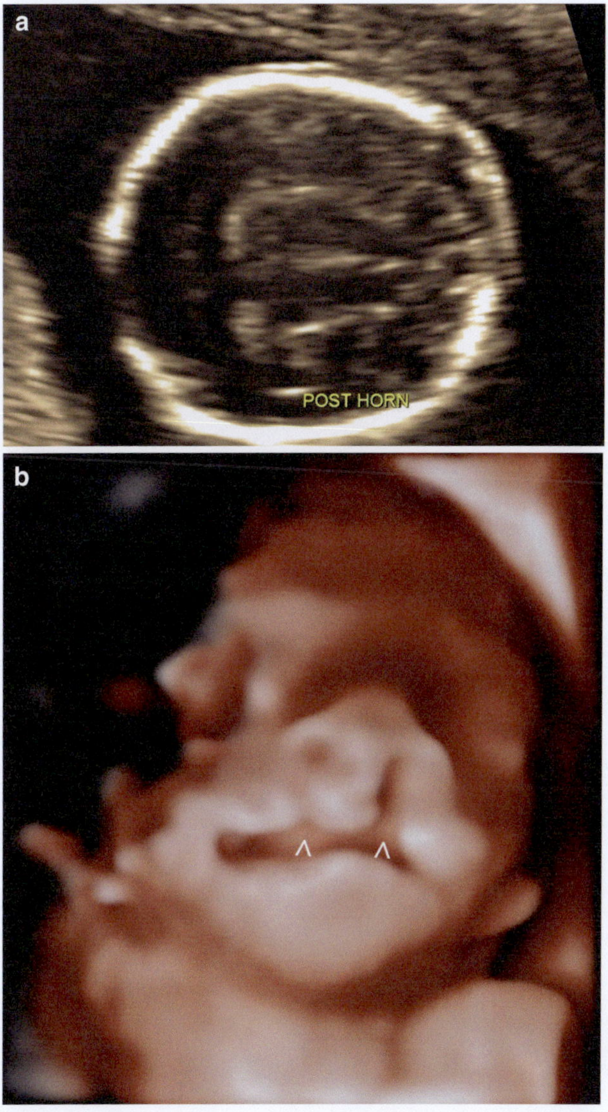

Fig. 13.2 Trisomy 13. (**a**) Semilobar holoprosencephaly. The posterior horns (*post horn*) of lateral ventricles are partially developed. (**b**) 3D surface rendering of fetal face showing bilateral cleft lip and palate (*arrowheads*). (**c**) Bilateral microphthalmia. Note that one eye is severely underdeveloped compared to the other (*arrows*). (**d**) Postaxial polydactyly

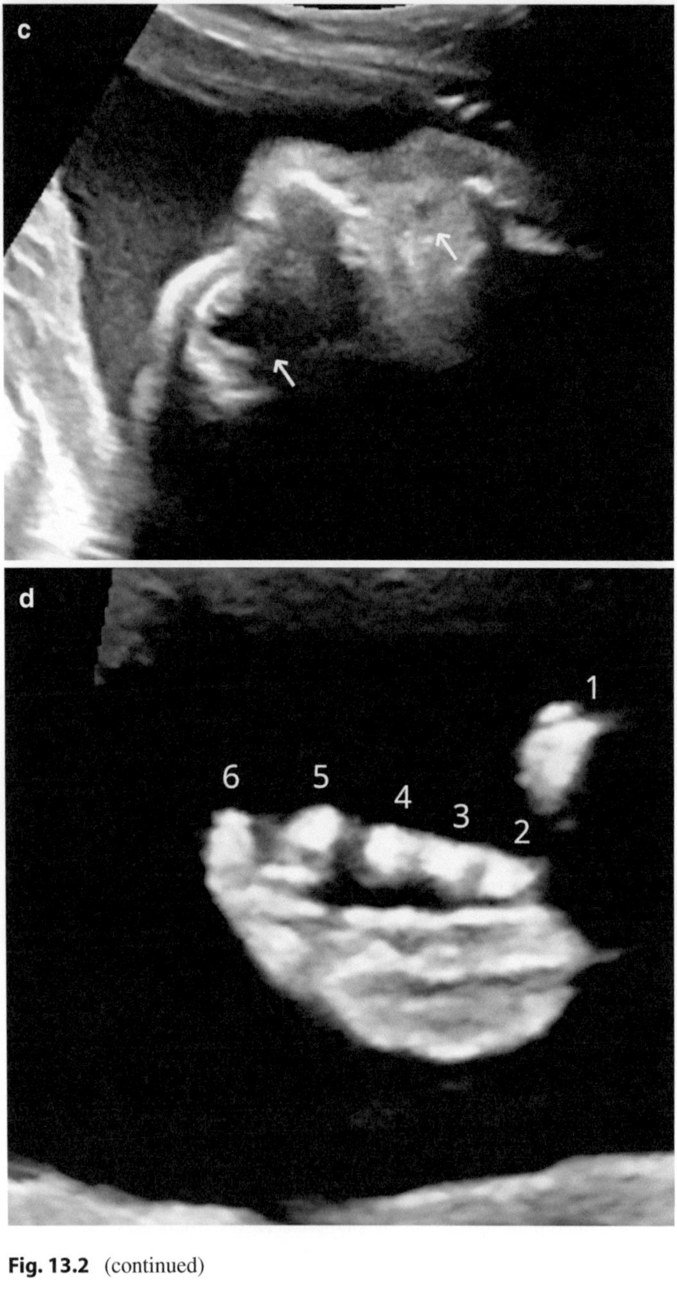

Fig. 13.2 (continued)

NIPT has a lower sensitivity for trisomy 13 compared to that for trisomy 21 (91% versus 99%), and a higher false-positive rate [18]. This is because of a lower guanine and cytosine (GC) content of chromosome 13, which increases sequencing errors. Other possible reasons include confined placental mosaicism and an undiagnosed vanishing twin with trisomy 13.

13.3.5 Natural History and Obstetric Management

Half of all fetuses with a prenatal diagnosis of trisomy 13 die in utero. Out of the live-born individuals, only 20% are alive at the end of the first month and only 3% at the end of the first year [19]. Survival beyond infancy is rare. In those rare cases without structural abnormalities, severe developmental delay is the rule. Blindness and epilepsy are frequently associated.

13.3.6 Risk of Recurrence

Risk of recurrence in the next pregnancy is expected to be 1%. As a quarter of cases result from a Robertsonian translocation, parental karyotyping is mandatory following a diagnosis of Patau syndrome in the fetus or neonate. When either parent shows a translocation, the risk of recurrence is high.

13.4 Monosomy X: Turner Syndrome

Turner syndrome is the commonest sex chromosomal abnormality with an incidence of 1 in 2500–3000 females at birth [20]. Turner syndrome has a wide range of genotypes and phenotypes. There can be a complete or partial loss of the second sex chromosome, or mosaicism. Mosaic individuals have a near-normal phenotype, and may sometimes go undetected until late adulthood. Affected individuals typically have a short stature, obesity, a broad chest, and a webbed neck. In addition, they may have a high-arched palate, cubitus valgus, low-set ears, and drooping eyelids. Associated conditions include deafness, renal problems, osteoporosis, hypertension, cardiac problems (commonest being coarctation of aorta), and primary ovarian failure.

13.4.1 Genetic Basis

Nondisjunction is the commonest mechanism responsible for monosomy X, most cases being paternal in origin.

- *Complete monosomy X:* Half of all cases are caused by a complete absence of a sex chromosome. These patients have typical features and manifest with primary ovarian failure.
- *Structural alterations:* In approximately 15–20% of cases, structural abnormalities of sex chromosomes are noted. The commonest is the formation of isochromosome X, a single chromosome formed by the fusion of two long arms. Other abnormalities include ring formation and deletion of either short or long arms.
- *Mosaicism:* Nearly one-third of cases of Turner syndrome are mosaics having both normal and abnormal cell lines. The abnormal cell lines may only be confined to certain tissues and may escape detection by peripheral blood karyotype. Low-level mosaicism can present with a history of oligomenorrhoea, poor ovarian reserve, infertility, and recurrent miscarriages.

13.4.2 Ultrasound Findings

Abnormal ultrasound findings are present in 92% of 45,X fetuses but only 55% of mosaics. One-third of cases are detected in the first trimester [21].

A cluster of first-trimester ultrasound findings is suggestive of monosomy X:

- Significantly increased NT with a median value of 7.8 mm.
- Septated cystic hygroma (Fig. 2.10b-d), fetal hydrops (Fig. 13.3a).
- Tachycardia.

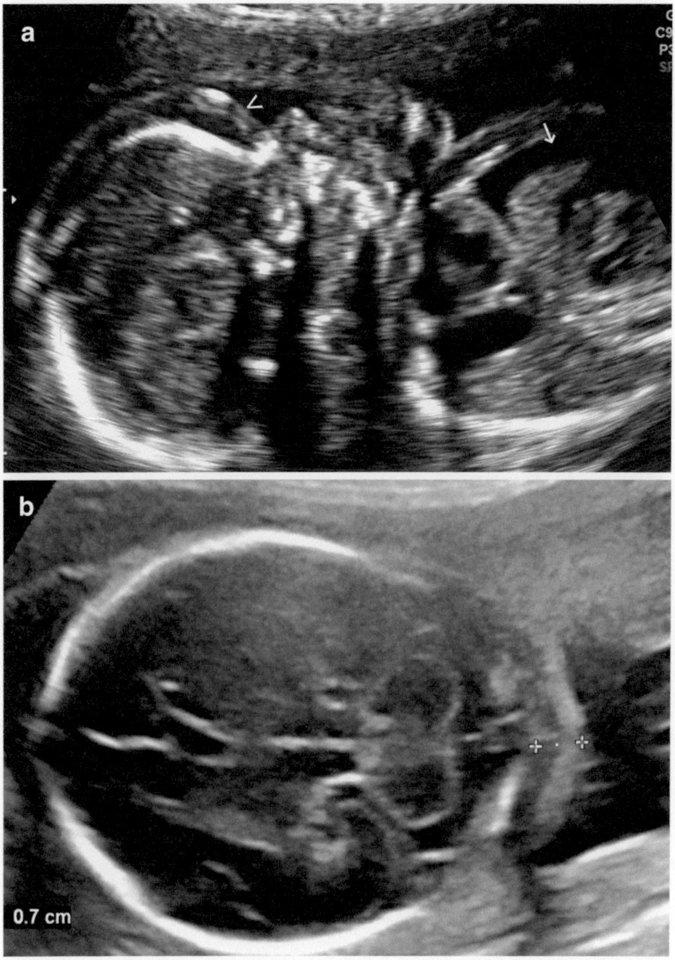

Fig. 13.3 Turner syndrome. (**a**) Diffuse hydrops. Note the prefrontal edema (*arrowhead*) and pleural effusion (*arrow*). (**b**) Transcerebellar section showing a thickened nuchal fold measuring 7 mm. (**c**) Coronal section of fetal trunk showing a horseshoe kidney (*hand icons*). (**d**) Aortic coarctation: three-vessel view showing a narrow aortic arch (*Ao*) with reversal of blood flow on color Doppler

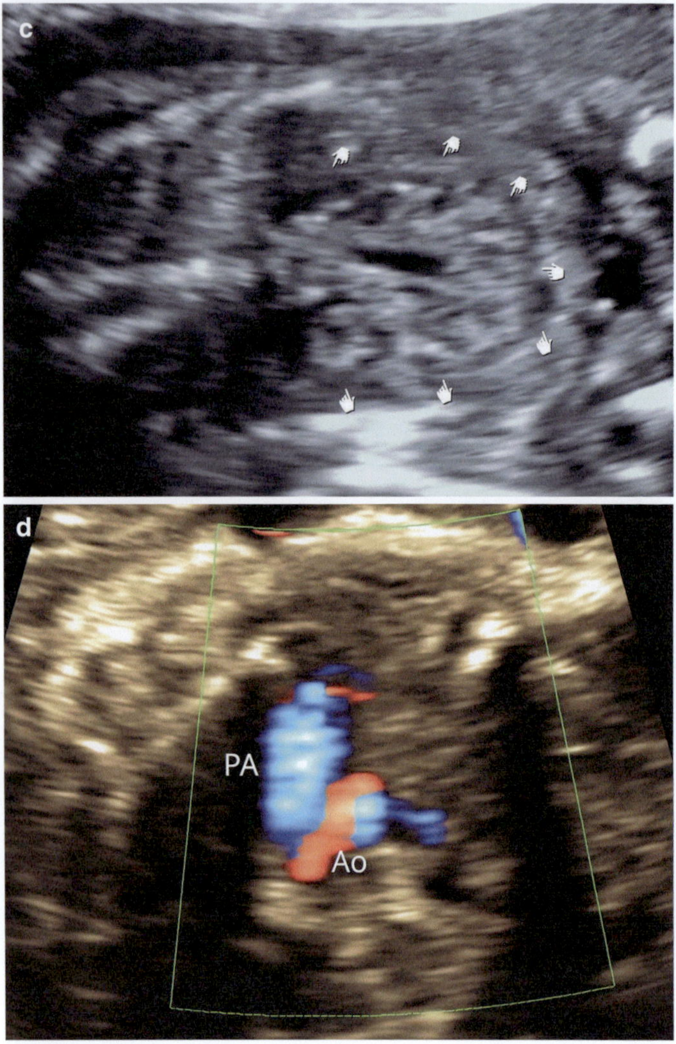

Fig. 13.3 (continued)

Additional second-trimester findings are:

- Nuchal edema (Fig. 13.3b).
- Short femur.
- Horseshoe kidney (Fig. 13.3c).
- Aortic arch abnormalities (Fig. 13.3d).
- Ventriculomegaly.

13.4.3 Maternal Screening

The risk of monosomy X does not increase with maternal age. Levels of PAPP-A and uE3 levels are frequently reduced and β-hCG and inhibin A levels are raised in cases of hydrops. Turner syndrome is not included as a part of maternal serum screening due to low sensitivity. Noninvasive prenatal testing can detect monosomy X with a sensitivity of 90.3% for an FPR of 0.23% [18]. Importantly, false-positive NIPT results can occur because of undiagnosed maternal mosaicism. As with other aneuploidies, a screen-positive NIPT result for monosomy X should always be confirmed by amniocentesis.

13.4.4 Natural History and Obstetric Management

Intrauterine demise occurs in over 90% fetuses having a 45,X genotype, usually following hydrops. Mortality is 100% in live-born babies with hydrops. In the absence of cardiac defects, long-term survivors have a good quality of life. Prenatal survival and long-term prognosis are significantly better in mosaic cases.

13.4.5 Risk of Recurrence

Risk of recurrence in the next pregnancy is not increased compared to the general population.

13.5 Triploidy

Triploidy refers to the presence of an extra haploid set of chromosomes, with each cell having 69 chromosomes instead of 46. Triploidy is the cause of 15–18% of all spontaneous early losses, and the incidence is approximately 1 in 10,000 at birth. Triploidy has a uniformly poor outcome and is not compatible with postnatal survival beyond a few hours [22].

13.5.1 Genetic Basis

The karyotype of triploid fetuses is 69, XXX or 69, XXY. Rarely, it may be 69, XYY. The extra chromosome set can be of maternal origin (digynic triploidy), or paternal origin (diandric triploidy). Most triploid pregnancies are diandric, caused by the fertilization of an ovum with either two sperms or a single diploid sperm. Digynic triploidy results from errors in meiosis II.

13.5.2 Ultrasound Findings

Each type of triploidy has a specific pattern of abnormal findings on ultrasound. However, variations exist in the phenotypic presentation, and molar changes in the placenta in paternally derived triploidy may not be appreciated at an early gestation. Table 13.1 lists the typical findings seen in diandric and digynic triploidy (Figs. 13.4a-d).

In addition, structural abnormalities are present in both types:

- *Head:* Agenesis of corpus callosum, holoprosencephaly, ventriculomegaly, Dandy-Walker malformation.
- *Face:* Microphthalmia, macrophthalmia, micrognathia.
- *Heart:* Septal defects.
- *Limbs:* Syndactyly.
- *Urogenital:* Renal dysplasia.

Table 13.1 Features of digynic and diandric triploidy

Finding	Digynic (maternal) triploidy	Diandric (paternal) triploidy
Growth	Small abdomen compared to head (>2 weeks discrepancy)	Short crown-rump length, symmetrical growth restriction
NT	Normal	Increased
Placenta	Small	Large with molar changes
B-hCG levels	Low	Very high
Maternal ovaries	Normal	May enlarge in response to high β-hCG levels
Liquor	Reduced	Reduced

Rarely, a dizygotic twin pregnancy (with a normal fetus and a complete mole) or placental mesenchymal dysplasia may mimic the findings seen in diandric triploidy.

13.5.3 Maternal Screening

The incidence of triploidy is not related to maternal age. Levels of PAPP-A are lower than normal in both types of triploidy. However, β-hCG levels are determined by the origin of the extra set of chromosomes. While maternal triploidy is associated with low levels of β-hCG, paternal triploidy results in very high levels of β-hCG. Maternal serum screening does not have an acceptable sensitivity for screening triploidy.

In triploidy, as an entire haploid set of chromosomes is duplicated, the relative ratios of each chromosome remain the same. Therefore, NIPT by next-generation sequencing (NGS) cannot be used, as this technique depends on an alteration in chromosome ratios. Single nucleotide polymorphism (SNP)-based NIPT can identify triploidy of paternal origin. A paternal blood sample can improve the detection rate. Overall, there is a lack of robust data regarding sensitivity and positive predictive value of this test. Digynic triploidy of maternal origin cannot be detected on NIPT.

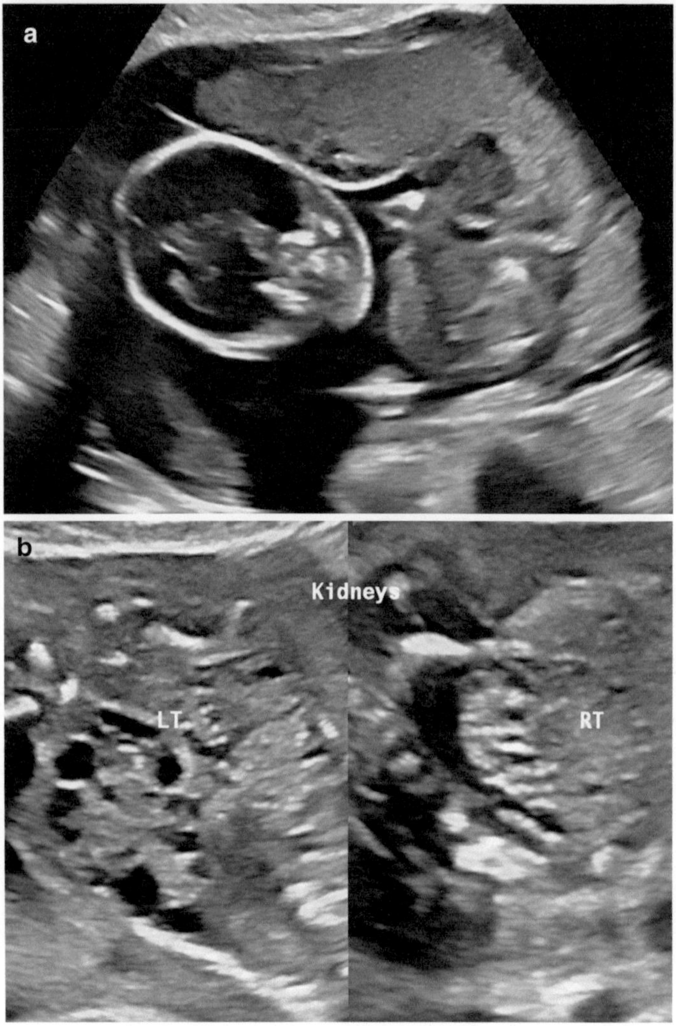

Fig. 13.4 Triploidy. (**a**) Severe asymmetrical growth restriction in digynic triploidy. Both the head and abdomen are seen in the same image. (**b**) Cystic renal dysplasia with severe oligohydramnios (*LT* left kidney, *RT* right kidney). (**c**) Molar changes in the placenta in diandric triploidy. (**d**) Maternal ovarian hyperstimulation in diandric triploidy

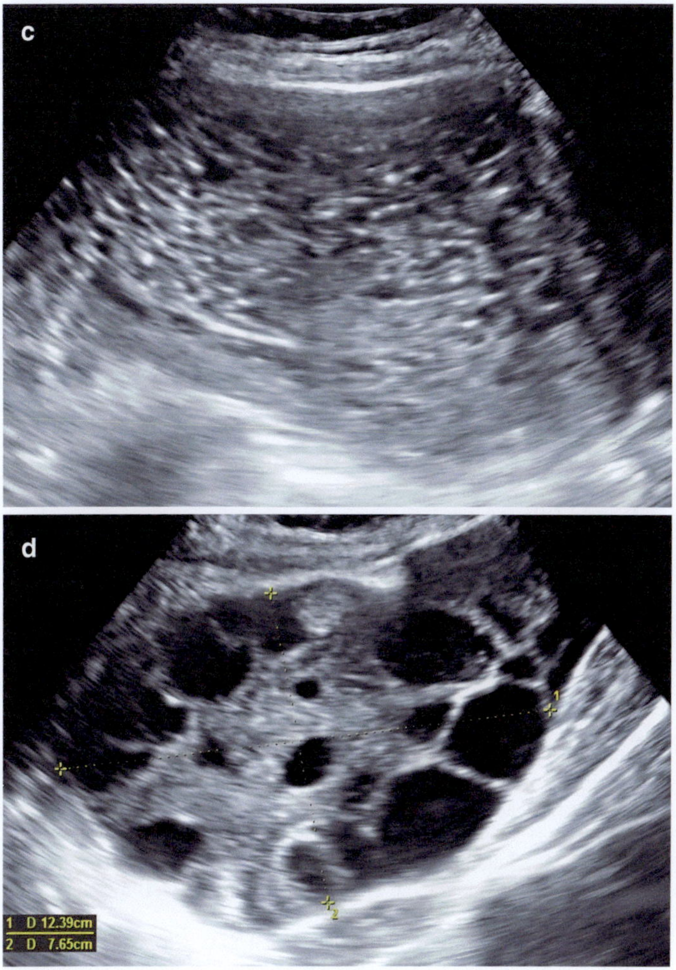

Fig. 13.4 (continued)

13.5.4 Natural History and Obstetric Management

Nearly all triploid fetuses die in utero, with a majority of them being lost in the early first trimester. In the rare instance of a live birth, death occurs within a few hours.

13.5.5 Risk of Recurrence

Risk of recurrence in the next pregnancy is not increased compared to the general population.

References

1. Cereda A, Carey JC. The trisomy 18 syndrome. Orphanet J Rare Dis. 2012;7:81.
2. Wagner P, Sonek J, Hoopmann M, Abele H, Kagan KO. First-trimester screening for trisomies 18 and 13, triploidy and turner syndrome by detailed early anomaly scan. Ultrasound Obstet Gynecol. 2016;48(4):446–51.
3. Breathnach FM, Malone FD, Lambert-Messerlian G, Cuckle HS, Porter TF, Nyberg DA, Comstock CH, Saade GR, Berkowitz RL, Klugman S, Dugoff L, Craigo SD, Timor-Tritsch IE, Carr SR, Wolfe HM, Tripp T, Bianchi DW, D'Alton ME. First and second trimester evaluation of risk (FASTER) research consortium. First- and second-trimester screening: detection of aneuploidies other than down syndrome. Obstet Gynecol. 2007;110(3):651–7.
4. Kazerouni NN, Currier RJ, Flessel M, Goldman S, Hennigan C, Hodgkinson C, Lorey F, Malm L, Tempelis C, Roberson M. Detection rate of quadruple-marker screening determined by clinical follow-up and registry data in the statewide California program, July 2007 to February 2009. Prenat Diagn. 2011;31(9):901–6.
5. Mackie FL, Hemming K, Allen S, Morris RK, Kilby MD. The accuracy of cell-free fetal DNA-based non-invasive prenatal testing in singleton pregnancies: a systematic review and bivariate meta-analysis. BJOG. 2017;124(1):32–46.
6. Bundy AL, Saltzman DH, Pober B, Fine C, Emerson D, Doubilet PM. Antenatal sonographic findings in trisomy 18. J Ultrasound Med. 1986;5(7):361–4.
7. Yeo L, Guzman ER, Day-Salvatore D, Walters C, Chavez D, Vintzileos AM. Prenatal detection of fetal trisomy 18 through abnormal sonographic features. J Ultrasound Med. 2003;22(6):581–90.
8. Bronsteen R, Lee W, Vettraino IM, Huang R, Comstock CH. Second-trimester sonography and trisomy 18. J Ultrasound Med. 2004;23(2):233–40.
9. Yang JH, Chung JH, Shin JS, Choi JS, Ryu HM, Kim MY. Prenatal diagnosis of trisomy 18: report of 30 cases. Prenat Diagn. 2005;25(2):119–22.
10. Watson WJ, Miller RC, Wax JR, Hansen WF, Yamamura Y, Polzin WJ. Sonographic findings of trisomy 18 in the second trimester of pregnancy. J Ultrasound Med. 2008;27(7):1033–8.

11. Lai S, Lau WL, Leung WC, Lai FK, Chin R. Is ultrasound alone enough for prenatal screening of trisomy 18? A single Centre experience in 69 cases over 10 years. Prenat Diagn. 2010;30(11):1094–9.
12. Becker DA, Tang Y, Jacobs AP, Biggio JR, Edwards RK, Subramaniam A. Sensitivity of prenatal ultrasound for detection of trisomy 18. J Matern Fetal Neonatal Med. 2019;32(22):3716–22.
13. Chen CP, Hsu TY, Tsai CC, Chern SR, Chen SW, Wu FT, Wu PS, Lee CC, Chen LF, Pan CW, Wang W. Mosaic trisomy 18 at amniocentesis associated with a favorable fetal outcome in a pregnancy. Taiwan J Obstet Gynecol. 2022;61(4):690–4.
14. Burke AL, Field K, Morrison JJ. Natural history of fetal trisomy 18 after prenatal diagnosis. Arch Dis Child Fetal Neonatal Ed. 2013;98(2): F152–4.
15. Kosho T, Nakamura T, Kawame H, Baba A, Tamura M, Fukushima Y. Neonatal management of trisomy 18: clinical details of 24 patients receiving intensive treatment. Am J Med Genet A. 2006;140(9):937–44.
16. Papp C, Beke A, Ban Z, Szigeti Z, Toth-Pal E, Papp Z. Prenatal diagnosis of trisomy 13: analysis of 28 cases. J Ultrasound Med. 2006;25(4): 429–35.
17. Santorum M, Wright D, Syngelaki A, Karagioti N, Nicolaides KH. Accuracy of first-trimester combined test in screening for trisomies 21, 18 and 13. Ultrasound Obstet Gynecol. 2017;49(6):714–20.
18. Gil MM, Quezada MS, Revello R, Akolekar R, Nicolaides KH. Analysis of cell-free DNA in maternal blood in screening for fetal aneuploidies: updated meta-analysis. Ultrasound Obstet Gynecol. 2015;45(3):249–66.
19. Vendola C, Canfield M, Daiger SP, Gambello M, Hashmi SS, King T, Noblin SJ, Waller DK, Hecht JT. Survival of Texas infants born with trisomies 21, 18, and 13. Am J Med Genet A. 2010;152A(2):360–6.
20. Morgan T. Turner syndrome: diagnosis and management. Am Fam Physician. 2007;76(3):405–10.
21. Papp C, Beke A, Mezei G, Szigeti Z, Bán Z, Papp Z. Prenatal diagnosis of turner syndrome: report on 69 cases. J Ultrasound Med. 2006;25(6): 711–7.
22. Kolarski M, Ahmetovic B, Beres M, Topic R, Nikic V, Kavecan I, Sabic S. Genetic counseling and prenatal diagnosis of Triploidy during the second trimester of pregnancy. Med Arch. 2017;71(2):144–7.

14 Screening for Preeclampsia

14.1 Introduction

Preeclampsia (PE) is the prodromal syndrome which precedes eclampsia, and has been classically defined as a new onset of hypertension and proteinuria developing in the second half of pregnancy and resolving after delivery. PE complicates 4.6% of all pregnancies globally and causes 63,000 maternal deaths annually. Screening can be used to prevent early PE by administering low-dose aspirin to women at risk. Furthermore, it can be performed at the 11–13 + 6 weeks scan along with combined aneuploidy screening [1].

This chapter looks at the pathophysiology, risk factors, and current understanding of PE, and the interplay between abnormal placentation and maternal cardiovascular changes. It addresses the challenges associated with early detection and prevention of PE because of the complex nature of its etiology.

14.2 Definition

The current definition of PE by the International Society for the Study of Hypertension in Pregnancy (ISSHP) is as follows [2]:

© The Author(s), under exclusive license to Springer Nature Singapore Pte Ltd. 2023
A. Kamat, *Down Syndrome Screening*,
https://doi.org/10.1007/978-981-99-7758-1_14

- New onset hypertension arising after 20 weeks of gestation (systolic ≥140 mm Hg and/or diastolic ≥90 mm Hg).
- With one additional finding:
  - Proteinuria ≥300 mg/day or protein/creatinine ratio of ≥30 mg/mmol or dipstick showing 2+ or more.
  - Maternal organ dysfunction.
    Acute kidney injury.
    Liver involvement.
    Neurological complications.
    Hematological complications.
  - Uteroplacental dysfunction.
    Fetal growth restriction.
    Abnormal umbilical artery Doppler.
    Stillbirth.

The ISSHP definition places emphasis on two major points. First, proteinuria is no longer mandatory for the diagnosis. Second, the terms 'mild' and 'severe' to describe PE have been abandoned completely because the natural history of the disorder is not predictably linear. The term 'mild PE' can be falsely reassuring and underestimates the complications that can occur in these women. These points have been affirmed by the American College of Obstetricians and Gynecologists (ACOG), and the National Institute for Health and Care Excellence (NICE) [2–4].

The onset of PE can be early or late (with delivery before or after 34 weeks of gestation). Abnormal placentation is likely to be the primary pathology in early-onset PE, while late-onset PE is caused by an imbalance between maternal perfusion and feto-placental demands, resulting in maternal cardiovascular dysfunction.

14.3 Pathophysiology

Preeclampsia is a condition caused by maternal systemic response to impaired placentation. Incomplete trophoblastic invasion of spiral arteries and impaired placental perfusion lead to placental stress. This alters the production of angiogenic factors, leading to platelet activation and maternal endothelial cell dysfunction, resulting in a massive systemic immunological and inflammatory response. The third component is believed to be inadequate maternal cardiac and hemodynamic adaptation.

14.3.1 Role of Placenta

Humans possess a hemochorial placenta, which is characterized by a minimal cellular barrier between the mother and the fetus in order to optimize nutrient transport. The musculoelastic structure of the spiral arterial wall gets replaced by a fibrinoid material containing the endovascular trophoblasts, which differentiate and closely resemble endothelial cells. The result is the formation of several low-pressure vessels with a large diameter. Remodeling of vessels has a minor impact on the volume of blood flowing to the placenta. However, it significantly reduces the velocity and pulsatility of the inflowing maternal blood and prevents injury to the growing villi and microvilli [1, 5].

Failure of effective trophophoblast invasion and incomplete spiral artery transformation results in placental dysfunction, which manifests as pregnancy loss, preeclampsia, or fetal growth restriction. Spiral artery invasion by the trophoblasts occurs in 2 waves, the first wave at 8–10 weeks and the second wave at 16–18 weeks. These represent specific gestations for applying interventions to improve the pregnancy outcome.

14.3.2 Angiogenic Factors

Placental stress causes peripheral endothelial cell dysfunction, leading to systemic inflammatory response with an increase in the release of pro-inflammatory cytokines, cell-free DNA, and soluble fms-like tyrosine kinase-1 (sFlt-1). Conversely, levels of placental growth factor (PlGF) and pregnancy-associated plasma protein A (PAPP-A) are reduced.

Placental growth factor (PlGF) is a member of the vascular endothelial growth factor (VEGF) family. It plays an important role in the development of feto-placental circulation and trophoblast growth. It has a pro-angiogenic function and enhances the activity of VEGF by binding to the VEGFR1 receptor. Levels of PlGF are low in the first trimester and increase from 11 weeks onwards until approximately 30 weeks, followed by a gradual decline. This contrasts with sFlt-1 which increases during late pregnancy [6].

Low levels of PlGF at 11–13 + 6 weeks increase the risk of developing both PE and fetal growth restriction. A raised sFlt-1/PlGF ratio also predicts imminent PE and adverse pregnancy outcomes, but its significance is greater in the second half of pregnancy [6].

Pregnancy-associated plasma protein A (PAPP-A) is a glycoprotein derived from syncytiotrophoblasts, which enhances the mitogenic function of the insulin-like growth factors. Low levels of PAPP-A are associated with placental dysfunction, preeclampsia, fetal growth restriction, and stillbirth.

Soluble fms-like tyrosine kinase-1 (sFlt-1) is an extracellular truncated form of the VEGF receptor. It lacks transmembrane and intracellular components, and therefore freely circulates in maternal blood.

In a normal pregnancy, sFlt-1 is mainly produced by the placenta and promotes the development of placental vasculature. While sFlt-1 levels increase substantially in a normal pregnancy, the rise is two-fold greater in women who develop PE. This is likely caused by placental stress and hypoxia in the second half of pregnancy in these women. Women who develop PE continue to have elevated sFlt-1 levels for several months after delivery, suggesting an additional genetic basis for sFlt-1 expression. Raised sFlt-1 binds to VEGF and reduces its bioavailability to the maternal endothelial cells. This causes an impaired secretion of nitric oxide, resulting in vasoconstriction, and consequently, preeclampsia [7].

14.3.3 Maternal Cardiovascular Dysfunction

Maternal cardiovascular maladaptation to pregnancy has been cited as a major component in the development of PE. Even in the preclinical phase, there is evidence of mildly impaired vascular reactivity, hemodynamic indices, and left ventricular function. Echocardiography performed in women who develop early PE demonstrates abnormal findings in the cardiac index, total vascular resistance index, myocardial relaxation, and ventricular wall thickness. In late-onset PE, the findings are not so well defined, although there is definite evidence of left ventricular dysfunction [8].

In further support of the cardiovascular dysfunction theory, the fall in uterine artery resistance seen in normal pregnancies is also noted in abdominal pregnancies, where spiral artery remodeling by syncytiotrophoblasts does not occur. Also, in some women with early-onset preeclampsia, the diastolic dysfunction persists for more than a year after delivery. In these women, the lifetime risk of death because of cardiovascular causes is twofold. Nonetheless, these changes cannot be viewed in isolation from placental dysfunction, as the degree of cardiovascular compromise correlates with levels of sFlt-1 and PlGF [9].

14.4 Maternal Risk Factors

Maternal risk factors for PE can be subdivided into high-risk factors and moderate-risk factors. A formal assessment of every pregnant woman should be conducted on the first visit, and those deemed at risk of developing PE should be offered low-dose aspirin (LDA) and increased surveillance. National Institute for Health and Care Excellence (UK) suggests the following risk factors based on maternal history [10].

- High risk.
  - Hypertension during a previous pregnancy.
  - Chronic renal disease.
  - Autoimmune disease such as systemic lupus erythematosus or antiphospholipid antibody syndrome.
  - Type 1 or type 2 diabetes.
  - Chronic hypertension.
- Moderate risk.
  - Primigravida.
  - Age 40 years or older.
  - Inter-pregnancy interval of over 10 years.
  - Body mass index of 35 or more.
  - Family history of PE.
  - Multiple pregnancy.
- Women considered at risk of developing PE.
  - At least 1 high-risk factor, or.
  - At least 2 moderate-risk factors.

A similar guideline has been published by the US Preventive Services Task Force. The ACOG, the Society for Maternal-Fetal Medicine, and the American Diabetes Association have endorsed it [11, 12].

14.4.1 Performance as a Screening Test

Using maternal risk factors alone, the detection rates for all PE are 29% and 40% for a false positive rate (FPR) of 5% and 10% respectively. For PE requiring delivery before 34 weeks, the detection rates are 36% for a 5% FPR and 51% for a 10% FPR [13].

ACOG and NICE recommend using maternal risk factors to stratify at-risk women for administration of LDA. The Federation of Obstetric and Gynecological Societies of India (FOGSI) recommends risk assessment by using the 'HDP-Gestosis' score. Under this scoring system, each clinical risk factor is assigned a risk of 1,2, or 3. Women with an overall score of ≥3 are considered at a high risk for developing PE [3, 4, 14].

14.5 Mean Arterial Pressure

Increased blood pressure (BP) is a secondary manifestation of PE caused by reactive vasoconstriction. Therefore, maternal BP readings in the first and second trimesters of pregnancy strongly relate to PE risk.

14.5.1 Technique

Equipment: Measurement of BP using a mercury sphygmomanometer has been considered as a gold standard method. However, its subjective nature and equipment safety concerns have resulted in most centers using automated or semi-automated devices.

Measurement technique: The patient should sit in a relaxed posture with her back supported and legs uncrossed. Bladder should be empty. After resting for 5 minutes, blood pressure is measured in both arms simultaneously (supported at the level of the heart). Systolic and diastolic pressure should be measured with the correct cuff size, and mean arterial pressure (MAP) calculated. After 1 minute, the measurements from both arms should be repeated. The mean of the four measurements of MAP (two from each arm) should be considered. MAP can be calculated using the formula:

$$\text{MAP} = \frac{\text{Systolic BP} + (2 \times \text{Diastolic BP})}{3}$$

Factors affecting MAP: MAP is dependent on several factors, including age, height, weight, race, smoking, and past history or family history of preeclampsia or chronic hypertension. A composite maternal risk of developing PE should be calculated using the MoM values of MAP along with the maternal risk factors. Several online PE risk calculators are available for this purpose.

14.5.2 Performance as a Screening Test

Addition of MAP to maternal risk factors improves the detection rate (DR) of early-onset PE to 73% and all PE to 54% for a 10% FPR. This approach is useful in low-resource settings, where screening using uterine artery Doppler and maternal serum markers is not feasible [13].

14.6 Uterine Artery Doppler

Uterine artery Doppler has emerged as a powerful tool in PE screening, especially when combined with other variables. Its correct technique and interpretation are of utmost importance in order to gain valuable information about placental function and vascular resistance. Increased uterine artery resistance reflects inefficient spiral artery transformation.

14.6.1 Anatomy

The uterine arteries arise from the anterior division of the internal iliac arteries. They travel medially through the broad ligament, cross the ureters, and supply the uterus. At the isthmus, each artery divides into ascending and descending branches. The ascending uterine arteries subsequently branch into the arcuate arteries. Radial arteries arise from these arcuate arteries and give rise to the basal arteries supplying the endometrium. Spiral arteries arise from the basal arteries, and perfuse the endometrium during the luteal phase of the menstrual cycle and the placenta during pregnancy.

14.6.2 Transabdominal (TAS) Technique

- Maternal bladder should be partially full.
- The curvilinear ultrasound transducer is placed vertically on the maternal suprapubic region. A midsagittal section of the uterus is obtained, and the cervix is imaged in the midline.

- Color Doppler is switched on and the transducer is tilted gently to one side in the parasagittal plane to visualize the uterine artery, which is the largest pulsating vessel in the paracervical region (Fig. 14.1a).
- In the second trimester, the uterine arteries are easier to insonate more laterally, at the point of their crossover with the external iliac arteries.
- Pulse wave Doppler with a small sample gate (2–3 mm) is placed over the ascending branch of the uterine artery close to the internal os. The angle of insonation should be less than 30°.
- Sampling of the correct vessel is confirmed by a peak systolic velocity of >60 cm/s and an upright (antegrade) waveform (Fig. 14.1b).
- Pulsatility index (PI) is an automatic calculation performed by the ultrasound machine by tracing the waveform.
- The process is repeated on the other side.

14.6.3 Transvaginal (TVS) Technique

- Maternal bladder should be completely empty.
- The TVS probe is placed in the anterior fornix in the midline to visualize the cervix.
- Color Doppler is switched on and the probe is moved laterally toward the fornix. The uterine artery is imaged similar to the abdominal technique (Fig 14.2a).
- The uterine artery appears as a large pulsatile curved vessel. By sampling the appropriate portion of the curving artery, it is possible to get an insonation angle of less than 30 degrees (Fig 14.2b).
- Sampling of the correct vessel is confirmed by a peak systolic velocity of >60 cm/s and an upright (antegrade) waveform. The PI is automatically calculated as mentioned above, and the process is repeated on the other side.

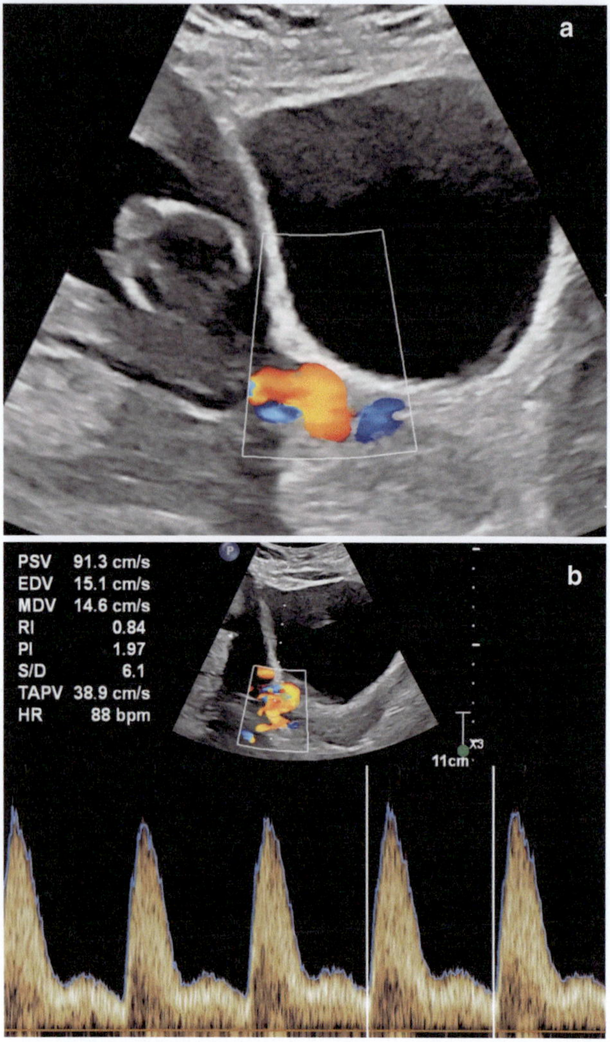

Fig. 14.1 TAS technique of performing the uterine artery Doppler. (**a**) Demonstration of the uterine artery on the left side of the maternal cervix using color Doppler (**b**) The uterine artery is sampled with pulsed Doppler, and the machine automatically calculates the PI by tracing the waveform. An upright waveform and a peak systolic velocity > 60 cm/s indicate that the correct vessel has been sampled

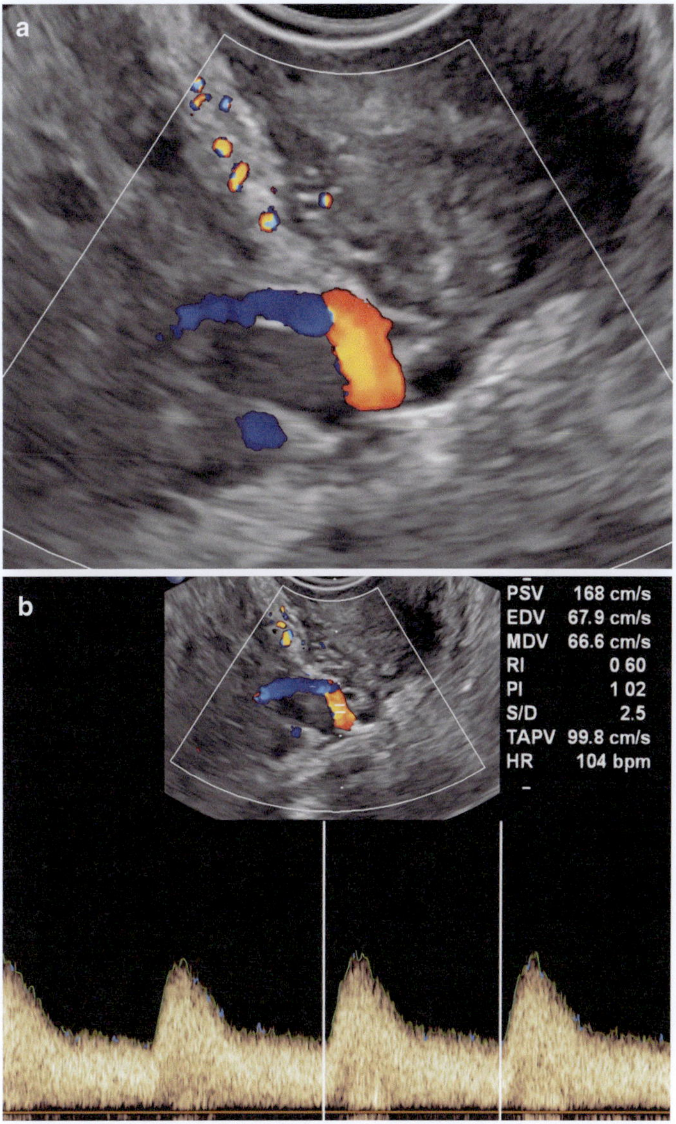

Fig. 14.2 TVS technique of performing the uterine artery Doppler. (**a**) Demonstration of the curved uterine artery in the parasagittal plane using color Doppler (**b**) By sampling the appropriate part of the vessel, it is possible to achieve an insonation angle of less than 30 degrees

14.6.4 Important Considerations

The ultrasound machine should be correctly set and fine-tuned. Ultrasound machines from different manufacturers use slightly different settings and terminology. Ideally, a separate preset for the uterine artery Doppler should be saved.

In brief, optimal sampling of uterine arteries requires a small color box, moderate color gain, and high color persistence. Pulse wave Doppler settings include a moderately high pulse repetition frequency (PRF) and wall motion filter. The PRF should be adjusted as required, such that the waveform height corresponds to approximately 75% of the designated area on the screen. The speed should be set to display 4–6 complete cardiac cycles on the screen. Either automatic or manual tracing of the waveform is acceptable.

If an inverse waveform is obtained, it is likely that the descending cervical branch is being erroneously sampled. In such cases, the vessel being sampled should be corrected.

14.6.5 Pulsatility Index

Doppler indices commonly used in obstetric practice are the systolic to diastolic ratio, resistance index, and pulsatility index (PI). Pulsatility index is the difference between the peak systolic velocity (PSV) and the end-diastolic velocity (EDV) divided by the mean velocity.

$$\mathrm{PI} = \frac{\mathrm{PSV} - \mathrm{EDV}}{\text{Mean velocity}}$$

The PI is preferred over other Doppler indices for several reasons. First, the PI is useful in all three trimesters. Second, the PI is calculated using the average of all maximum velocities throughout the waveform. Third, unlike the resistance index, the PI does not become infinite even in cases of absent end diastolic flow. Ultrasound machines can automatically calculate PI with a high intra-observer and inter-observer reproducibility.

Important points for using the uterine artery PI (UtPI):

1. The mean PI value of the two uterine arteries should be considered. High-resistance uterine artery flow is defined as PI above 95th percentile (see Table 14.1).
2. When the placental implantation site is the left or the right uterine wall, the PI on the contralateral side is usually raised. Unilateral high-resistance flow is not associated with an increased risk of PE.
3. The mean PI varies depending on the gestational age and the sampling route. Between 11 and 13 + 6 weeks, 95th percentile for mean uterine PI can be approximated as 2.35 when measured by the transabdominal approach.
4. The PI is higher when measured by TVS, likely because of a different anatomical site of sampling or a smaller angle of insonation. When measured transvaginally, the 95th percentile falls from 3.1 at 11 weeks to 2.36 at 13 + 6 weeks [15].
5. In the second trimester, the PI gradually falls with increasing gestation.

Table 14.1 Reference values for uterine artery PI (95th percentile) using transabdominal approach [16, 17]

Gestational age (weeks)	95th percentile for mean UtPI
11	2.35
12	2.35
13	2.35
14	2.24
15	2.11
16	1.99
17	1.88
18	1.79
19	1.70
20	1.61
21	1.54
22	1.47
23	1.41
24	1.35
25	1.30
26	1.25
27	1.21
28	1.17

14.6.6 Uterine Artery Notching

Presence of bilateral uterine artery notching in addition to a high PI further increases the likelihood of placental dysfunction. However, notching alone is a poor predictor for PE because of the following reasons:

1. Uterine artery notching is a subjective finding. Degree of fall in velocity at the notch does not correlate well with adverse pregnancy outcomes.
2. *Notching is present in more than half of normal pregnancies in the first trimester as the low-resistance vessels within the placenta are not completely developed.*
3. In the second trimester, it has a similar sensitivity to PI, but a higher FPR.

14.6.7 Performance as a Screening Test

First-trimester uterine artery Doppler has a moderate sensitivity of 42% for a 10% FPR for all PE. The sensitivity for early-onset PE is 75% for the same FPR. It performs better in the second trimester, with a sensitivity of 43% for all PE and 78% for early-onset PE < 34 weeks with a 5% FPR. The risk of preeclampsia is highest when high PI and bilateral notching persist from the first to the second trimester. Third-trimester assessment of uterine artery Doppler has an important role in the diagnosis of late-onset FGR. However, there is inadequate evidence showing its benefit in PE prediction and management [18, 19].

In 2019, the Indian Radiological and Imaging Association (IRIA) launched a nationwide program called 'Samrakshan' to reduce perinatal mortality in India. It involves training radiologists to perform a risk assessment for preterm PE and FGR at 11–14 weeks using maternal demographic factors, MAP and mean UtPI. The calculator provided by the Fetal Medicine Foundation is used to estimate the risk of developing early PE. Analysis of data of 4372 pregnant women over a 3-year period showed a sensitivity of 64% for a 10% FPR using a risk cutoff of 1:150. Daily administration of 150 mg of aspirin resulted in a 76.5% reduction in preterm PE in high-risk women. This approach may be useful for low-income and middle-income countries [20–22].

14.7 Combined Screening Using Serum Markers

Like Down syndrome screening, PE screening can be performed by using software algorithms combining maternal risk factors with MAP, mean UtPI, and serum markers (PlGF and PAPP-A). Such an approach aims to increase screening sensitivity and reduce the FPR compared to single-factor screening. Screening can be offered between 11 and 13 + 6 weeks when the woman presents for the NT scan [12].

Women who subsequently develop PE have a higher MAP and higher mean UtPI. Levels of PAPP-A and PlGF are lower, reflecting placental dysfunction. The software program converts each of these values into multiples of median (MoM) and integrates them to arrive at a risk estimate. Women who have a screen-positive result are offered low-dose aspirin (LDA) from the time of screening until delivery.

Second- and third-trimester screening with maternal factors and sFlt-1 levels or sFlt-1/PlGF ratio has been shown to be useful for predicting PE. Unfortunately, LDA started after 16 weeks has a very limited role. Second-trimester prediction is more useful for initiating increased surveillance, rather than for prevention.

14.7.1 Performance as a Screening Test

First-trimester levels of PlGF are significantly lower in women who subsequently develop early PE. PlGF alone has a sensitivity of 56% for early PE for a 9% FPR. This is significantly better than that of PAPP-A, which only has a 16% sensitivity when used alone. A combined risk assessment using maternal risk factors, MAP, UtPI, and PLGF can successfully predict 90% of early PE, 75% of preterm PE, and 41% of term PE, at a screen positive rate of 10% [23–25]. A contingent model has also been suggested. In this model, the whole population is screened using maternal risk factors and MAP, and those with intermediate risk (approximately 30%) undergo further screening with UtPI and PlGF.

Combined first-trimester screening is currently recommended as the most efficient screening model by the International Federation of Gynecology and Obstetrics (FIGO), International Society of Ultrasound in Obstetrics and Gynecology (ISUOG), and the Society of Obstetricians and Gynaecologists of Canada (SOGC) [12, 26, 27].

14.8 Limitations of PE Screening

Unlike Down syndrome screening, preeclampsia screening has not found universal acceptance for several reasons, as discussed below.

Positive predictive value (PPV): In order to achieve an acceptable detection rate with PE screening, the FPR needs to be at least 10%. The high FPR, in turn, reduces the PPV to only 20%. This implies that 80% of women deemed to be at high risk would not develop PE. The result would be unnecessary interventions and increased anxiety in these women, and an increased load on healthcare systems.

Combined screening: Combined screening provides a modest increase in sensitivity compared to maternal characteristics, MAP, and uterine Doppler. However, combined screening is based on the calculation of MoM values, which requires robust data for the local population. Unlike Down syndrome screening, data regarding PE screening is limited. Furthermore, women with risk factors for PE still require close surveillance in pregnancy, irrespective of their combined screening result.

Twin pregnancies: Multiple pregnancy is a moderate risk factor for PE. Conversely, the mean uterine artery PI is lower because of the larger size of the placenta. Unless twin-specific ranges are used, the sensitivity of the uterine artery Doppler is significantly lower.

Using a combined screening model, the detection rates for early PE, preterm PE, and term PE are 100%, 99%, and 97%, respectively. However, this is achieved at the cost of a staggeringly high 75% screen-positive rate. This would translate to administering LDA prophylaxis to three-fourths of all women with twin pregnancies [28].

Second- and third-trimester screening: The INSPIRE clinical trial was a randomized interventional study which used the sFlt-1/PlGF ratio in women who presented with suspected PE. For developing PE in the next 4 weeks, a ratio of >38 had a PPV of 36.7%, while a ratio of ≤38 had a negative predictive value (NPV) of 97%. While it improved the clinical precision in diagnosing PE, there was no difference in the total number of admissions or the perinatal outcome [29, 30].

Screening in the second half of pregnancy does not leave much room for preventive strategies to be applied. Rather, these women may benefit from monitoring for hypertension, proteinuria, and fetal growth restriction.

Late-onset PE: The prediction of late-onset PE remains elusive, irrespective of the screening method used. A scoping systematic review in 2023 concluded that no single biomarker had sufficient clinical sensitivity and specificity for screening late-onset and term PE. Multivariate models combining maternal risk factors with serum markers performed marginally better, but lacked validation data [31].

14.9 Low-Dose Aspirin

The entire premise of first-trimester screening for PE is based on the hope of preventing its occurrence or reducing its severity.

Aspirin or acetylsalicylic acid is a non-steroidal anti-inflammatory drug which inhibits the cyclooxygenase isoenzymes COX-1 and COX-2. In platelets, COX-1 is essential for the synthesis of thromboxane A2, which stimulates platelet aggregation and vasoconstriction. Vascular endothelial cells also express COX-1, which boosts prostacyclin production (causing vasodilatation). Low-dose aspirin (LDA) selectively inhibits platelet COX-1 reducing thromboxane A2 synthesis, while allowing prostacyclin synthesis by the endothelium. This has a net effect of vasodilatation. It is unlikely that the preventive mechanism of LDA is solely based on the alteration of thromboxane A2/prostacyclin ratio. Possibly, LDA also affects early placental perfusion and vascular remodeling [32].

14.9.1 Efficacy in PE Prevention

Starting aspirin before 16 weeks reduces the risk of preterm PE. Doses between 100 and 150 mg appear to be most effective, as some women show aspirin resistance at lower doses. There is evidence of a modest benefit even when aspirin is started between 16 and 28 weeks [33].

The ASPRE study was a multicenter, double-blind, placebo-controlled trial which randomized 1776 women with singleton pregnancy at high risk of preeclampsia to receive either 150 mg of aspirin or placebo from 11 to 14 weeks until 36 weeks of gestation. The result was a 62% risk reduction (from 4.3 to 1.6%) for preterm PE [34].

In multiple pregnancies, LDA has been shown to reduce the risk of developing mild PE, but not severe PE. Due to insufficient data, there is only limited evidence supporting its benefits [35].

14.9.2 Maternal and Fetal Risks

Continuation of LDA after the second trimester of pregnancy has not been shown to increase maternal risk of bleeding or placental abruption. Gestation at which it is discontinued also does not affect bleeding at the time of delivery. Aspirin need not be stopped in case of vaginal spotting, if it is self-limiting. LDA does not increase the risk of congenital anomalies, premature closure of ductus arteriosus, or fetal intracranial hemorrhage. Similarly, the risk of neonatal complications is not increased [12, 33, 34].

Table 14.2 Recommendations on preeclampsia screening and prevention. ACOG, American College of Obstetricians and Gynecologists; NICE, National Institute for Health and Care Excellence; FIGO, International Federation of Gynecology and Obstetrics; ISUOG, International Society of Ultrasound in Obstetrics and Gynecology; SOGC, Society of Obstetricians and Gynaecologists of Canada; FOGSI, Federation of Obstetric and Gynecological Societies of India; IRIA, Indian Radiological and Imaging Association [4, 12, 14, 22, 26, 27, 33]

Recommending bodies	Screening protocol for PE	LDA dose (mg/day)	Gestation to start	Gestation to stop[a]
ACOG	Maternal risk factors	81	12–28 weeks (ideally <16 weeks)	At delivery
NICE	Maternal risk factors	75–150	12 weeks	At delivery
FIGO, ISUOG	Combined screening[b]	100–150	11–15 weeks	36 weeks or at delivery
SOGC	Combined screening[b]	81–162	Before 16 weeks	36 weeks
FOGSI	Maternal risk factors	75–150	<12 weeks	2 days prior to delivery
IRIA	Maternal risk factors + MAP + UtPI	150	11–14 weeks	36 weeks

[a]In all cases, LDA should be stopped if preterm delivery occurs

[b]In low-resource settings, the minimum screening recommended is a combination of maternal risk factors and MAP

14.9.3 Recommendations for PE Screening and LDA Use

Recommendations by different medical organizations differ slightly as regards the recommended screening protocol and the dose of aspirin (Table 14.2).

14.9.4 Other Preventive Measures

Measures like salt restriction, rest, exercise, and antioxidants have not shown significant benefit in clinical trials. In women who are deficient in calcium, dietary supplementation may help reduce the PE risk [12, 14].

Since sFlt-1 is implicated to be a key biomarker in the causation of PE, therapeutic reduction of its levels should, in theory, result in alleviation of this syndrome and prolongation of pregnancy. At present, interventions to reduce maternal sFlt-1 levels, such as the drug pravastatin and plasma apheresis, are considered experimental.

14.10 Key Messages

1. PE results from maternal cardiovascular maladaptation to altered inflammatory and angiogenic mediator levels because of impaired placentation.
2. PE screening using maternal risk factors, MAP, UtPI, and PlGF has the highest sensitivity, but is resource intensive.
3. In lower resource settings, either maternal risk factors alone, or combined with MAP, with or without UtPI may be used.
4. All screening models are better at predicting early PE rather than late PE.
5. All PE screening models have a high FPR and a low PPV.
6. PE screening in multiple pregnancies has not been standardized or validated.
7. Treating high-risk singleton pregnancies with 100–150 mg aspirin from 12 weeks till term reduces the risk of severe PE by at least two-thirds.

References

1. Burton GJ, Redman CW, Roberts JM, Moffett A. Pre-eclampsia: pathophysiology and clinical implications. BMJ. 2019;366:l2381.
2. Brown MA, Magee LA, Kenny LC, Karumanchi SA, McCarthy FP, Saito S, Hall DR, Warren CE, Adoyi G, Ishaku S. International Society for the Study of hypertension in pregnancy (ISSHP). Hypertensive disorders of pregnancy: ISSHP classification, diagnosis, and management recommendations for international practice. Hypertension. 2018;72(1):24–43.
3. Gestational Hypertension and Preeclampsia. ACOG practice bulletin, number 222. Obstet Gynecol. 2020;135(6):e237–60.

4. National Institute for Health and Care Excellence. 2019. Hypertension in pregnancy: diagnosis and management [NICE Guideline No. 133]. https://www.nice.org.uk/guidance/ng133. Accessed 17 June 2023.
5. Soares MJ, Varberg KM, Iqbal K. Hemochorial placentation: development, function, and adaptations. Biol Reprod. 2018;99(1):196–211.
6. Chau K, Hennessy A, Makris A. Placental growth factor and preeclampsia. J Hum Hypertens. 2017;31(12):782–6.
7. Caillon H, Tardif C, Dumontet E, Winer N, Masson D. Evaluation of sFlt-1/PlGF ratio for predicting and improving clinical Management of Pre-eclampsia: experience in a specialized perinatal care center. Ann Lab Med. 2018;38(2):95–101.
8. Melchiorre K, Sharma R, Thilaganathan B. Cardiovascular implications in preeclampsia: an overview. Circulation. 2014;130(8):703–14.
9. Yagel S, Verlohren S. Role of placenta in development of pre-eclampsia: revisited. Ultrasound Obstet Gynecol. 2020;56(6):803–8.
10. National Institute for Health and Care Excellence. 2019. Hypertension in pregnancy: Quality standard [QS35]. https://www.nice.org.uk/guidance/qs35. Accessed 17 June 2023.
11. LeFevre ML, U.S. Preventive Services Task Force. Low-dose aspirin use for the prevention of morbidity and mortality from preeclampsia: U.S. preventive services Task Force recommendation statement. Ann Intern Med. 2014;161(11):819–26.
12. Poon LC, Shennan A, Hyett JA, Kapur A, Hadar E, Divakar H, McAuliffe F, da Silva CF, von Dadelszen P, McIntyre HD, Kihara AB, Di Renzo GC, Romero R, D'Alton M, Berghella V, Nicolaides KH, Hod M. The International Federation of Gynecology and Obstetrics (FIGO) initiative on pre-eclampsia: a pragmatic guide for first-trimester screening and prevention. Int J Gynaecol Obstet. 2019;145(Suppl 1(Suppl 1)):1–33.
13. Wright D, Akolekar R, Syngelaki A, Poon LC, Nicolaides KH. A competing risks model in early screening for preeclampsia. Fetal Diagn Ther. 2012;32(3):171–8.
14. The Federation of Obstetric and Gynecological Societies of India. 2019. Hypertensive Disorders in Pregnancy [Good Clinical Practice Recommendations]. https://www.fogsi.org/fogsi-hdp-gcpr-2019. Accessed 17 June 2023.
15. Plasencia W, Barber MA, Alvarez EE, Segura J, Valle L, Garcia-Hernandez JA. Comparative study of transabdominal and transvaginal uterine artery Doppler pulsatility indices at 11-13 + 6 weeks. Hypertens Pregnancy. 2011;30(4):414–20.
16. Martin AM, Bindra R, Curcio P, Cicero S, Nicolaides KH. Screening for pre-eclampsia and fetal growth restriction by uterine artery Doppler at 11-14 weeks of gestation. Ultrasound Obstet Gynecol. 2001;18(6):583–6.
17. Gómez O, Figueras F, Fernández S, Bennasar M, Martínez JM, Puerto B, Gratacós E. Reference ranges for uterine artery mean pulsatility

index at 11-41 weeks of gestation. Ultrasound Obstet Gynecol. 2008;32(2):128–32.
18. Akolekar R, Syngelaki A, Poon L, Wright D, Nicolaides KH. Competing risks model in early screening for preeclampsia by biophysical and biochemical markers. Fetal Diagn Ther. 2013;33(1):8–15.
19. Yu CK, Smith GC, Papageorghiou AT, Cacho AM, Nicolaides KH. Fetal Medicine Foundation second trimester screening group. An integrated model for the prediction of pre-eclampsia using maternal factors and uterine artery Doppler velocimetry in unselected low-risk women. Am J Obstet Gynecol. 2006;195(1):330.
20. Choorakuttil RM, Patel H, Bavaharan R, Devarajan P, Kanhirat S, Shenoy RS, Tiwari OP, Sodani RK, Sharma LK, Nirmalan PK. Samrakshan: an Indian radiological and imaging association program to reduce perinatal mortality in India. Indian J Radiol Imaging. 2019;29(4):412–7.
21. The Fetal Medicine Foundation. Risk assessment—Risk for preeclampsia [Internet]. https://fetalmedicine.org/research/assess/preeclampsia/first-trimester. Assessed 17 June 2023.
22. Choorakuttil RM, Rajalingam B, Satarkar SR, Sharma LK, Gupta A, Baghel A, Jain N, Dhankar S, Aneja K, Chhajer G, Dwivedi S, Patekar TY, Rajput E, Nirmalan PK. Effectiveness of the first trimester Samrakshan protocol for the identification of pregnant women at high risk for preterm Pre-eclampsia. Indian J Radiol Imaging. 2022;33(1):98–100.
23. Zhong Y, Zhu F, Ding Y. Serum screening in first trimester to predict pre-eclampsia, small for gestational age and preterm delivery: systematic review and meta-analysis. BMC Pregnancy Childbirth. 2015;15:191.
24. Morris RK, Bilagi A, Devani P, Kilby MD. Association of serum PAPP-A levels in first trimester with small for gestational age and adverse pregnancy outcomes: systematic review and meta-analysis. Prenat Diagn. 2017;37(3):253–65.
25. Tan MY, Syngelaki A, Poon LC, Rolnik DL, O'Gorman N, Delgado JL, Akolekar R, Konstantinidou L, Tsavdaridou M, Galeva S, Ajdacka U, Molina FS, Persico N, Jani JC, Plasencia W, Greco E, Papaioannou G, Wright A, Wright D, Nicolaides KH. Screening for pre-eclampsia by maternal factors and biomarkers at 11-13 weeks' gestation. Ultrasound Obstet Gynecol. 2018;52(2):186–95.
26. Sotiriadis A, Hernandez-Andrade E, da Silva CF, Ghi T, Glanc P, Khalil A, Martins WP, Odibo AO, Papageorghiou AT, Salomon LJ, Thilaganathan B, ISUOG CSC Pre-eclampsia Task Force. ISUOG practice guidelines: role of ultrasound in screening for and follow-up of pre-eclampsia. Ultrasound Obstet Gynecol. 2019;53(1):7–22.
27. Magee LA, Smith GN, Bloch C, Côté AM, Jain V, Nerenberg K, von Dadelszen P, Helewa M, Rey E. Guideline No. 426: hypertensive disor-

ders of pregnancy: diagnosis, prediction, prevention, and management. J Obstet Gynaecol Can. 2022;44(5):547–571.e1.

28. Francisco C, Wright D, Benkő Z, Syngelaki A, Nicolaides KH. Competing-risks model in screening for pre-eclampsia in twin pregnancy according to maternal factors and biomarkers at 11-13 weeks' gestation. Ultrasound Obstet Gynecol. 2017;50(5):589–95.
29. Cerdeira AS, O'Sullivan J, Ohuma EO, Harrington D, Szafranski P, Black R, Mackillop L, Impey L, Greenwood C, James T, Smith I, Papageorghiou AT, Knight M, Vatish M. Randomized interventional study on prediction of preeclampsia/eclampsia in women with suspected preeclampsia: INSPIRE. Hypertension. 2019;74(4):983–90.
30. Cerdeira AS, O'Sullivan J, Ohuma EO, James T, Papageorghiou AT, Knight M, Vatish M. Ruling out preeclampsia in the next 4 weeks using a soluble fms-like tyrosine kinase 1/placental growth factor ratio ≤38: secondary analysis of the interventional study on prediction of preeclampsia/eclampsia in women with suspected preeclampsia. Am J Obstet Gynecol. 2022;226(3):443–5.
31. Han L, Holland OJ, Da Silva CF, Perkins AV. Potential biomarkers for late-onset and term preeclampsia: a scoping review. Front Physiol. 2023;14:1143543.
32. Atallah A, Lecarpentier E, Goffinet F, Doret-Dion M, Gaucherand P, Tsatsaris V. Aspirin for prevention of preeclampsia. Drugs. 2017;77(17):1819–31.
33. ACOG Committee Opinion No 743. Low-dose aspirin use during pregnancy. Obstet Gynecol. 2018;132(1):e44–52.
34. Rolnik DL, Wright D, Poon LC, O'Gorman N, Syngelaki A, de Paco MC, Akolekar R, Cicero S, Janga D, Singh M, Molina FS, Persico N, Jani JC, Plasencia W, Papaioannou G, Tenenbaum-Gavish K, Meiri H, Gizurarson S, Maclagan K, Nicolaides KH. Aspirin versus placebo in pregnancies at high risk for preterm preeclampsia. N Engl J Med. 2017;377(7):613–22.
35. Bergeron TS, Roberge S, Carpentier C, Sibai B, McCaw-Binns A, Bujold E. Prevention of preeclampsia with aspirin in multiple gestations: a systematic review and meta-analysis. Am J Perinatol. 2016;33(6):605–10.

Screening for Open Spina Bifida

15

15.1 Introduction

Every year, over 3,00,000 children are born with a neural tube defect (NTD), only outnumbered by those with congenital heart defects [1]. Open neural tube defects (ONTDs) are characterized by an absence of skin cover, and therefore have a poor prognosis compared to closed NTDs. Widespread use of folic acid supplementation has reduced their prevalence in the last few decades. Unfortunately, the neural tube is one of the earliest structures to develop, and forms at a time when the woman may not even be aware of her pregnancy. Hence, improved antenatal detection will go a long way in further lowering the burden of ONTDs. While anencephaly is readily diagnosed on ultrasound, cases of open spina bifida (OSB) may present with less obvious findings, increasing the likelihood of missed diagnoses. This chapter examines the evolving approach in the detection of open spina bifida from serum screening to first-trimester imaging.

15.2 Open Neural Tube Defects

The brain and spine develop from the neural tube, which is formed by the folding of the neural plate, a flat sheet of neuroepithelial cells. The formation of the neural tube occurs during the 3–4 weeks

© The Author(s), under exclusive license to Springer Nature Singapore Pte Ltd. 2023
A. Kamat, *Down Syndrome Screening*,
https://doi.org/10.1007/978-981-99-7758-1_15

following fertilization. It begins in the cervical region and extends cranially and caudally. Failure of closure of the cranial end of the neural tube results in anencephaly or craniorachischisis (anencephaly + contiguous spinal defect), while non-closure of the caudal end leads to OSB.

Over two hundred genes are involved in the process of neurulation. ONTDs have a multi-factorial etiology, with both genetic and environmental influences. Besides trisomy 13, trisomy 18, and triploidy, an ONTD can be a part of several syndromes caused by deletions, duplications, and single-gene defects.

Folic acid and vitamin B12 deficiencies are strongly linked to the occurrence of isolated non-syndromic ONTDs. Drugs which lower folic acid levels or interfere with folic acid metabolism (e.g., valproic acid) have a similar effect. Women with methylenetetrahydrofolate reductase (MTHFR) gene polymorphism are also at a slightly higher risk, however, routine screening of this mutation has no demonstrable benefits. *Folic acid is the only type of folate known to help prevent ONTDs. There is no evidence that other folates like methyl-tetrahydrofolate have a beneficial role* [2].

Other risk factors include diabetes, obesity, and hyperthermia in early pregnancy. Geographical, racial, and ethnic influences may also play a role.

15.2.1 Open Spina Bifida (OSB)

Spina bifida can present as an open neural tube defect (ONTD) or a closed neural tube defect. Most cases of spina bifida occur in the lumbosacral region. Open spina bifida (also called 'open spinal dysraphism') is associated with a skin defect overlying the NTD, causing neural elements to be exposed to the exterior and leakage of cerebrospinal fluid (CSF). Approximately 80% of cases of spina bifida are open. Loss of CSF produces characteristic changes in the fetal brain (the Chiari malformation type 2), which makes the OSB far easier to diagnose compared to the closed one. Absent skin cover also results in the leakage of alpha-fetoprotein (AFP) and acetylcholinesterase in the amniotic fluid, which can be detected by amniocentesis, and (in the case of AFP) by maternal serum screening.

OSB can be of three types:

- Meningocele: Only the meninges protrude through the spinal defect forming a cystic mass filled with CSF.
- Meningomyelocele: Neural elements also herniate through the spinal defect, and can be demonstrated within the dorsal sac.
- Myeloschisis: This is the most severe form in which the neural placode is not covered by meninges, and therefore directly exposed to the exterior. Often, the neural placode is flush with the skin, making direct visualization difficult if the fetal back is posterior.

Prognosis depends on the level and size of the defect, severity of the Chiari II malformation, and the presence or absence of hydrocephalus. Approximately 15% of affected children die within the first 5 years, the figure increasing to 35% in those with brainstem disorders. Approximately 80% of patients require shunt placement to prevent complications. Lesions above spinal level L2 typically result in paraplegia. Over 50% of affected individuals experience bowel or bladder incontinence. In-utero repair of OSB is associated with better survival and neurological outcomes, at least in the short term [3].

Closed spina bifida (or 'closed spinal dysraphism') is characterized by normal skin covering the NTD. Closed NTDs are classified into defects with a subcutaneous mass (meningocele/lipoma) or defects without a subcutaneous mass (diastematomyelia). In either case, prenatal diagnosis is relatively difficult because of the subtle spinal findings and the absence of cranial signs. They cannot be detected by amniocentesis or maternal serum screening, as there is no CSF leak, and the maternal serum AFP levels remain unchanged. As brain herniation does not occur, neurological outcomes are vastly better.

15.3 Maternal Serum Alpha-Fetoprotein (MSAFP)

Alpha-fetoprotein (AFP) is a glycoprotein secreted by the yolk sac and fetal liver (see Chap. 3). It was first discovered in 1956, when protein electrophoresis of fetal serum produced a new band which was not present in adults. By the late 1970s, it was recognized that open neural tube defects and fetal abdominal wall defects led to higher levels of AFP in amniotic fluid. Subsequently, MSAFP was recognized as a screening test for ONTDs because of its correlation with amniotic fluid AFP levels [4, 5].

15.3.1 Alpha-Fetoprotein and Fetal Defects

Fetal serum concentration of AFP is approximately 2000 μg/mL, while the amniotic fluid concentration is 100 times lower (20 μg/mL). Amniotic fluid AFP levels are very high in ONTDs and abdominal wall defects, because of leakage of fetal fluids into the amniotic cavity. Raised amniotic fluid AFP is therefore considered a diagnostic test for these anomalies [5].

Maternal serum concentration of AFP is 100 times lower than that of amniotic fluid. It also depends on transplacental transfer of AFP. Therefore, raised MSAFP is suggestive, but not diagnostic of an ONTD. Conversely, raised MSAFP in the absence of an ONTD is a marker for placental dysfunction [5].

15.3.2 Performance and Limitations of MSAFP Screening

Levels of MSAFP are expressed as multiples of median (MoM), and a single cutoff of >2.5 MoM is considered screen-positive for risk of ONTD. Screening by MSAFP is most sensitive between 16 and 18 weeks; the quadruple marker test should ideally be performed at this gestation to optimize the detection rates of OSB along with aneuploidy. Maternal serum screening for OSB has a sensitivity of approximately 65%–80% for a false positive rate of

1%–3%. The sensitivity increases when the pregnancy is dated by the biparietal diameter (BPD), as these fetuses have a smaller head size [6].

Serum screening for fetal ONTDs was proposed when fetal imaging was still in its infancy. With high-resolution USG machines, the detection rate far exceeds that of MSAFP screening. Today, the detection rate of OSB at the 20-week targeted anomaly scan is over 95%. Several factors can affect MSAFP levels. MSAFP levels in twins are usually between 4.0 and 5.0 MoM. Rarer conditions raising MSAFP levels are congenital nephrotic syndrome and Beckwith-Wiedemann syndrome. Importantly, closed NTDs do not raise MSAFP levels, because the intact skin cover prevents leakage of AFP into amniotic fluid.

15.3.3 Current Role of MSAFP as a Screening Test

As of today, two-dimensional ultrasonography is the gold standard for diagnosing NTDs. MSAFP may still have a role in select cases [7]. Obese patients may be offered MSAFP screening along with a second-trimester ultrasound to increase detection rates of OSB. MSAFP may also help to differentiate between open and closed defects when spina bifida is associated with an overlying mass but no cranial findings. In such cases, the estimation of AFP and acetylcholinesterase in the amniotic fluid may confirm the diagnosis. This is rarely, if ever, required in contemporary clinical practice.

15.3.4 Raised MSAFP with a Structurally Normal Fetus

If the maternal serum screening shows an increased risk of ONTD because of high AFP levels, a targeted ultrasound scan should be performed by an expert sonologist. In structurally normal fetuses, raised MSAFP should be considered a marker for placental dysfunction. This occurs because of an increased trans-placental leakage into maternal circulation rather than overproduction.

When both raised MSAFP and low PAPP-A are present, their effect is synergistic. These women are at a significant risk of pre-eclampsia, fetal growth restriction, preterm birth, and stillbirth.

15.4 Second-Trimester Ultrasound

Second-trimester ultrasound is the gold standard for diagnosis of OSB. The demonstration of the spinal defect is possible in nearly all cases, provided a systematic examination of the spine is performed. In the not-so-obvious cases, the identification of secondary cranial signs (the Chiari II malformation) usually leads the sonographer to the spinal defect.

15.4.1 Demonstration of the Spinal Defect

Visualization of the spine may be hampered by an unfavorable fetal position. If the spine is posterior, it is a sound practice to re-scan the patient after the fetus turns. As fetuses tend to move relatively less in the third trimester, the woman may need to be called in again after a day or two.

The spinal defect can be demonstrated in three planes:

Sagittal plane: The normal spine appears as two parallel rows of echoes (anterior and posterior ossification centers) which diverge slightly at the cervical region and converge at the sacral end (Fig. 15.1a). The coccyx is not ordinarily ossified in the fetus. The sagittal view can demonstrate the size of the defect and the presence or absence of skin cover (Fig. 15.1b). It is possible to determine the level of the defect by counting from the last rib (T12) or the iliac crest (L5/S1). Associated abnormalities like kyphosis (gibbus deformity) can also be noted (Fig. 15.1c).

Coronal plane: In a posterior coronal plane, the spine appears as two parallel rows corresponding to the posterior vertebral arch on each side (Fig 15.2a). In a slightly anterior section, only one row of ossification centers is seen corresponding to the vertebral bodies (Fig 15.2b). In spina bifida, there is a widening of the spine caused by splaying of the lateral processes (Fig. 15.2c). The mar-

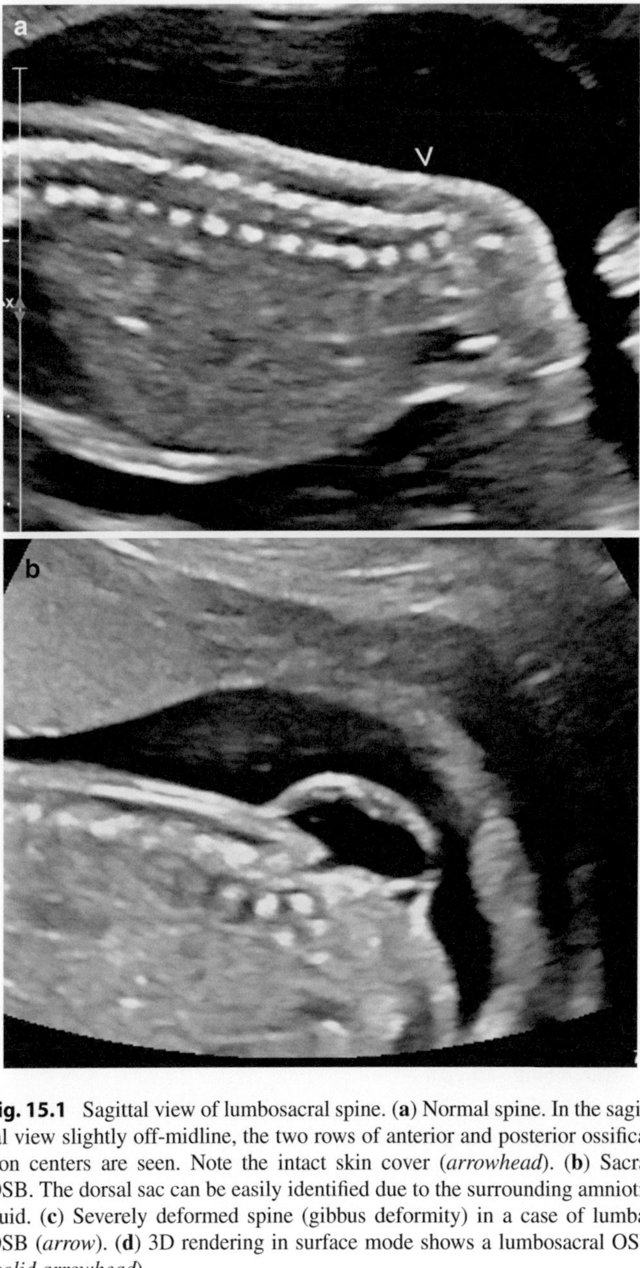

Fig. 15.1 Sagittal view of lumbosacral spine. (**a**) Normal spine. In the sagittal view slightly off-midline, the two rows of anterior and posterior ossification centers are seen. Note the intact skin cover (*arrowhead*). (**b**) Sacral OSB. The dorsal sac can be easily identified due to the surrounding amniotic fluid. (**c**) Severely deformed spine (gibbus deformity) in a case of lumbar OSB (*arrow*). (**d**) 3D rendering in surface mode shows a lumbosacral OSB (*solid arrowhead*)

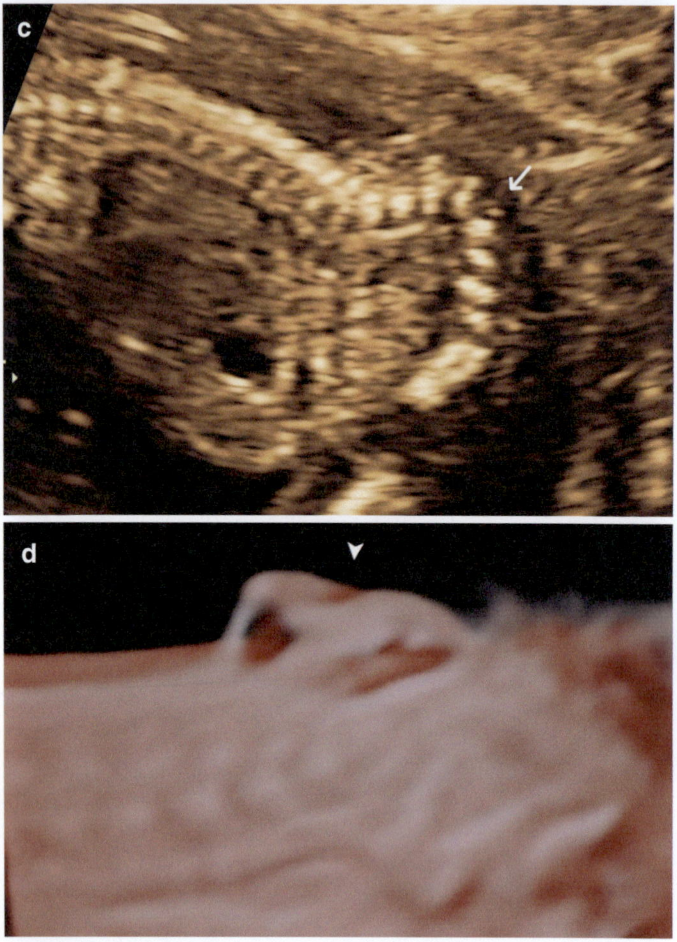

Fig. 15.1 (continued)

gins of the dorsal sac and the exposed placode can be well demonstrated (Fig. 15.2d).

Axial plane: This view shows the body and the lamina enclosing the spinal canal, represented by three echoes in a circular configuration (Fig 15.3a). In ONTD, the affected vertebrae have a 'V' or a 'U' shape due to the splaying of dorsal arches (Figs. 15.3b-d).

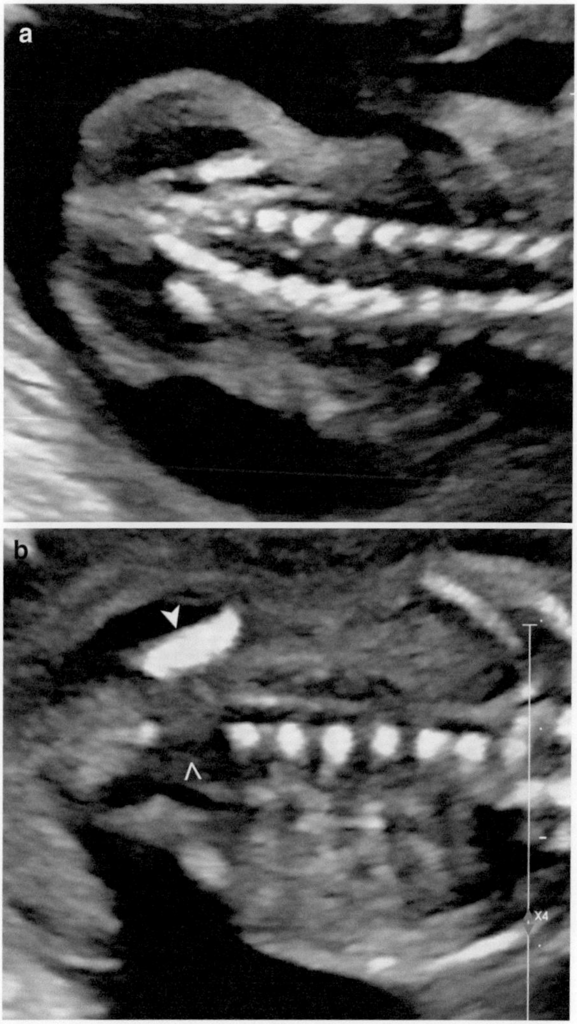

Fig. 15.2 Coronal view of lumbosacral spine. (**a**) Posterior coronal view of normal spine. The spine gives a 'railroad tracks' appearance caused by the posterior ossification centers. (**b**) Anterior coronal view of the normal spine. A single row of ossification centers is noted, corresponding to the vertebral bodies. A few sacral ossification centers are not visible (*arrowhead*) due to acoustic shadowing by the iliac bone (*solid arrowhead*). (**c**) Open spina bifida. Widening of the lumbar canal with exposed neural placode (*hand icons*). (**d**) Coronal section through the dorsal sac. The exposed neural placode is seen (*arrowhead*)

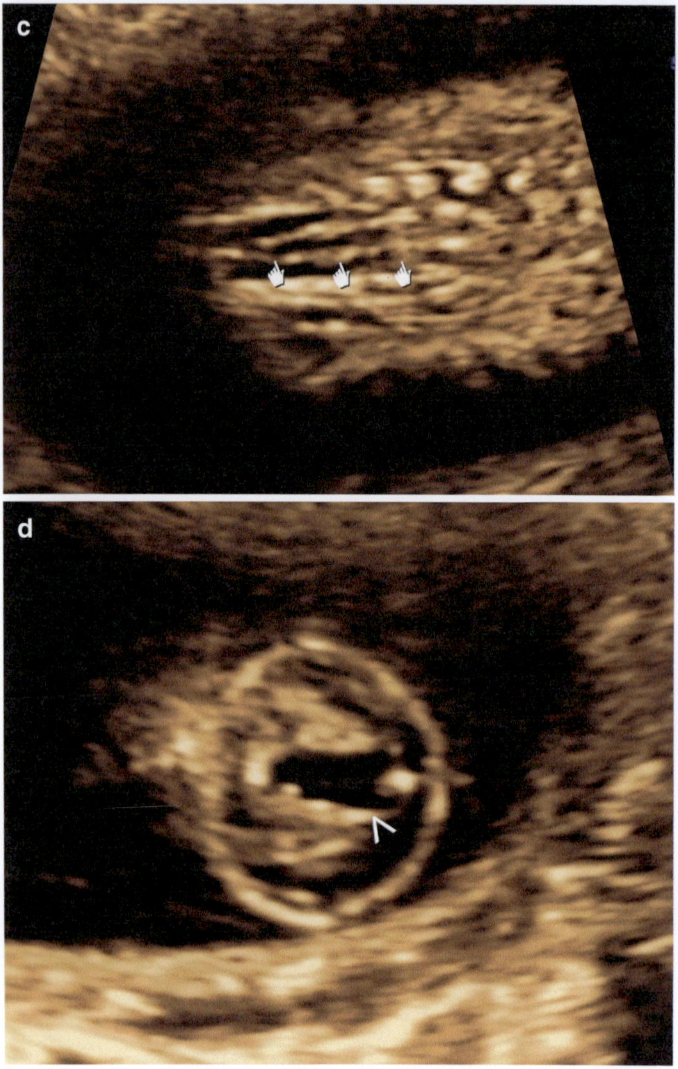

Fig. 15.2 (continued)

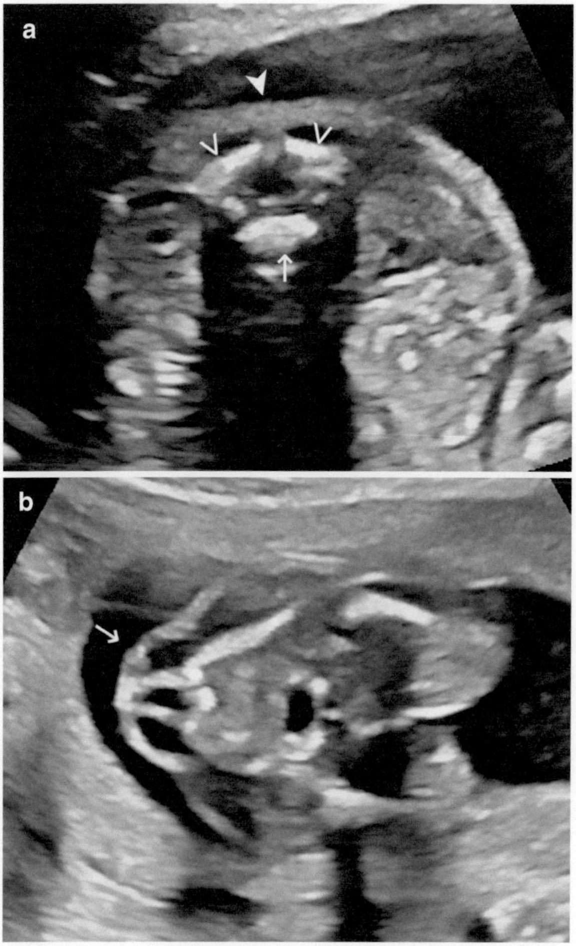

Fig. 15.3 Axial view of lumbar spine. (**a**) Normal spine. One anterior ossification center (*arrow*) and two posterior ossification centers (*arrowheads*) are seen. Note the intact dorsal skin cover (*solid arrowhead*). (**b**) Axial section showing sacral myelomeningocele (*arrow*). (**c**) Axial section showing lumbar myeloschisis. Note the splaying of posterior arches and absence of dorsal sac (*hand icon*). (**d**) 3D rendering showing myeloschisis (*solid arrowhead*)

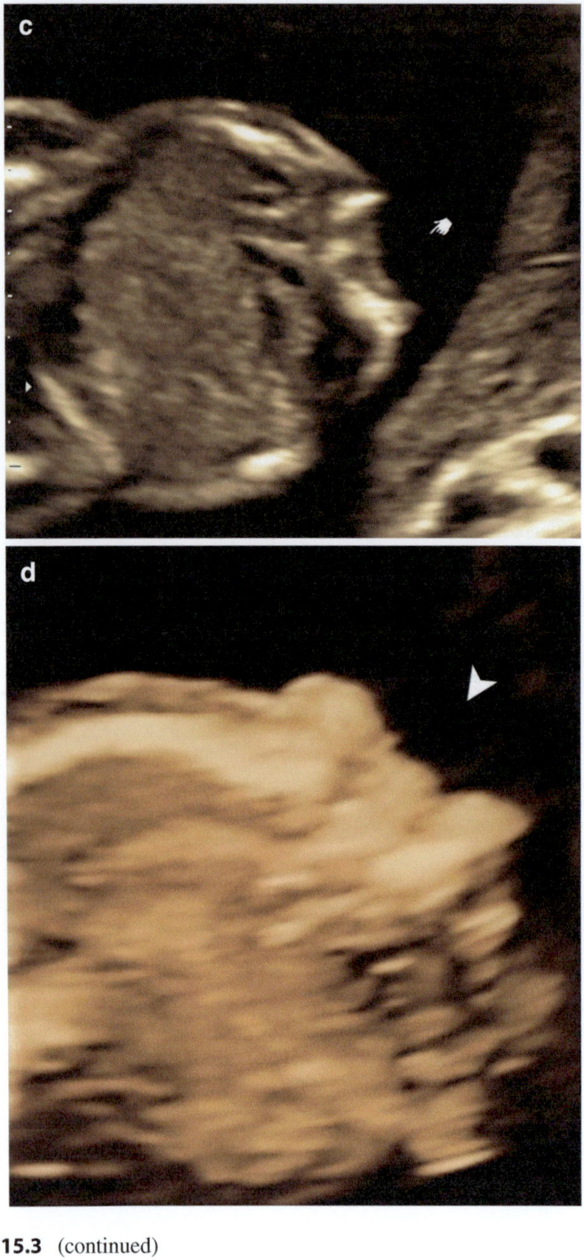

Fig. 15.3 (continued)

15.4.2 Chiari II Malformation

The Chiari II malformation (Arnold Chiari type 2 malformation) is a series of changes in the brain caused by the leakage of CSF through the OSB. Initially, there is downward displacement of the vermis, brainstem, and fourth ventricle into the foramen magnum. As a result, the posterior fossa does not adequately expand to accommodate the growing cerebellum and brainstem, causing these structures to herniate through the cervical canal. The following signs are seen on ultrasound:

Lemon sign: This refers to the scalloping of frontal bones, causing the skull to have the shape of a lemon (Fig. 15.4). It is present in about half the cases of OSB, usually disappears in the third trimester, and is considered nonspecific in the absence of other signs.

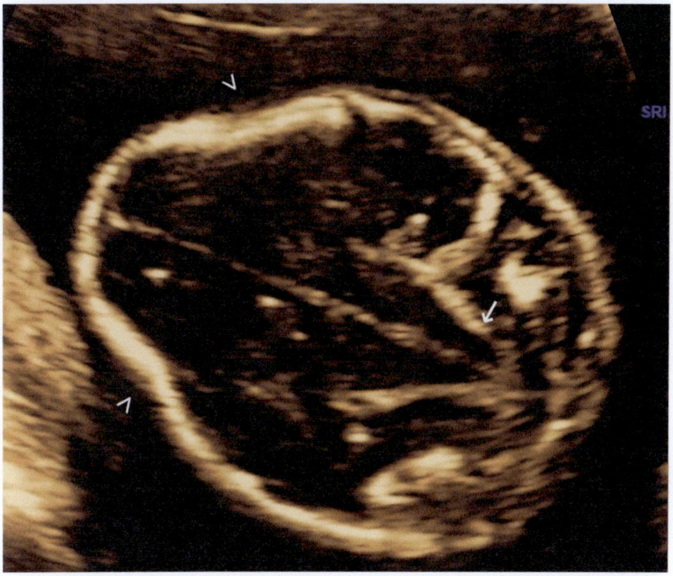

Fig. 15.4 Intracranial signs in OSB: Scalloping of frontal bones – the lemon sign (*arrowheads*), and beaking of the tectum (*arrow*)

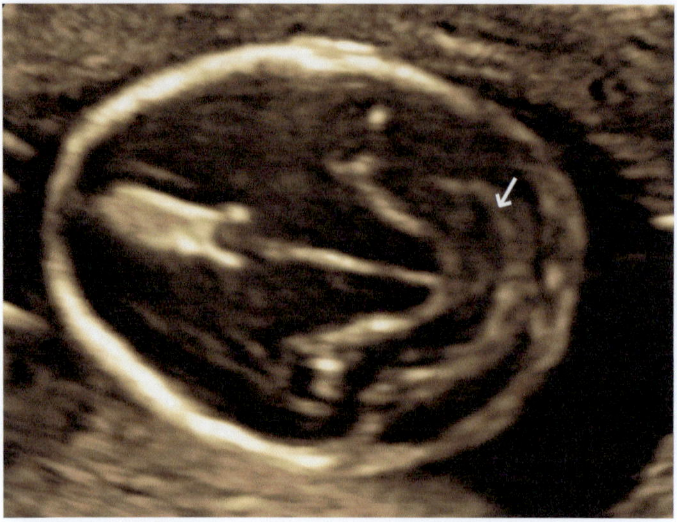

Fig. 15.5 The banana sign (*arrow*). Compare the shape of the cerebellum in this case with that of a normal dumbbell-shaped cerebellum shown in Fig. 6.12

Banana sign: The small and dysmorphic cerebellum, which is pushed posteriorly and inferiorly, has an abnormal curved shape resembling a banana (Fig. 15.5).

Ventriculomegaly: Ventriculomegaly occurs late in pregnancy and is either due to the obstruction of CSF flow through the fourth ventricle or due to the associated aqueductal stenosis (Fig. 15.6). OSB complicated by hydrocephalus is associated with a worse outcome.

15.4.3 Newer Ultrasound Signs

Newer ultrasound findings in the axial plane have been described that were previously identified only on MRI [8–10].

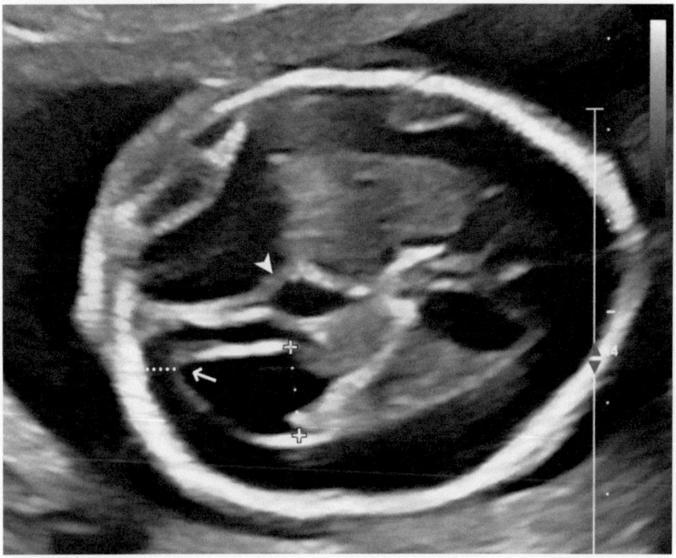

Fig. 15.6 Ventricular signs in OSB: Ventriculomegaly (*calipers*), ventricular pointing (*arrow*), and cavum veli interpositi cyst – diamond sign (*solid arrowhead*). Also note the proximity of the posterior horn to the occipital bone (*dotted line*)

Ventricular pointing: In normal fetuses, the posterior horns of the lateral ventricles are smoothly rounded. Conversely, fetuses with OSB have sharply pointed posterior horns (Fig. 15.6).

Tectal beaking: The tectum or the quadrigeminal plate is the dorsal part of midbrain, which can be visualized superior and anterior to the cerebellum. In OSB, the tectum assumes an elongated or a beak-shaped configuration, unlike its normal square or round shape (Fig. 15.4).

Interhemispheric cyst (non-specific sign): OSB can be associated with midline cysts like arachnoid cysts, pineal cysts, and cavum veli interpositi cysts. Cavum veli interpositi cyst presents as a midline diamond-shaped cyst, hence referred to as the *diamond sign* (Fig. 15.6).

15.4.4 Three-Dimensional Ultrasound and Fetal MRI

Three-dimensional USG allows the simultaneous visualization of the spinal defect in all three planes and makes it easier to identify its exact location and extent (Fig. 15.1d). The splaying of lateral vertebral processes and widening of the spinal canal can be demonstrated by rendering in maximum mode (Fig. 15.3d). The fetal spine needs to be anterior at the time of volume acquisition to capture adequate information and permit detailed evaluation.

Fetal MRI has a limited role in the diagnosis of ONTDs because of the high sensitivity and specificity of USG alone. It has a greater role in the characterization of closed neural tube defects.

15.5 First-Trimester Ultrasound

The 11–13 + 6 weeks scan has emerged as the first screening window for structural malformations. Early suspicion of OSB allows for a confirmatory scan around 15–16 weeks, making termination of affected pregnancies easier and safer. Early diagnosis also allows adequate time for prenatal genetic testing in women who opt for continuation of pregnancy and in-utero repair of the OSB.

Second-trimester cranial findings, such as the banana sign and the lemon sign, are not visible in the first trimester. In 2002, Buisson and coworkers described a narrowing of the frontal bones and parallel cerebral peduncles in first-trimester fetuses with OSB. Following this, several other investigators described other cranial findings with the potential to serve as ultrasound markers. Among these, the most widely accepted sign is the intracranial translucency, which can be evaluated in the same plane as the nuchal translucency. All secondary cranial findings are a manifestation of the posterior and inferior displacement of the brain. Knowledge about the different cranial findings improves the detection rate of OSB as affected fetuses may display only a few of the many related signs [11, 12].

15.5.1 Demonstration of the Spinal Defect

The certain diagnosis of OSB can only be made by the indisputable demonstration of the spinal defect in three orthogonal planes. In the first trimester, this requires a combination of a high-end ultrasound machine, a high-resolution probe, and transvaginal imaging. Presence of secondary cranial signs usually directs the examination toward a detailed evaluation of the spine. Even in expert hands, the actual demonstration of spina bifida may be difficult before 13 weeks (Fig 15.7a, b). In such cases, it is prudent to repeat the scan at 15–16 weeks and demonstrate the spinal defect clearly before taking irrevocable decisions.

15.5.2 Intracranial Translucency

Section: Midsagittal

When the fetus is examined in the mid-sagittal view of the face (also used for measuring nuchal translucency), two echogenic lines are visible in the posterior part of the fetal brain, forming an equal sign (=). The anterior line represents the dorsal limit of the brainstem and the posterior line represents the choroid plexus of the fourth ventricle. The space between these two lines is called the intracranial translucency (IT) which is the developing fourth ventricle. A smaller space between the posterior line and the occipital bone is the developing cisterna magna (CM) (Fig. 15.8). The mean anteroposterior diameter of the IT is approximately 1.5 mm at 11 weeks, increasing to 2.5 mm at 14 weeks [12].

In OSB, the CSF leakage results in the caudal displacement of the brain, leading to a compression of the fourth ventricle. This can be seen on ultrasound as obliteration of the IT (Fig. 15.9a).

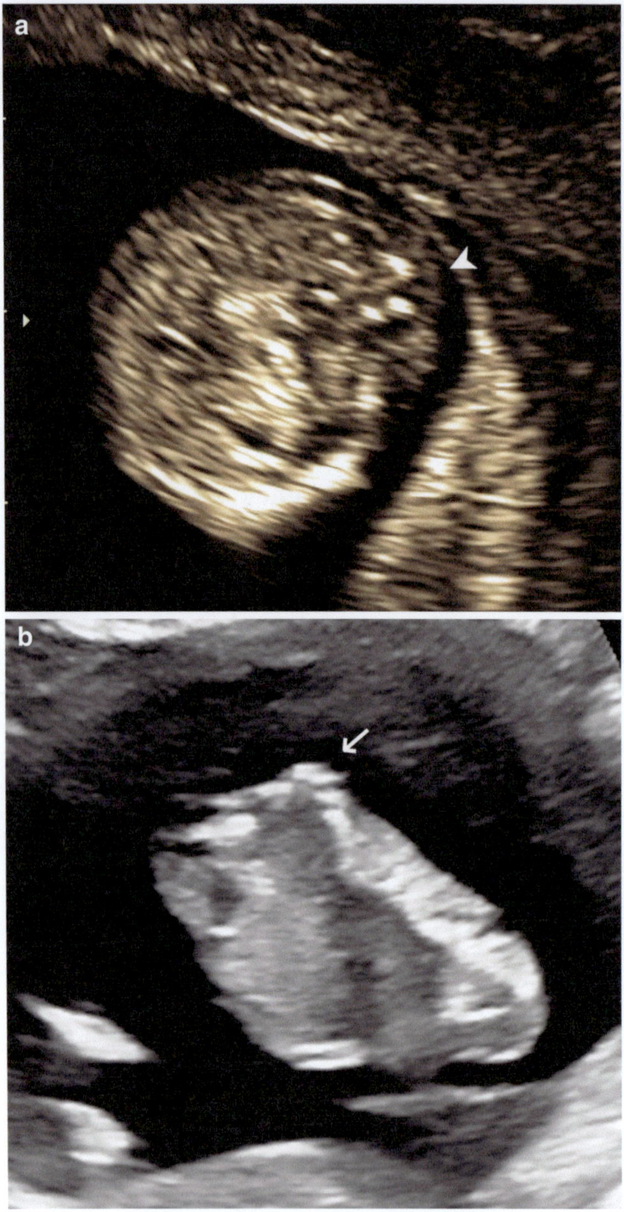

Fig. 15.7 Spinal defects in two first-trimester fetuses with OSB. (**a**) Axial section showing lumbar OSB (*solid arrowhead*). Note that the defect is less conspicuous than in the second trimester. (**b**) Severe kyphosis of the lumbar spine (*arrow*)

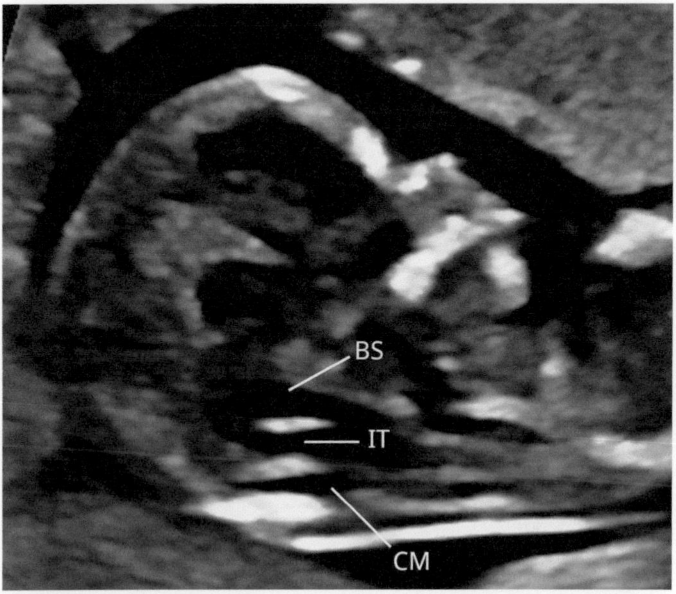

Fig. 15.8 Midsagittal view of the head in a normal fetus at 13 weeks. Note the equal sign (=) formed by the echogenic posterior border of the brainstem (*BS*) anteriorly and the choroid plexus of the fourth ventricle posteriorly. The space between the two echogenic lines is the intracranial translucency (*IT*). The space posterior to the equal sign is the cisterna magna (*CM*)

15.5.3 Cisterna Magna Obliteration

Section: Midsagittal

The developing cisterna magna can be seen in the standard midsagittal section as a space posterior to the choroid plexus of the fourth ventricle (Fig. 15.8). Cisterna magna obliteration is seen either as a disruption of the IT, or the equal sign touching the occipital bone (Fig. 15.9b). This is a more sensitive marker for OSB compared to IT obliteration [13].

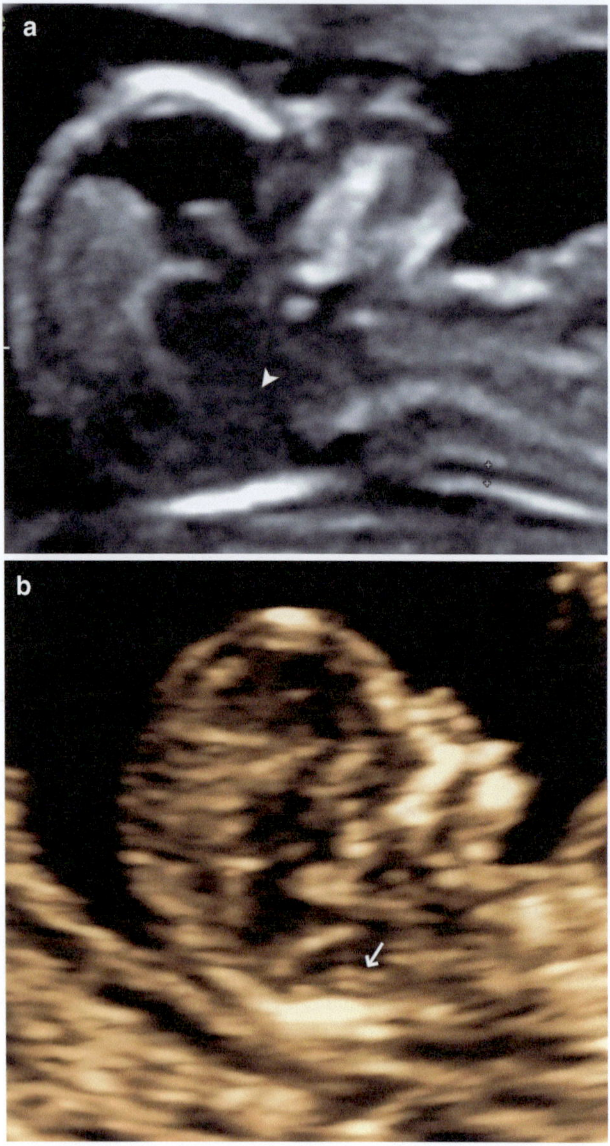

Fig. 15.9 Midsagittal views of the head in two fetuses with OSB. (**a**) There is shifting of brain toward the occiput, causing brainstem to appear enlarged (*solid arrowhead*). The equal sign (=) corresponding to the IT is not seen. (**b**) The IT is pushed toward the occipital bone, with obliteration of the cisterna magna (*arrow*)

15.5.4 Crash Sign

Section: Axial

This refers to the posterior displacement of the midbrain and the aqueduct of Sylvius, causing it to 'crash' against the occipital bone in the axial view (Fig. 15.10b). It is so named as it resembles the back of a car that has crashed into a wall. Its strength lies in the fact that it can be identified simply by pattern recognition in the transthalamic plane that is used to measure BPD. As the BPD image is usually stored for all fetuses, retrospective evaluation for the crash sign is possible [14].

15.5.5 Crushed Butterfly Sign

Section: Axial

In a normal fetus, the two choroid plexuses together form the shape of a butterfly with lateral concavities (Fig. 15.11a). In fetuses with OSB, the choroid plexuses are deformed, often with lateral convexities. The space between the choroid and the skull is also reduced due to loss of CSF (Fig 15.11b).

15.5.6 Biometric Ratios Suggestive of OSB

Altered biometric ratios within the fetal cranium can increase the sensitivity for the detection of OSB. However, they require exact ultrasound sections as described by the original author and a comparison with established reference ranges. Except for BPD, these measurements and ratios are not meant to be used in routine clinical practice.

Biparietal Diameter *(Axial section)*: A BPD value lower than expected for CRL, or a BPD smaller than the transverse abdominal diameter, increases the probability of an OSB.

Brainstem-to-occipital bone diameter (*Midsagittal section)*: In the open spina bifida group, the brain stem diameter is increased and the brainstem-to-occipital bone diameter (BSOB) diameter is reduced. As a result, the brain stem to BSOB ratio is significantly increased (Fig. 15.12). The BS/BSOB ratio serves as an objective method for evaluating the posterior fossa.

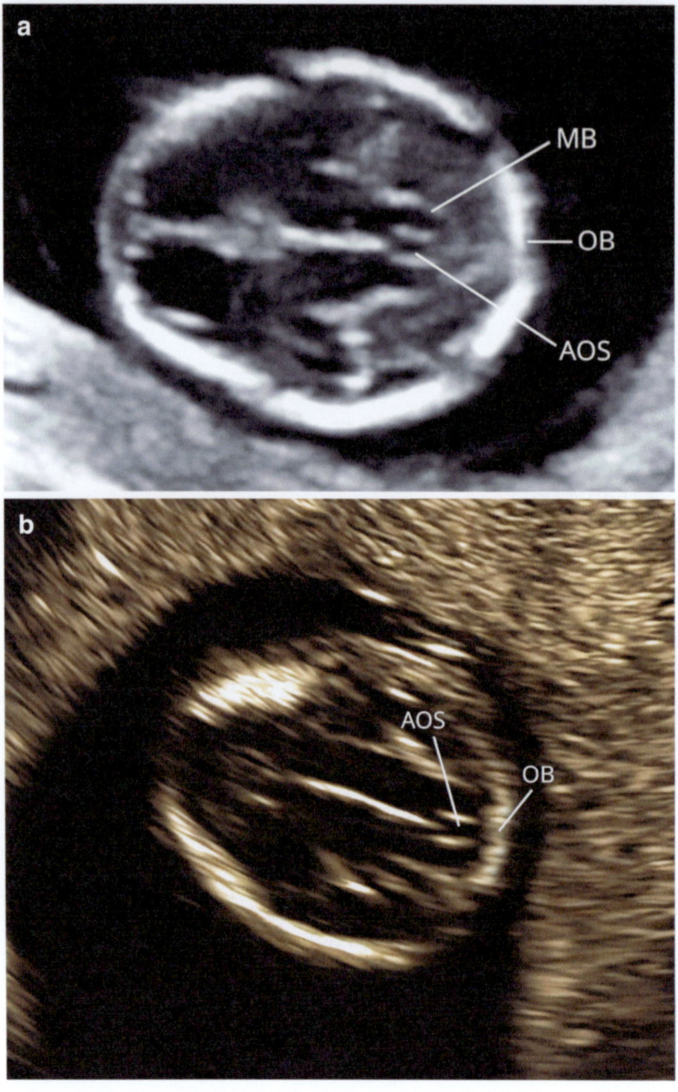

Fig. 15.10 Axial view of the head at the level of the midbrain (**a**) In a normal fetus, the midbrain (*MB*) and the aqueduct of Sylvius (*AOS*) are distant from the occipital bone (*OB*). (**b**) In a fetus with OSB, the posterior displacement of the midbrain causes it to 'crash' against the occipital bone. The AOS-to-OB distance is reduced

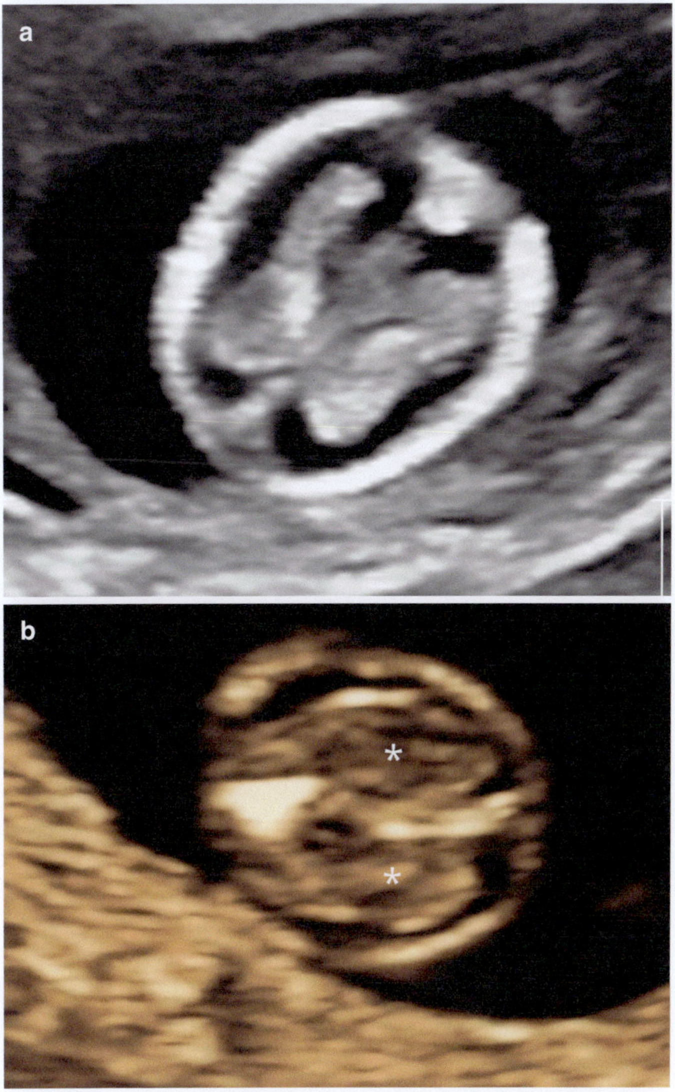

Fig. 15.11 Crushed butterfly sign. (**a**) In a normal fetus, the two choroid plexuses form the shape of a butterfly (**b**) In a fetus with OSB, the choroid plexuses (*) are deformed with lateral convexities. Also note the reduced space between the choroid plexuses and the skull

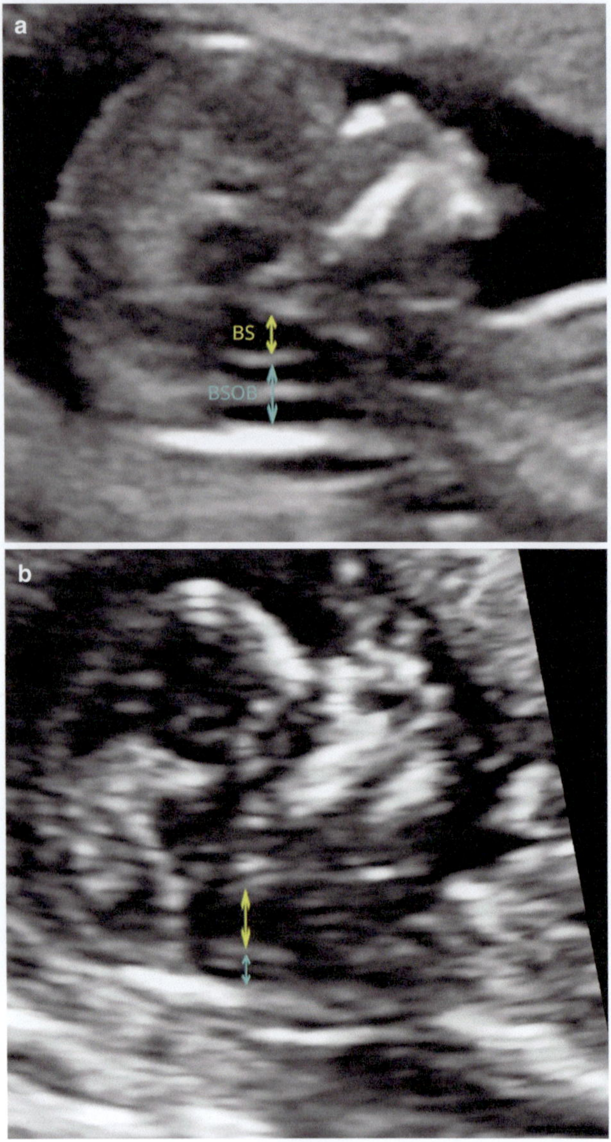

Fig. 15.12 Midsagittal view of the face and head. (**a**) In a normal fetus, the brainstem diameter (*BS, yellow double-sided arrow*) is smaller than the brainstem to occipital bone distance (*BSOB, cyan double-sided arrow*). (**b**) In a fetus with OSB, the BS > BSOB, and the BS/BSOB ratio is increased

Aqueduct of Sylvius to occipital bone distance *(Axial section):* The aqueduct of Sylvius (AOS) to occipital bone distance is the mathematical equivalent of the crash sign (Fig. 15.10). In normal fetuses, the mean ranges from 2.3 mm at 11 weeks to 5.7 mm at 14 weeks. Fetuses with open spinal defects have an AOS-to-occiput distance below the lower limit of normal (defined as mean minus 2 standard deviations) [15].

Frontomaxillary facial angle (FMF angle) *(Midsagittal section):* This refers to the angle between the frontal bone and the upper surface of the palate in the mid-sagittal view of the fetal face (Fig. 15.13). In normal fetuses, its mean value is 84.0° at 11 weeks, and gradually reduces to 76.5° at 13 + 6 weeks. In fetuses with OSB, the caudal displacement of the fetal brain results in backward tilting of the forehead. Therefore, the fronto-maxillary angle is approximately 10 degrees lower [16].

15.5.7 Performance of First-Trimester Signs

While first-trimester ultrasound presents an exciting vista for early detection of OSB, its performance remains sub-par compared to the 20 weeks scan.

In a retrospective review of 200 scans at 11–13 weeks, IT was found to detect 4/8 fetuses with OSB giving a sensitivity of only 50%. A systematic review and meta-analysis in 2016 showed similar results. The specificity, however, was 99%. Despite the high specificity, false-positive results still occur, leading to unnecessary parental anxiety [17, 18].

In a series of 260 mid-sagittal first-trimester ultrasound images using IT, caudal brainstem displacement, and obliteration of cisterna magna, the detection rate for OSB was 50–90% depending on the observer. Interestingly, obliteration of cisterna magna was the best-performing sign, while the absence of IT was associated with a lower detection rate [19].

In a large prospective, multicenter longitudinal 'Berlin-IT study,' more than 16,000 fetuses with 11 cases of OSB were examined in the first trimester. Each fetus was evaluated for IT, brain stem, cisterna magna, BSOB, and BS/BSOB ratio. The detection rate was only 18% for the complete non-visualization of

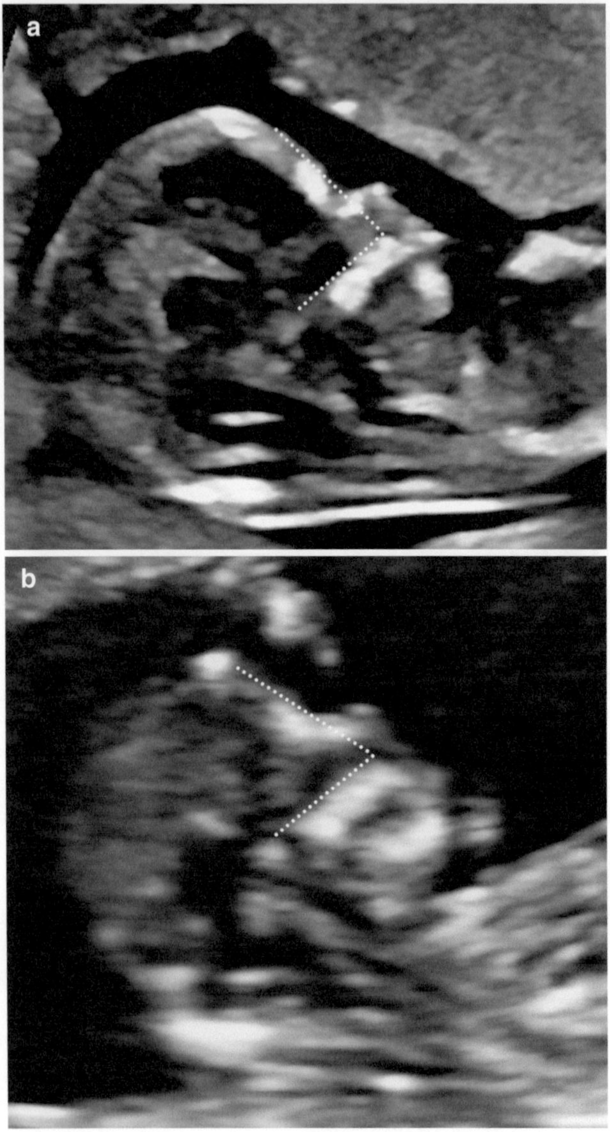

Fig. 15.13 Midsagittal view of the face and head. (**a**) In a normal fetus, the frontomaxillary angle is close to 90 degrees (*dotted lines*). (**b**) In a fetus with OSB, the FMF angle is markedly reduced due to backward tilting of the forehead caused by posterior displacement of the brain

IT and 45% using cutoff values. For the cisterna magna size, the detection rate was 64% for the absence of cisterna magna and 73% using cutoff values. The other measurements were inconclusive. Finally, using a combination of all signs resulted in a 100% detection rate, either at the primary visit or a scheduled second visit following suspicion of ONTD [20].

Importantly, several cases of OSB have been reported with normal cranial anatomy in the first trimester. Ultrasound machine resolution and maternal habitus also influence the first-trimester detection rates.

15.6 Key Messages

1. MSAFP has a limited role in screening for OSB, as the second-trimester ultrasound detection rate is over 95% with modern machines.
2. Elevated MSAFP in the absence of an ONTD is a marker for placental dysfunction.
3. Cisterna magna obliteration has the highest sensitivity among all the first-trimester ultrasound signs of OSB.
4. More than two-thirds of OSB can be detected at the 11–13 + 6 weeks scan using a combination of ultrasound signs.
5. Folic acid is the only type of folate with a proven benefit in the prevention of ONTDs.

References

1. Christianson A, Howson C, Modell B. March of Dimes global report on birth defects: the hidden toll of dying and disabled children. The March of Dimes Birth Defects Foundation 2006. https://dev.marchofdimes.org/mission/march-of-dimes-global-report-on-birth-defects.aspx. Accessed 25 June 2023.

2. Centers for Disease Control and Prevention. MTHFR Gene, Folic Acid, and Preventing Neural Tube Defects. 2022. https://www.cdc.gov/ncbddd/folicacid/mthfr-gene-and-folic-acid.html. Accessed 25 June 2023.
3. Adzick NS. Fetal myelomeningocele: natural history, pathophysiology, and in-utero intervention. Semin Fetal Neonatal Med. 2010;15(1):9–14.
4. Milunsky A. Prenatal detection of neural tube defects. VI. Experience with 20,000 pregnancies. JAMA. 1980;244(24):2731–5.
5. Palomaki GE, Bupp C, Gregg AR, Norton ME, Oglesbee D, Best RG. ACMG biochemical genetics Subcommittee of the Laboratory Quality Assurance Committee. Laboratory screening and diagnosis of open neural tube defects, 2019 revision: a technical standard of the American College of Medical Genetics and Genomics (ACMG). Genet Med. 2020;22(3):462–74.
6. Knight GJ, Palomaki GE. Epidemiologic monitoring of prenatal screening for neural tube defects and down syndrome. Clin Lab Med. 2003;23(2):531–51.
7. Norem CT, Schoen EJ, Walton DL, Krieger RC, O'Keefe J, To TT, Ray GT. Routine ultrasonography compared with maternal serum alpha-fetoprotein for neural tube defect screening. Obstet Gynecol. 2005;106(4):747–52.
8. Wax JR, Pinette MG, Cartin A, Michaud J, Blackstone J. Fetal cerebral ventricular pointing as a marker of spina bifida: incidence and observational agreement. J Ultrasound Med. 2009;28(3):317–20.
9. Kunpalin Y, Richter J, Mufti N, Bosteels J, Ourselin S, De Coppi P, Thompson D, David AL, Deprest J. Cranial findings detected by second-trimester ultrasound in fetuses with myelomeningocele: a systematic review. BJOG. 2021;128(2):366–74.
10. Callen AL, Stengel JW, Filly RA. Supratentorial abnormalities in the Chiari II malformation, II: tectal morphologic changes. J Ultrasound Med. 2009;28(1):29–35.
11. Buisson O, De Keersmaecker B, Senat MV, Bernard JP, Moscoso G, Ville Y. Sonographic diagnosis of spina bifida at 12 weeks: heading towards indirect signs. Ultrasound Obstet Gynecol. 2002;19(3):290–2.
12. Chaoui R, Benoit B, Mitkowska-Wozniak H, Heling KS, Nicolaides KH. Assessment of intracranial translucency (IT) in the detection of spina bifida at the 11-13-week scan. Ultrasound Obstet Gynecol. 2009;34(3):249–52.
13. Kose S, Altunyurt S, Keskinoglu P. A prospective study on fetal posterior cranial fossa assessment for early detection of open spina bifida at 11-13 weeks. Congenit Anom (Kyoto). 2018;58(1):4–9.
14. Ushakov F, Sacco A, Andreeva E, Tudorache S, Everett T, David AL, Pandya PP. Crash sign: new first-trimester sonographic marker of spina bifida. Ultrasound Obstet Gynecol. 2019;54(6):740–5.
15. Finn M, Sutton D, Atkinson S, Ransome K, Sujenthiran P, Ditcham V, Wakefield P, Meagher S. The aqueduct of Sylvius: a sonographic land-

mark for neural tube defects in the first trimester. Ultrasound Obstet Gynecol. 2011;38(6):640–5.

16. Lachmann R, Picciarelli G, Moratalla J, Greene N, Nicolaides KH. Frontomaxillary facial angle in fetuses with spina bifida at 11-13 weeks' gestation. Ultrasound Obstet Gynecol. 2010;36(3):268–71.
17. Fong KW, Toi A, Okun N, Al-Shami E, Menezes RJ. Retrospective review of diagnostic performance of intracranial translucency in detection of open spina bifida at the 11-13-week scan. Ultrasound Obstet Gynecol. 2011;38(6):630–4.
18. Maruotti GM, Saccone G, D'Antonio F, Berghella V, Sarno L, Morlando M, Giudicepietro A, Martinelli P. Diagnostic accuracy of intracranial translucency in detecting spina bifida: a systematic review and meta-analysis. Prenat Diagn. 2016;36(11):991–6.
19. Mangione R, Dhombres F, Lelong N, Amat S, Atoub F, Friszer S, Khoshnood B, Jouannic JM. Screening for fetal spina bifida at the 11-13-week scan using three anatomical features of the posterior brain. Ultrasound Obstet Gynecol. 2013;42(4):416–20.
20. Chen FC, Gerhardt J, Entezami M, Chaoui R, Henrich W. Detection of spina bifida by first trimester screening—results of the prospective multicenter Berlin IT-study. Ultraschall Med. 2017;38(2):151–7.

MIX
Papier aus verantwortungsvollen Quellen
Paper from responsible sources
FSC® C105338

If you have any concerns about our products,
you can contact us on
ProductSafety@springernature.com

In case Publisher is established outside the EU,
the EU authorized representative is:
Springer Nature Customer Service Center GmbH
Europaplatz 3, 69115 Heidelberg, Germany

Printed by Libri Plureos GmbH
in Hamburg, Germany